Metabolic Bone Diseases

Pauline M. Camacho
Editor

Metabolic Bone Diseases

A Case-Based Approach

Springer

Editor
Pauline M. Camacho
Division of Endocrinology and Metabolism
Loyola University Medical Center
Maywood
IL
USA

ISBN 978-3-030-03693-5 ISBN 978-3-030-03694-2 (eBook)
https://doi.org/10.1007/978-3-030-03694-2

Library of Congress Control Number: 2019930837

This Springer imprint is published by the registered company Springer Nature Switzerland AG
The registered company address is: Gewerbestrasse 11, 6330 Cham, Switzerland

Contents

Contributors

Lily Agrawal, MD Department of Medicine, Division of Endocrinology and Metabolism, Edward Hines Jr. VA Hospital, Hines, Illinois, USA

Rod Marianne Arceo-Mendoza, MD Division of Endocrinology and Metabolism, Loyola University Medical Center, Loyola University Osteoporosis and Metabolic Bone Disease Center, Maywood, IL, USA

Anne Margarette Bacal, MD Division of Endocrinology and Metabolism, Loyola University Medical Center, Loyola University Osteoporosis and Metabolic Bone Disease Center, Maywood, IL, USA

Pauline M. Camacho, MD, FACE Division of Endocrinology and Metabolism, Loyola University Medical Center, Loyola University Osteoporosis and Metabolic Bone Disease Center, Maywood, IL, USA

Gerald Charnogursky, MD Department of Medicine, Division of Endocrinology and Metabolism, Loyola Medicine, Maywood, IL, USA

Bart L. Clarke, MD Mayo Clinic, Rochester, MN, USA

Megan R. Crawford, DO Department of Endocrinology, Diabetes and Metabolism, Cleveland Clinic Foundation, Cleveland, OH, USA

Mary Ann Emanuele, MD Department of Medicine, Division of Endocrinology and Metabolism, Loyola University Medical Center, Maywood, IL, USA

Nicholas Emanuele, MD Endocrinology Section, Hines VA Hospital, Loyola University of Chicago Stritch School of Medicine, Hines, IL, USA

Allison Hahr, MD Division of Endocrinology, Metabolism and Molecular Medicine, Northwestern University Feinberg School of Medicine, Chicago, IL, USA

Daniel L. Hurley, MD Department of Medicine and Division of Endocrinology, Diabetes, Metabolism and Nutrition, Mayo Clinic College of Medicine, Mayo Clinic, Rochester, MN, USA

Sumeet Jain, MD Division of Endocrinology and Metabolism, Loyola University Medical Center, Maywood, IL, USA

Sina Jasim, MD, MPH Department of Internal Medicine and Division of Endocrinology, Metabolism and Lipid Research, Washington University School of Medicine, St. Louis, MO, USA

Susan Karam, MD Department of Endocrinology, Metabolism and Molecular Medicine, Northwestern Memorial Hospital, Chicago, IL, USA

Leila Khan, MD Department of Endocrinology, Diabetes and Metabolism, Cleveland Clinic Foundation, Cleveland, OH, USA

Anupam Kotwal, MBBS Department of Medicine and Division of Endocrinology, Diabetes, Metabolism and Nutrition, Mayo Clinic College of Medicine, Mayo Clinic, Rochester, MN, USA

Joshua A. Levine, MD, PhD Division of Endocrinology, Metabolism and Molecular Medicine, Northwestern University Feinberg School of Medicine, Chicago, IL, USA

E. Michael Lewiecki MD, FACP, FACE New Mexico Clinical Research & Osteoporosis Center, Albuquerque, NM, USA

Angelo Licata, MD, PhD Department of Endocrinology, Diabetes and Metabolism, Cleveland Clinic Foundation, Cleveland, OH, USA

Alaleh Mazhari, DO Department of Medicine, Division of Endocrinology and Metabolism, Loyola University Medical Center, Maywood, IL, USA

Farah Meah, DO Department of Medicine, Division of Endocrinology and Metabolism, Edward Hines Jr. VA Hospital, Hines, Illinois, USA

Clare O'Connor, MD Division of Endocrinology, Metabolism and Molecular Medicine, Northwestern University Feinberg School of Medicine, Chicago, IL, USA

Ruchita Patel, DO Department of Medicine, Division of Endocrinology and Metabolism, Loyola University Medical Center, Maywood, IL, USA

Namratha Reddy, MD Department of Medicine, Loyola University Medical Center, Maywood, Illinois, USA

Mark Anthony Sandoval, MD, FPCP, FPSEDM Department of Physiology and Section of Endocrinology, Diabetes and Metabolism, Department of Medicine, College of Medicine and Philippine General Hospital, University of the Philippines Manila, Manila, Philippines

Jad G. Sfeir, MD Department of Medicine and Division of Endocrinology, Diabetes, Metabolism and Nutrition, Mayo Clinic College of Medicine, Mayo Clinic, Rochester, MN, USA

Vinita Singh, MD Department of Medicine, Division of Endocrinology and Metabolism, Loyola University Medical Center, Maywood, IL, USA

Robert Wermers, MD Department of Medicine and Division of Endocrinology, Diabetes, Metabolism and Nutrition, Mayo Clinic College of Medicine, Mayo Clinic, Rochester, MN, USA

Susan E. Williams, MS, RD, MD Department of Endocrinology, Diabetes and Metabolism, Cleveland Clinic Foundation, Cleveland, OH, USA

Chapter 1
Osteoporosis

E. Michael Lewiecki

Case Presentation and Discussion

A 58-year-old woman has a screening bone density test with dual-energy X-ray absorptiometry (DXA) that shows a T-score of −2.9 at the left femoral neck. She is generally healthy except for episodic diarrhea and constipation, which has been attributed to irritable bowel syndrome and treated with a high-fiber diet. She has a family history osteoporosis (mother with hip fracture at age 82 years). She has no known fracture and has never received pharmacological therapy to reduce fracture risk. A diagnosis of osteoporosis is made, and she is started on treatment with a generic oral bisphosphonate. Eighteen months later she has a repeat bone density test at the same facility using the same instrument. She is reported to have a decrease in bone mineral density (BMD) compared with the baseline study. Detailed discussion suggests she is taking medication regularly and correctly with no recognizable adverse effects. What should be done now?

Before starting treatment for osteoporosis, every patient should have a laboratory evaluation for factors contributing to skeletal fragility, to guide the management plan, and assure the safety of proceeding with treatment. As examples, a finding of severe chronic kidney disease would lead to avoidance of bisphosphonates for treatment, and a finding of a monoclonal antibody might necessitate referral to an oncologist. In this patient, a thorough baseline evaluation was not done. Laboratory studies now revealed several abnormalities of importance. A 24-h urine collection showed low calcium of 35 mg while having an adequate calcium intake and normal renal function. Subsequently testing show high levels of celiac antibodies. A diagnosis of celiac disease was confirmed by small bowel biopsy. She was placed on a gluten-free diet and maintained on the same oral bisphosphonate. A follow-up bone density test 1 year later showed substantial improvement in BMD consistent with a beneficial effect of therapy.

The original version of this chapter was revised. A correction to this chapter can be found at https://doi.org/10.1007/978-3-030-03694-2_16

E. M. Lewiecki (✉)
New Mexico Clinical Research & Osteoporosis Center, Albuquerque, NM, USA

P. M. Camacho (ed.), *Metabolic Bone Diseases*,
https://doi.org/10.1007/978-3-030-03694-2_1

Introduction

Osteoporosis is a systemic skeletal disease characterized by low bone strength leading to an increased risk of fracture. Bone strength is determined by BMD and other skeletal properties that include bone architecture, remodeling, mineralization, and damage accumulation. A 2004 report of the US Surgeon General on bone health in America identified osteoporosis as a major public health problem that affected about 10 million Americans over the age of 50 years [1]. Worldwide, about 200 million individuals are afflicted with osteoporosis, with 1 in 3 women and 1 in 5 men over the age of 50 years expected to experience an osteoporotic fracture in their remaining lifetimes [2]. The consequences of osteoporotic fractures are serious, including disability, loss of independence, and death. After a hip fracture, 40% of patients cannot walk independently, and 10–20% require permanent nursing home care [2]. The economic burden is high, with healthcare costs of about €37 billion per year in the EU and $19 billion USD per year in the USA [2].

Excellent clinical tools are now available to diagnose osteoporosis and assess fracture risk. A wide range of pharmacological agents have been tested and approved for treatment of to reduce fracture risk. Clinical practice guidelines to assist clinicians in managing osteoporosis patients have been developed. And yet, osteoporosis remains a disease that is underdiagnosed and undertreated. The osteoporosis treatment gap, the difference between those who could benefit from treatment but do not receive it, has reached crisis proportions [3]. This is an update of our current understanding of osteoporosis, opportunities to reduce fracture risk, and challenges in managing patients with this disease.

Diagnosis

BMD is classified as osteoporosis, osteopenia (low bone mass), or normal according to criteria established by the World Health Organization (WHO) [4] and refined for use in clinical practice by the International Society for Clinical Densitometry (ISCD) [5]. A DXA T-score of −2.5 or below (i.e., BMD at least 2.5 standard deviations (SD) less than the mean BMD of a young-adult reference population) is consistent with a diagnosis of osteoporosis (Table 1.1). However, the finding of a T-score ≤ -2.5 can also be due to other disorders, such as osteomalacia. It is the responsibility of the clinician to evaluate the patient for all factors that might be responsible for the low T-score and address those that are relevant. Recent guidance from the ISCD states that femoral neck and total hip T-scores calculated from two-dimensional (2-D) projections of quantitative computed tomography (QCT) data are equivalent to the corresponding DXA T-scores for diagnosis of osteoporosis using the WHO criteria [5].

A diagnosis of osteoporosis may also be made in the presence of a fragility fracture, independently of BMD. The US National Bone Health Alliance (NBHA) has

Table 1.1 The World Health Organization classification of bone mineral density measured by dual-energy X-ray absorptiometry [4]

Classification	T-score
Normal	−1.0 and above
Osteopenia (low bone mass)	Between −1.0 and −2.5
Osteoporosis	−2.5 and below
Severe osteoporosis	−2.5 and below and fragility fracture

Table 1.2 Criteria for the diagnosis of osteoporosis from NBHA and AACE/ACE [6, 7]

Method of diagnosis	Criteria	Applicability
Bone density	T-score ≤−2.5 at lumbar spine, total hip, femoral neck, or 33% radius	Worldwide
Fracture	Low trauma hip fracture regardless of BMD; low trauma vertebral, proximal humerus, pelvis, or some distal forearm fractures with T-score between −1.0 and −2.5	USA
Fracture risk	FRAX 10-year probability of major osteoporotic fracture ≥20% or hip fracture ≥3% (corresponds to thresholds for treatment with the guidelines of the National Osteoporosis Foundation)	USA

identified types of fractures leading to a diagnosis of osteoporosis and also recommended that a high fracture probability by the WHO fracture risk algorithm (FRAX) is sufficient for a diagnosis of osteoporosis [6]. Table 1.2 summarizes the recommendations of the NBHA for a clinical diagnosis of osteoporosis, which are supported by the American Association of Clinical Endocrinologists (AACE)/American College of Endocrinology (ACE) and other professional societies.

BMD Measurement

DXA measurements of BMD are used to diagnose osteoporosis, monitor changes in BMD, and estimate fracture risk. DXA utilizes ionizing radiation with photon beams of two different energy levels, resulting in a 2-D projection of the bone and soft tissue that is visualized on a computer monitor. The difference in attenuation of the photon beams passing through body tissues with variable composition provides a quantitative measurement of areal BMD in grams per square centimeter (g/cm^2). A "central" DXA system consists of a table supporting the patient, a radiation source below the table, a radiation detector above the table, and a computer to acquire and analyze the data (Fig. 1.1). DXA is the standard technology for measuring BMD in clinical practice because of BMD by DXA is strongly correlated with bone strength in biomechanical studies, epidemiological studies show a strong relationship with fracture risk, WHO classification of BMD is based primarily on

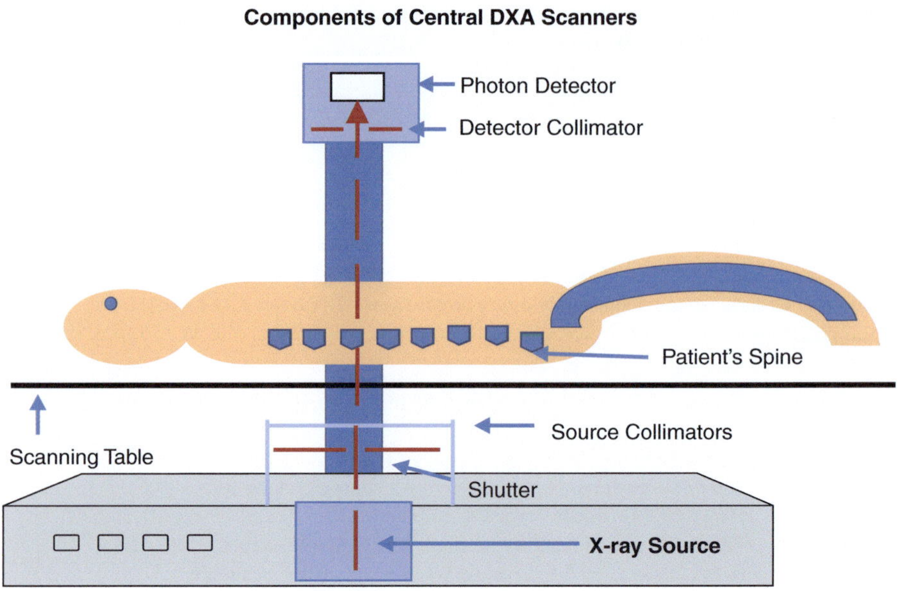

Fig. 1.1 Components of central DXA scanners. (Image courtesy of S. Bobo Tanner, MD. Used with permission)

reference data obtained by DXA, and enrollment of subjects in registration clinical trials is based entirely or partly on DXA measurements. In addition, precision and accuracy of DXA is excellent and the radiation dose is low. DXA measurements have non-BMD applications, including vertebral fracture assessment (VFA), analysis of body composition, hip structural analysis (HSA), and trabecular bone score (TBS) determination. Quantitative ultrasound (QUS) can be used to measure properties of bone that correlate well with fracture risk, although QUS cannot be used to diagnose osteoporosis and parameters measured by QUS respond poorly and/or slowly to treatment [8].

The clinical utility of BMD testing is highly dependent on the quality of the measurement, especially for serial BMD measurements with quantitative comparisons. When BMD measurements are correct and interpretation is consistent with well-established standards, clinicians are best equipped to make proper clinical decision. Poor quality acquisition, analysis, or interpretation of DXA data can mislead healthcare providers. This may be followed by unnecessary tests, failure to do needed tests, inappropriate treatment, or failure to treat. Best use of limited healthcare resources and appropriate patient management is optimized when DXA facilities follow recommended procedures for instrument calibration, acquisition, analysis, interpretation, and reporting of results. For these reasons, the ISCD has developed Official Positions [5] and DXA best practices [9]. Strict adherence to these standards assures referring clinicians that the DXA results are a reliable source of information to aid in making treatment decisions. Indications for BMD testing from the US National Osteoporosis Foundation (NOF) are provided in Table 1.3.

Table 1.3 Indications for bone density testing from the US National Osteoporosis Foundation [10]

Women age 65 and older and men age 70 and older
Postmenopausal women and men above age 50–69, based on risk factor profile
Postmenopausal women and men age 50 and older who have had an adult age fracture, to diagnose and determine degree of osteoporosis

Fracture Risk Assessment

Measurement of BMD is a powerful tool for estimating fracture risk. The lower the BMD, the greater is the risk of fracture. For every SD decrease in BMD at the hip measured by DXA, there is about a 2.6-fold increase in hip fracture risk and a 1.6-fold increase in the risk of any fracture [11]. However, BMD combined with clinical risk factors (CRFs) predicts fracture risk better than BMD or CRFs alone [12]. FRAX is a computer-based algorithm that estimates 10-year fracture probability in untreated men and women from age 40 to 90 years by combining CRFs and femoral neck BMD, when available. CRFs included in the FRAX algorithm are previous fracture, parent with hip fracture, current smoking, glucocorticoid therapy, rheumatoid arthritis, secondary osteoporosis, and alcohol intake of three or more units per day. A "yes" or "no" response is allowed for each of these CRFs, not allowing for gradation of risk according to dose, severity, or duration of the risk. Secondary osteoporosis is a "dummy" risk factor that does not change the risk estimation unless femoral neck BMD is not entered. A FRAX calculator is included in current DXA software, available online at http://www.shef.uk/FRAX, and can be purchased for use with handheld electronic devices. FRAX provides a quantitative estimate of the 10-year probability of major osteoporotic fracture (clinical spine, forearm, hip, shoulder fracture) and the 10-year probability of hip fracture. When BMD is not available, FRAX can be used without BMD, and in some countries, it is used to determine which patients qualify for DXA. Since many or most patients with a hip fracture do not have T-scores in the osteoporosis range [13], the use of T-scores alone will lead to missed opportunities for interventions to reduce fracture risk.

Evaluation

Osteoporosis is often classified as primary (i.e., due to postmenopausal estrogen deficiency or aging in women and men), secondary (i.e., due to factors such nutritional deficiencies and medications with harmful skeletal effects), or idiopathic (osteoporosis in children or young adults without identifiable cause). A patient may have both primary and secondary osteoporosis. It is essential for all patients at risk for fracture to be evaluated for secondary osteoporosis prior to starting treatment. Previously unrecognized causes of osteoporosis are common. The prevalence of

Table 1.4 Laboratory tests to consider in the evaluation for secondary causes of osteoporosis

For all patients
Complete blood count (CBC)
Chemistry levels (including calcium, phosphorus, renal function, liver function, alkaline phosphatase)
25-OH-vitamin D
24-h urine for calcium
For selected patients
Thyroid test for patients on thyroid medication or with symptoms or signs of thyroid disease
Parathyroid hormone (PTH) when abnormalities are suspected
Total testosterone and gonadotropin in younger men
Bone turnover markers
Serum protein electrophoresis (SPEP) or serum immunofixation electrophoresis
Serum kappa/lambda free light chains
Celiac antibodies
Homocysteine
Prolactin
Tryptase
Urinary free cortisol level
Urinary histamine

Adapted from Cosman et al. [10]

secondary osteoporosis also varies according to the extent of evaluation and the cutoffs for distinguishing normal from abnormal. Evaluation of a patient with osteoporosis includes a thorough bone-related medical history, physical exam with accurate height measurement and falls assessment, laboratory tests (Table 1.4), and sometimes imaging studies [14]. The benefits of such an evaluation include the identification of previously unrecognized conditions affecting skeletal health that may require different or additional therapy and assessment of factors that could influence treatment decisions. The case presented at the opening of this chapter is an example of a disease (celiac disease) that requires additional treatment with a gluten-free diet. A history of esophageal stricture should lead to avoidance of oral bisphosphonates, and a history of a clotting disorder suggests that raloxifene and estrogen should not be prescribed. Historical loss of height (height measured with a wall-mounted stadiometer >1.5 in. less than historical maximum height) suggests possible vertebral fracture and usually warrants spine imaging for further evaluation.

The finding of a previously unrecognized vertebral fracture could lead to a change in diagnostic classification, enhance fracture risk stratification, and possibly lead to a change in treatment decisions [15]. The ISCD has developed recommendations for vertebral imaging with VFA by DXA or conventional radiography (Table 1.5). VFA is lateral spine imaging by DXA that offers an opportunity for point-of-service care done at the same visit as for BMD testing by DXA, with lower cost and less radiation than spine X-rays. Image resolution is not as good as with X-ray, but some vertebral fractures are more easily identified due to less parallax effect.

Table 1.5 Indications for spine imaging to identify vertebral fractures from the International Society for Clinical Densitometry [5]

Lateral spine imaging with standard radiography or densitometric VFA is indicated when T-score is <−1.0 and one or more of the following is present:
Women age ≥70 years or men ≥ age 80 years,
Historical height loss >4 cm (>1.5 in.),
Self-reported but undocumented prior vertebral fracture,
Glucocorticoid therapy equivalent to ≥5 mg of prednisone or equivalent per day for ≥3 months

Table 1.6 Indications (US-specific) for pharmacological therapy to reduce fracture risk from the US National Osteoporosis Foundation [10]

Treatment recommendation may vary by country depending on healthcare priorities, cost, and availability of healthcare resources
In those with hip or vertebral (clinical or asymptomatic) fractures
In those with T-scores ≤−2.5 at the femoral neck, total hip, or lumbar spine by DXA
In postmenopausal women and men age 50 and older with low bone mass (T-score between −1.0 and −2.5) at the femoral neck, total hip, or lumbar spine by DXA and a 10-year hip fracture probability ≥3% or a 10-year major osteoporosis-related fracture probability ≥20% based on the USA-adapted WHO absolute fracture risk model (FRAX)

Treatment

Advances in understanding the pathophysiology of osteoporosis have led to the development of a broad range of medications (e.g., bisphosphonates [alendronate, risedronate, ibandronate, zoledronic acid], raloxifene, denosumab, salmon calcitonin, teriparatide and abaloparatide) that strengthen bone and reduce fracture risk [16]. The cost of some of these, especially the oral bisphosphonates, is very low. Clinical trials have shown that the balance of benefits and risks is highly favorable in appropriately selected patients. Abaloparatide [17], a synthetic analog of parathyroid hormone related peptide (PTHrP[1–34]) with skeletal anabolic effects, received regulatory approval in 2017 for the treatment of postmenopausal women with osteoporosis at high risk of fracture. Romosozumab [18] is a humanized monoclonal protein that blocks the action of sclerostin, a naturally occurring inhibitor of osteoblastic bone formation. Phase 3 clinical trials with romosozumab have been completed. It appears to be a promising agent for the treatment of women with postmenopausal osteoporosis, but it has not received regulatory approval at the time of this writing.

Table 1.6 shows indications for pharmacological therapy in the USA. Treatment decisions must be individualized considering all available clinical information, including patient preference. AACE/ACE has recommendations for choosing initial medication (Table 1.7). After any treatment is started, patients should be monitored to assess tolerance and adherence to therapy. Patients who are suboptimal respond-

Table 1.7 Recommendations for initial treatment of osteoporosis from AACE/ACE [7]

Approved agents with efficacy to reduce hip, nonvertebral, and spine fractures including alendronate, risedronate, zoledronic acid, and denosumab are appropriate as initial therapy for most patients at high risk of fracture
Teriparatide, denosumab, or zoledronic acid should be considered for patients unable to use oral therapy and as initial therapy for patients at especially high fracture risk
Raloxifene or ibandronate may be appropriate initial therapy in some cases where patients requiring drugs with spine-specific efficacy

ers to therapy, by virtue of having a decline in BMD, failure of bone turnover markers to respond as expected, or multiple fractures on therapy, should be reevaluated to identify contributing factors. Suboptimal response to therapy could be due to circumstances such as poor absorption of an oral bisphosphonate, even when taken regularly and correctly, or development of a new disease or condition, such as multiple myeloma or vitamin D deficiency.

Osteoporosis Treatment Gap

Despite the availability of medications to reduce fracture risk, most patients who could benefit from these medications are not taking them [19]. Of those who are prescribed a medication, some do not fill the prescription, do not take medication regularly or correctly (proper administration is especially important with oral bisphosphonates), or do not take it long enough to achieve the desired reduction of fracture risk [20]. The net result is a large osteoporosis treatment gap, resulting in a high personal and economic burden from fractures that might have been prevented by treatment. Many factors contribute to the osteoporosis treatment gap. For some, it is the misperception that osteoporosis is a normal part of aging and not a treatable disease. Others may believe that osteoporosis only affects women. BMD testing is not universally available or affordable. Clinical practice guidelines for osteoporosis treatment are sometimes confusing or conflicting. Physicians and their patients sometimes have a poor understanding of the balance of benefits and risks with osteoporosis treatment. There is often limited time during encounters with patients to address osteoporosis issues. Patients who have had a fracture may not appreciate the high risk of future fractures. There are few osteoporosis specialists with advanced levels of expertise in managing patients with osteoporosis.

Many patients are afraid to take drugs that might help them. Fear of osteoporosis drugs was assessed in a recent study conducted by the NOF with their "online community" of about 28,000 individuals, with 853 (3%) responding [21]. Thirty-eight percent of responders had been prescribed a medication they did not take, with 79% of these stating that fear of side effects was the reason for not taking it. Forty-three percent felt that the risk of side effects with osteoporosis treatment was greater than the benefit. The findings of the NOF survey are consistent with the clinical experience that many patients who might benefit from an osteoporosis medication are afraid to take it.

The osteoporosis treatment gap appears to be worsening, with concern that more hip fractures than expected have been occurring in the USA in recent years [22]. The gap has been termed as crisis by the American Society for Bone and Mineral Research (ASBMR) [3], with a call to action to find ways to reduce the treatment gap.

New Concepts in Osteoporosis Care

How Long to Treat Long-term bisphosphonate therapy has been associated with rare adverse effects such as osteonecrosis of the jaw [23] and atypical femur fractures [24]. Discontinuing treatment appears to reduce the risk of these very unlikely events. Since bisphosphonates have a long skeletal retention time with persistence of antiresorptive effects and perhaps anti-fracture effects when long-term therapy is stopped, the concept of a bisphosphonate "holiday" has emerged. The rationale is that for patients no longer at high risk of fracture who have taken a bisphosphonate for 3–5 years, temporarily withholding treatment will allow continuing benefit while reducing the risk of adverse events. Although there is little evidence to guide clinical decisions, the evidence that is available has been carefully reviewed by an ASBMR task force that recently reported their findings (Table 1.8), which are similar to recommendations from AACE/ACE. Drug holidays apply only to bisphosphonates, as other osteoporosis medications, such as denosumab, rapidly lose their beneficial effects with discontinuation [26]. Patients who are started on a drug holiday should be monitored periodically with the thought of resuming treatment when fracture risk is once again high.

Table 1.8 Managing patients on long-term bisphosphonate therapy from an ASBMR task force [25]. AACE/ACE guidelines are similar with a slightly different terminology: consider a "bisphosphonate holiday" after 5 years of stability with oral bisphosphonate therapy in moderate-risk patients and after 6–10 years of stability in higher-risk patients; for intravenous (IV) zoledronic acid, consider a drug holiday after three annual doses in moderate-risk patients and after six annual doses in higher-risk patients [7]

For postmenopausal women treated with an oral bisphosphonate for ≥5 years or an intravenous bisphosphonate for ≥3 years, consider treatment decisions based on fracture risk stratification, as follows:
Low fracture risk
Definition: hip T-score >–2.5 and no hip, spine, or multiple osteoporotic fracture before or during therapy
Suggestion: consider drug holiday of 2–3 years
High fracture risk
Definition: hip T-score ≤–2.5 or hip, spine, or multiple osteoporotic fracture before or during therapy
Suggestion: consider continuing oral bisphosphonate up to 10 years and intravenous bisphosphonate up to 6 years

Treat-to-Target The concept of treat-to-target is based on the premise that a response to therapy is not necessarily the same as achieving an acceptable level of fracture risk [27, 28]. While a response to therapy is necessary in order to reduce fracture risk, it is not always sufficient to bring fracture risk to a level that is desirable. Since treatment targets are common clinical practice for some other chronic diseases, such as diabetes mellitus and hypertension, and might be useful in the care of patients with osteoporosis, an ASBMR-NOF working group was formed with the charge of exploring the feasibility of treat-to-target for osteoporosis. The findings were recently reported [29]. It was suggested that baseline risk stratification be performed and that a treatment target be identified before treatment is started. The choice of initial treatment should be one that is likely to reach the target. When treatment is started according to a T-score ≤−2.5, then the target should be at least a T-score > 2.5, above the threshold for starting treatment with the NOF guidelines. A target T-score >−2.0 allows for the variability of DXA measurements and the LSC. These suggestions were primarily based on expert opinion, recognizing the need for more data to confirm or reject the clinical utility of osteoporosis treatment targets.

Fracture Liaison Service Secondary fracture prevention by coordinator-based systematic identification and management of patients with fractures may help to close the osteoporosis treatment gap [30–32]. The concept of a fracture liaison service (FLS) has been emerging worldwide. Uptake of FLS seems to be best in countries with a national healthcare system and in the USA for large integrated health systems that have financial incentives to reduce healthcare costs. With fee-for-service medical care, the adoption of FLS has been slower. A study with a Markov state-transition computer simulation model nevertheless found potential economic benefit with FLS in the USA [33]. This may encourage further use of FLS in the USA.

Education by Teleconferencing The idea that every primary care provider would be willing and able to manage the vast majority of patients with osteoporosis has not been successful, thereby contributing to the osteoporosis treatment gap. An alternative strategy is to find a single healthcare provider or a small group in each community with a special interest in osteoporosis and then elevate their level of knowledge to near-expert level through the use of teleconferencing technology. Project ECHO (Extension for Community Healthcare Outcomes), developed at the University of New Mexico in Albuquerque, New Mexico, USA, has been shown to improve the care of chronic hepatitis C in rural New Mexico [34]. The same concept has been applied to Bone Health TeleECHO to improve the care of osteoporosis in underserved communities [35, 36]. Weekly videoconferences are held to link faculty and learners anywhere that an electronic link is available. Learning is primarily through case-based discussions with brief weekly didactic presentations. Preliminary results have been favorable, with a very large effect size for self-confidence in osteoporosis patient care responsibilities.

Summary

Osteoporosis is a common disease that weakens bones and increases the risk of fractures. The consequences of osteoporotic fractures include disability, loss of independence, and death. Effective and safe medications have been proven effective at reducing fracture risk, but are currently underutilized, resulting in a large osteoporosis treatment gap. New strategies with the potential of reducing the treatment gap are being developed.

Disclosure In the past year, E. Michael Lewiecki has received institutional grant/research support from Amgen, Merck, and Eli Lilly; he has served on scientific advisory boards for Amgen, Merck, Eli Lilly, Radius Health, Shire, AbbVie, and Alexion; he serves on the speakers' bureau for Shire and Alexion.

References

1. US Department of Health and Human Services. Bone health and osteoporosis: a report of the surgeon general. Rockville: US Department of Health and Human Services, Office of the Surgeon General; 2004.
2. International Osteoporosis Foundation. Osteoporosis. http://www.iofbonehealth.org/osteoporosis. Accessed 30 Nov 2016.
3. Khosla S, Shane EA. Crisis in the treatment of osteoporosis. J Bone Miner Res. 2016;31(8):1485–7.
4. WHO Study Group on Assessment of Fracture Risk and its Application to Screening for Postmenopausal Osteoporosis. Assessment of fracture risk and its application to screening for postmenopausal osteoporosis. Geneva: World Health Organization; 1994.
5. Shepherd JA, Schousboe JT, Broy SB, Engelke K, Leslie WD. Executive summary of the 2015 ISCD position development conference on advanced measures from DXA and QCT: fracture prediction beyond BMD. J Clin Densitom. 2015;18(3):274–86.
6. Siris ES, Adler R, Bilezikian J, Bolognese M, Dawson-Hughes B, Favus MJ, et al. The clinical diagnosis of osteoporosis: a position statement from the National Bone Health Alliance Working Group. Osteoporos Int. 2014;25(5):1439–43.
7. Camacho PM, Petak SM, Binkley N, Clarke BL, Harris ST, Hurley DL, et al. American Association of Clinical Endocrinologists and American College of Endocrinology Clinical Practice Guidelines for the Diagnosis and Treatment of Postmenopausal Osteoporosis – 2016 – executive summary. Endocr Pract. 2016;22(9):1111–8.
8. Krieg MA, Barkmann R, Gonnelli S, Stewart A, Bauer DC, Del Rio BL, et al. Quantitative ultrasound in the management of osteoporosis: the 2007 ISCD Official Positions. J Clin Densitom. 2008;11(1):163–87.
9. Lewiecki EM, Binkley N, Morgan SL, Shuhart CR, Camargos BM, Carey JJ, et al. Best practices for dual-energy X-ray absorptiometry measurement and reporting: International Society for Clinical Densitometry Guidance. J Clin Densitom. 2016;19(2):127–40.
10. Cosman F, de Beur SJ, LeBoff MS, Lewiecki EM, Tanner B, Randall S, et al. Clinician's guide to prevention and treatment of osteoporosis. Osteoporos Int. 2014;25(10):2359–81.
11. Marshall D, Johnell O, Wedel H. Meta-analysis of how well measures of bone mineral density predict occurrence of osteoporotic fractures. BMJ. 1996;312(7041):1254–9.

12. De Laet C, Oden A, Johansson H, Johnell O, Jonsson B, Kanis JA. The impact of the use of multiple risk indicators for fracture on case-finding strategies: a mathematical approach. Osteoporos Int. 2005;16(3):313–8.
13. Wainwright SA, Marshall LM, Ensrud KE, Cauley JA, Black DM, Hillier TA, et al. Hip fracture in women without osteoporosis. J Clin Endocrinol Metab. 2005;90(5):2787–93.
14. Lewiecki EM. Evaluation of the patient at risk for osteoporosis. In: Marcus R, Feldman D, Dempster DW, Luckey M, Cauley JA, editors. Osteoporosis, vol. 2. 4th ed. Waltham: Elsevier; 2013. p. 1481–504.
15. Lewiecki EM, Laster AJ. Clinical applications of vertebral fracture assessment by dual-energy X-ray absorptiometry. J Clin Endocrinol Metab. 2006;91(11):4215–22.
16. Drake MT, Clarke BL, Lewiecki EM. The pathophysiology and treatment of osteoporosis. Clin Ther. 2015;37(6):1837–50.
17. Miller PD, Hattersley G, Riis BJ, Williams GC, Lau E, Russo LA, et al. Effect of abaloparatide vs placebo on new vertebral fractures in postmenopausal women with osteoporosis: a randomized clinical trial. JAMA. 2016;316(7):722–33.
18. Cosman F, Crittenden DB, Adachi JD, Binkley N, Czerwinski E, Ferrari S, et al. Romosozumab treatment in postmenopausal women with osteoporosis. N Engl J Med. 2016;375(16):1532–43.
19. Solomon DH, Johnston SS, Boytsov NN, McMorrow D, Lane JM, Krohn KD. Osteoporosis medication use after hip fracture in U.S. patients between 2002 and 2011. J Bone Miner Res. 2014;29(9):1929–37.
20. Cramer JA, Gold DT, Silverman SL, Lewiecki EM. A systematic review of persistence and compliance with bisphosphonates for osteoporosis. Osteoporos Int. 2007;18(8):1023–31.
21. National Osteoporosis Foundation. Bone health index survey final report. Unpublished data; Arlington, VA, USA. 2016.
22. Lewiecki EM, Adler RA, Curtis JR, Gagel R, Saag KG, Singer AJ, et al. Hip fractures and declining DXA testing: at a breaking point? J Bone Miner Res. 2016;31(Suppl):S26.
23. Khosla S, Burr D, Cauley J, Dempster DW, Ebeling PR, Felsenberg D, et al. Bisphosphonate-associated osteonecrosis of the jaw: report of a task force of the American Society for Bone and Mineral Research. J Bone Miner Res. 2007;22(10):1479–89.
24. Shane E, Burr D, Abrahamsen B, Adler RA, Brown TD, Cheung AM, et al. Atypical subtrochanteric and diaphyseal femoral fractures: second report of a task force of the American Society for Bone and Mineral Research. J Bone Miner Res. 2014;29(1):1–23.
25. Adler RA, El-Hajj Fuleihan G, Bauer DC, Camacho PM, Clarke BL, Clines GA, et al. Managing osteoporosis in patients on long-term bisphosphonate treatment: report of a task force of the American Society for Bone and Mineral Research. J Bone Miner Res. 2016;31(1):16–35.
26. McClung MR. Cancel the denosumab holiday. Osteoporos Int. 2016;27(5):1677–82.
27. Lewiecki EM, Cummings SR, Cosman F. Treat-to-target for osteoporosis: is now the time? J Clin Endocrinol Metab. 2013;98(3):946–53.
28. Cummings SR, Cosman F, Eastell R, Reid IR, Mehta M, Lewiecki EM. Goal-directed treatment of osteoporosis. J Bone Miner Res. 2013;28(3):433–8.
29. Cummings SR, Cosman F, Lewiecki EM, Schousboe JT, Bauer DC, Black DM, et al. Goal-directed treatment for osteoporosis: a progress report from the ASBMR-NOF working group on goal-directed treatment for osteoporosis. J Bone Miner Res. 2017;32(1):3–10.
30. National Bone Health Alliance. Fracture prevention central 2016 [updated March 28, 2016]. Available from: www.nbha.org/fpc.
31. International Osteoporosis Foundation. Capture the fracture 2016 [updated March 28, 2016]. Available from: www.capturethefracture.org.
32. Tosi LL, Gliklich R, Kannan K, Koval KJ. The American Orthopaedic Association's "Own the Bone" initiative to prevent secondary fractures. J Bone Joint Surg Am. 2008;90(1):163–73.
33. Solomon DH, Patrick AR, Schousboe J, Losina E. The potential economic benefits of improved postfracture care: a cost-effectiveness analysis of a fracture liaison service in the US health-care system. J Bone Miner Res. 2014;29(7):1667–74.

34. Arora S, Thornton K, Murata G, Deming P, Kalishman S, Dion D, et al. Outcomes of treatment for hepatitis C virus infection by primary care providers. N Engl J Med. 2011;364(23):2199–207.
35. Lewiecki EM, Boyle JF, Arora S, Bouchonville MF 2nd, Chafey DH. Telementoring: a novel approach to reducing the osteoporosis treatment gap. Osteoporos Int. 2017;28(1):407–11.
36. Lewiecki EM, Bouchonville MF 2nd, Chafey DH, Bankhurst A, Arora S. Bone Health ECHO: telementoring to improve osteoporosis care. Women's Health (Lond Engl). 2016;12(1):79–81.

E. Michael Lewiecki, MD, is Director of New Mexico Clinical Research & Osteoporosis Center, Clinical Assistant Professor of Medicine at University of New Mexico Health Sciences Center, and Director of Bone Health TeleECHO in Albuquerque, New Mexico, USA. He is a clinical researcher with a consulting practice in osteoporosis and metabolic bone diseases. He serves on the Board of Trustees of the National Osteoporosis Foundation and the Board of Directors of the International Society for Clinical Densitometry.

Chapter 2
Primary Hyperparathyroidism

Clare O'Connor, Joshua A. Levine, and Allison Hahr

Case

A 22-year-old man presented to the endocrine clinic for evaluation of presumed polyostotic fibrous dysplasia that had been previously diagnosed at a different hospital. He had a history of a motor vehicle accident at age 15 that led to discovery of a lesion on his left humerus. This lesion was subsequently removed with diagnosis of fibrous dysplasia as per histopathology report. He then had femoral epiphysis slipping requiring bilateral stabilization with screws as well as multiple fractures of his left clavicle, ribs, and right wrist over several years. Imaging had shown multiple sclerotic lesions in his calvarium. He reported chronic polydipsia/polyuria and fluctuating mood due to his chronic bone pain. Review of systems was otherwise negative for headache, weight loss/gain, abdominal pain, nausea, constipation/diarrhea, edema, or skin lesions. There was no reported family history of endocrine disorders.

Workup at his initial visit showed a serum calcium of 13 mg/dL (8.3–10.5 mg/dL), parathyroid hormone (PTH) 583 pg/mL (12–88 pg/mL), albumin 4.7 g/dL, 25 hydroxy vitamin *D* < 13 ng/mL (30–100 ng/mL), phosphorus 1.7 mg/dL (2.5–5.0 mg/dL), and alkaline phosphatase 184 unit/L (34–104). Twenty-four-hour urine calcium was elevated at 475 mg in 2950 mL (100–300 mg). Initially,

C. O'Connor · A. Hahr (✉) · J. A. Levine
Division of Endocrinology, Metabolism and Molecular Medicine,
Northwestern University Feinberg School of Medicine, Chicago, IL, USA
e-mail: a-hahr@northwestern.edu

P. M. Camacho (ed.), *Metabolic Bone Diseases*,
https://doi.org/10.1007/978-3-030-03694-2_2

a CT chest was ordered to evaluate for extent of disease of his polyostotic fibrous dysplasia. The CT showed multiple bone lesions and ectopic tissue in the left paratracheal space. Multiple expansile bone lesions and sclerotic foci were noted in the ribs as well as bilateral humeral neck and heads (Fig. 2.1). Based on this workup, a diagnosis of primary hyperparathyroidism (PHPT) was made. Subsequent parathyroid ultrasound showed a 3.2 × 1.7 × 1.5 cm soft tissue nodule inferior to the left thyroid lobe compatible with a parathyroid adenoma (Fig. 2.2).

The patient's skeletal disease was due to osteitis fibrosa cystica from PHPT and not fibrous dysplasia as previously diagnosed; fibrous dysplasia does not present

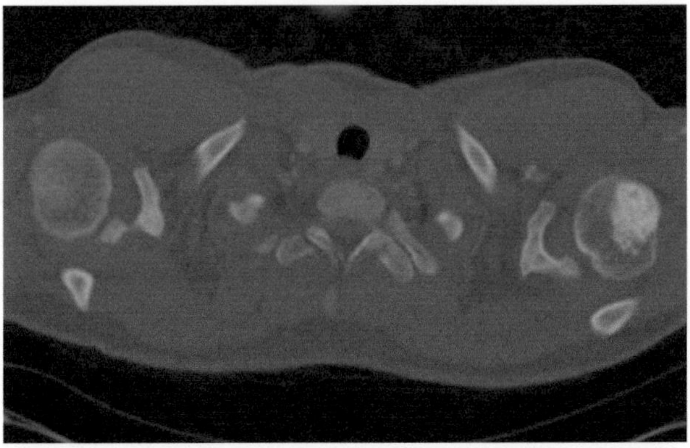

Fig. 2.1 Sclerotic expansile bone lesion of the left humerus seen on CT

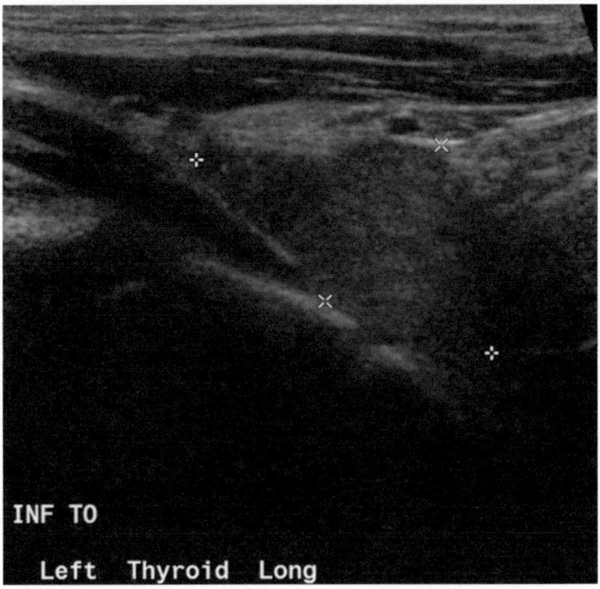

Fig. 2.2 Parathyroid ultrasound showing 3.2 × 1.7 × 1.5 cm soft tissue nodule in the left paratracheal region compatible with a parathyroid adenoma

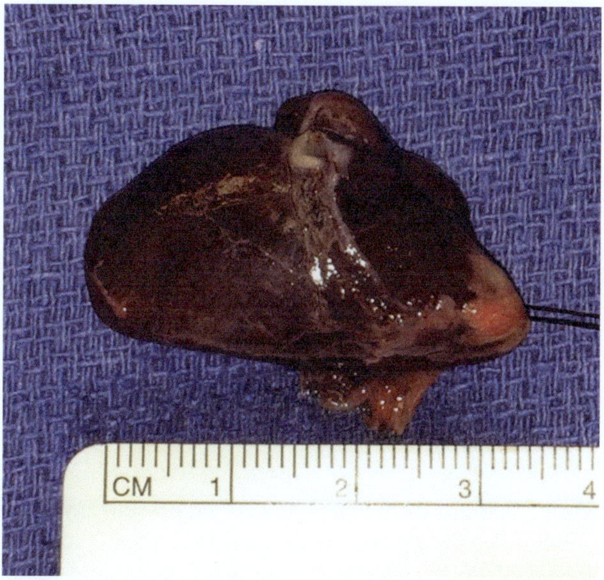

Fig. 2.3 Parathyroid adenoma weighing 4.3 g

with an elevated PTH and hypercalcemia. The patient underwent a parathyroidectomy with a 4.3 g adenoma removed and pathology showing hypercellular parathyroid tissue (Fig. 2.3). Intraoperatively, his highest baseline PTH level was 1686 which fell to 149 at 5 min, 90 at 10 min, and 56 at 20 min after resection. Postoperatively, the PTH levels were in the normal range, and his calcium has remained within normal limits. His bone pain completely resolved. He did not have any hypocalcemia postoperatively.

Introduction

This case illustrates an uncommon presentation of primary hyperparathyroidism, a common endocrine disorder, and the most common cause of hypercalcemia. Incidence of PHPT has been reported as an average of 21.6 per 100,000 person-years [1] (from Rochester MN predominantly Caucasian population). There is higher incidence in women (average incidence 65.5 per 100,000 person-years for women vs. 24.7 per 100,000 person-years for men) [2], those over 50 years old, and certain races (black women found to have highest incidence of PHPT followed by white women) [2]. Hypercalcemia is due to autonomous release of parathyroid hormone (PTH) from one or more parathyroid glands. The source of elevated PTH is most often a solitary parathyroid adenoma (80%) and less often four-gland hyperplasia (10–15%). It is important to think of genetic causes in patients with a strong family history of PHPT and in young patients, such as the patient profiled in our case, especially if four-gland hyperplasia is present.

Clinical Manifestations

Most cases of PHPT today are asymptomatic at the time of diagnosis and are diagnosed incidentally based on lab findings revealing an elevated serum calcium level. However, most patients are not truly asymptomatic on close evaluation. In the past, PHPT often presented as a symptomatic disease due to the prolonged effect of elevated PTH at various sites and symptoms of hypercalcemia ("bones, stones, abdominal groans, and psychiatric overtones"). Although overtly symptomatic disease may be less common, it is important for the clinician to be aware of these manifestations.

Skeletal Manifestations

Skeletal effects from PHPT most often present asymptomatically with reduced bone mineral density (BMD) at cortical-rich sites (such as forearm) and relatively preserved BMD at cancellous bone sites (spine and femoral neck). Therefore, guidelines suggest assessing BMD with dual-energy X-ray absorptiometry (DXA) using three sites (lumbar spine, hip, and distal 1/3 radius) for initial evaluation and monitoring [3]. In fact, the forearm was the only osteoporotic site involved in 11.2% of patients in a PHPT cohort study. Including the forearm BMD measurement increased the number of patients with asymptomatic PHPT meeting surgical criteria [4].

Interestingly, despite mostly preserved BMD at cancellous bone sites (such as lumbar spine and femoral neck), there is evidence of globally increased fracture risk at both non-vertebral (cortical) and vertebral (cancellous/trabecular) sites in postmenopausal women with PHPT compared to controls [5]. This suggests there is more than BMD involved in determining fracture risk in patients with PHPT, especially in the postmenopausal state. Further studies have looked at bone microarchitecture and bone quality with trabecular bone score as described in a review by Walker and Silverberg [6]. Several studies outlined in this review have shown that PHPT leads to deteriorated microarchitecture at the spine, radius, and tibia which may help explain the globally increased fracture risk in PHPT despite fairly preserved BMD at spine and femoral neck [6]. Parathyroidectomy has been shown to lead to improved BMD at the lumbar spine and total hip at 6 months and at the femoral neck at 12 months; however there were no changes noted at the distal 1/3 radius, and no significant changes in trabecular bone score following parathyroidectomy [7].

The case presented above highlights that the initial presenting feature can be symptomatic skeletal abnormalities such as osteitis fibrosa cystica. This is the initial presentation in <5% of cases in the United States, but is still a common presentation in other parts of the world [6, 8]. When a patient presents with a lytic bone lesion and hypercalcemia as the patient above did, it is important to consider PHPT in the differential diagnosis. Osteitis fibrosa cystica is often associated with bone pain (as described with the patient in this case), subperiosteal bone resorption, osteolysis of distal clavicles, "salt and pepper" appearance of the skull, bone cysts, and brown tumors of bones (due to hemosiderin deposition) [8, 9].

Of note, skeletal manifestations of PHPT are often significantly worse if there is concomitant vitamin D deficiency as in this case. Vitamin D deficiency is very common in PHPT and often leads to higher PTH levels compared to PHPT patients without vitamin D deficiency [10]. It is thought that these higher PTH levels lead to increased catabolic effect in cortical bone (cortical thinning) and increased anabolic effects in trabecular bone (higher cancellous bone volume), although more studies are needed to better understand this mechanism [10].

Renal Manifestations

Renal complications related to PHPT have been decreasing over the past years. Common renal manifestations related to PHPT include nephrolithiasis (15–20%) [9] and nephrocalcinosis (calcium phosphate deposits in the parenchyma) [3, 11]. The 2014 guidelines for the management of asymptomatic primary hyperparathyroidism from the Fourth International Workshop now suggest a more extensive renal evaluation as part of initial workup to screen for these renal manifestations (see below) [3]. Hypercalciuria is also a common finding in PHPT that correlates with plasma calcium levels. While hypercalciuria is thought to be a risk factor for development of nephrolithiasis in general, the relationship of hypercalciuria and the risk of developing nephrolithiasis in PHPT are not fully understood. In a review by Rejnmark on this subject, they report studies show mixed findings, with only some studies showing an association between increased urinary calcium levels in PHPT patients with nephrolithiasis, whereas other studies have not found that association [11]. The same review did find that male gender and young age at diagnosis of PHPT did increase risk of nephrolithiasis [11].

Neuropsychiatric Manifestations

Several vague neuropsychiatric symptoms have been described in the literature (fatigue, weakness, depression, cognitive dysfunction, decreased quality of life) that have been associated with PHPT. Studies evaluating whether parathyroidectomy reverses these symptoms have been inconsistent [6]. For example, one prospective case-control study did find that parathyroidectomy improved depressive symptoms (compared to patients that had thyroidectomy) [12]. However, there have been several other small case-control studies evaluating depression that have been inconsistent [13]. Due to the inconsistent results, the 2014 guidelines do not recommend parathyroidectomy in patients with neuropsychiatric complaints if they do not otherwise meet criteria for surgical intervention [3].

Gastrointestinal Manifestations

High plasma calcium levels are associated with constipation; however constipation is not usually seen today as a symptom of PHPT due to early detection and mild hypercalcemia on initial presentation. Past literature has identified higher incidences of peptic ulcer disease and pancreatitis in PHPT; however these associations are difficult to assess due to high use of proton pump inhibitors and early detection of PHPT [14]. The pathophysiology link between peptic ulcer disease and PHPT is also unclear, except in the rare cases of multiple endocrine neoplasia type 1 (MEN1) which can present with both features [9].

Cardiovascular Manifestations

There are possible cardiovascular manifestations associated with PHPT reported that include hypertension, endothelial dysfunction (early atherosclerosis marker), arrhythmias, and glucose metabolism impairment [15]. Cardiac mortality does appear to be increased in severe disease, but not in mild disease [13]. Hypertension is often seen even in asymptomatic sporadic PHPT (not part of MEN syndrome) [13]. However, a randomized controlled trial of parathyroidectomy versus observation did not find a between-group difference in blood pressure [16]. Overall, there have been inconsistent results on cardiovascular outcomes after parathyroidectomy [15]. Therefore, the 2014 guidelines do not recommend assessing for cardiovascular dysfunction as part of PHPT evaluation and do not recommend parathyroidectomy as a way to improve cardiovascular outcomes if abnormalities are seen [3].

Clinical Evaluation and Diagnosis

Most often PHPT is diagnosed by incidentally discovered mild hypercalcemia (adjusted if there is any abnormality in albumin levels), with coinciding elevated PTH or inappropriately normal PTH (PTH in mid-upper normal range in setting of hypercalcemia). Most other causes of hypercalcemia will have suppressed PTH (PTH-independent processes). Other PTH-dependent processes to consider and rule out before diagnosing PHPT include tertiary hyperparathyroidism (autonomous parathyroid gland due to prolonged ESRD/secondary hyperparathyroidism). Concomitant secondary hyperparathyroidism (elevated PTH with normal calcium value or hypocalcemia) should also be considered and further evaluated as indicated below. Additionally, it is important to consider familial hypocalciuric hypercalcemia (FHH) in the differential.

PHPT can also occur with normal calcium values. This can be found during the initial laboratory evaluation for secondary causes of osteoporosis where hyperparathyroidism is assessed as a cause of osteoporosis. Normocalcemic PHPT by definition occurs in the setting of normal vitamin D levels, normal urinary calcium excretion (not low), and normal renal function, with exclusion of all secondary causes of hyperparathyroidism. Medications that can cause a rise in parathyroid hormone levels such as bisphosphonates, denosumab, thiazides, and lithium should be taken into consideration. Management of normocalcemic PHPT is not quite clear due to lack of data and guidelines, but many physicians tend to use the same guidelines as for patients with asymptomatic hypercalcemic PHPT where applicable [17].

It is important to obtain a 24-h urine calcium and creatinine collection when indicated to distinguish familial hypocalciuric hypercalcemia (FHH) from PHPT, as the management is different. To help distinguish between the two, calculating the ratio of calcium clearance to creatinine clearance can be helpful. A value less than 0.01 in a patient with hypercalcemia who is vitamin D replete with normal renal function suggests FHH as the cause [18]. Typically values in PHPT are much higher. The ratio can be calculated using serum calcium (Ca_s), serum creatinine (Cr_s), urine calcium (Ca_u), and urine creatinine (Cr_u): $Ca_{Cl}/Cr_{Cl} = (Ca_u \text{ x } Cr_s)/(Ca_s \text{ x } Cr_u)$. A ratio of 0.01–0.02 warrants consideration of genetic testing for FHH [19].

PHPT must be distinguished from secondary and tertiary hyperparathyroidism. Secondary hyperparathyroidism is associated with normal (or low) calcium values in the setting of an appropriate parathyroid stimulus such as low vitamin D or chronic kidney disease. Tertiary hyperparathyroidism results from autonomous parathyroid overproduction, from long-standing stimulation similar to secondary hyperparathyroidism, most often seen in the setting of long-standing chronic kidney/end-stage renal disease. In contrast to secondary hyperparathyroidism, tertiary hyperparathyroidism is associated with hypercalcemia.

Once the diagnosis of PHPT is made, the 2014 PHPT guidelines suggest further laboratory and imaging evaluation in asymptomatic patients with PHPT to help identify patients that meet criteria for parathyroidectomy. They recommend a biochemistry panel (calcium, phosphate, alkaline phosphatase, BUN, creatinine), 25(OH)D, and PTH [3]. Phosphorus is often either low or in the low-normal range in PHPT. Vitamin D deficiency is common in PHPT and can exacerbate symptoms/disease and lead to increased PTH levels.

It is recommended to obtain a DXA to evaluate BMD that includes lumbar spine, hip, and distal 1/3 radius measurements as well as a vertebral spine assessment due to the abovementioned globally increased fracture risk for both vertebral and peripheral fractures in patients with PHPT. Additionally, it is recommended to obtain abdominal imaging (X-ray, ultrasound, or CT scan) to assess for asymptomatic nephrolithiasis or nephrocalcinosis [3].

Parathyroid imaging has no role in diagnosing primary hyperparathyroidism as the diagnosis must be made biochemically, but imaging can be obtained after decision is made to proceed with parathyroidectomy to help guide operative planning. Options for imaging include cervical ultrasound and/or sestamibi or four-dimensional CT [20].

Etiologies of Primary Hyperparathyroidism

The vast majority of cases of PHPT are idiopathic in nature. Sporadic parathyroid adenomas do not appear to have many somatic variants, with the most common being MEN1 and cyclin D1 (genes regulating the cell cycle) [6, 21, 22]. Iatrogenic causes of PHPT include chronic lithium use and external radiation to the neck. Lithium has been associated with hyperparathyroidism and is not an uncommon side effect for patients on long-standing lithium. It can cause both single parathyroid disease and multiple-gland parathyroid disease [23].

Familial forms of PHPT also occur, are much less common than idiopathic or iatrogenic cases, and represent about 5–10% of cases of PHPT [6]. These inherited forms should be suspected if patients present at a young age or have a strong family history of PHPT or other endocrine disorders. Multiple endocrine neoplasia type 1 (MEN1) is an autosomal dominant genetic disorder associated with genetic mutations in *MEN1*, the gene encoding for menin. Parathyroid tumors are one of the most common features, present in >90% of individuals with MEN1 between ages 20 and 25 and developing hypercalcemia by age 50 (high penetrance) [24]. These patients can also present with pituitary adenomas and pancreatic neuroendocrine tumors. Another familial cause of PHPT, multiple endocrine neoplasia type 2A (MEN2A), is another autosomal dominant genetic disorder. These patients, who have mutations in *RET*, can also have PHPT, although at a much lower rate of occurrence (20–30%) [25]. MEN2A patients are at high risk for medullary thyroid cancer and pheochromocytoma. Hyperparathyroid-jaw tumor syndrome is an autosomal dominant disorder associated with mutations in *CDC73*. Germline variants in *CDC73* typically present with single-gland parathyroid adenomas (70%), ossifying maxillary/mandibular fibromas (25–50%), or parathyroid carcinoma (15%) [25]. These patients can also have uterine tumors and renal anomalies [25].

Clinical Management of Hyperparathyroidism

Parathyroidectomy remains the only method of cure for PHPT. In patients with mild PHPT that were followed for 15 years without surgery, PHPT progressed in one third of individuals over 15 years (met one or more new guidelines for surgery), suggesting that PHPT can often remain fairly stable over a long time period [26].

In the short term, severe hypercalcemia can warrant medical therapy, including intravenous fluids, diuretics, calcitonin, bisphosphonates, and dialysis. Calcitonin should not be used for more than 48 hours as there is a risk for tachyphylaxis. If able to use (no significant heart failure or renal insufficiency), intravenous fluids are the first-line treatment. In general, diuretics should be avoided. Bisphosphonates should not be used if a parathyroidectomy is anticipated in the near future as patients will be at increased risk for hungry bone disease and associated hypocalcemia postoperatively. While these therapies can provide short-term relief for symptomatic hypercalcemia, parathyroidectomy should be performed in all surgical candidates.

All patients with symptomatic hypercalcemia from PHPT should be offered a parathyroidectomy. In contrast, surgery is not recommended for all asymptomatic patients with PHPT. In 2014, the Endocrine Society published updated guidelines for the management of asymptomatic PHPT. The goal of a parathyroidectomy is either to reverse or prevent the secondary effects of elevated PTH and hypercalcemia. Patients under the age of 50 should undergo surgery as hypercalcemia over decades can lead to nephrolithiasis, renal dysfunction, and osteoporosis. Patients with serum calcium levels >1 mg/dL above the upper limit of normal should also undergo parathyroidectomy. Osteoporosis is a known outcome of PHPT, and thus, patients with osteoporosis (defined as T-score ≤ -2.5 at the lumbar spine, total hip, femoral neck, or distal 1/3 of the radius, or the presence of a vertebral fracture on imaging, or a Z-score ≤ -2.5 in premenopausal women or men <50 years old) should undergo surgery to prevent progression and improve bone mineral density. As mentioned above, there are data on improved BMD after parathyroidectomy. However, despite this improvement in bone mineral density, there is a paucity of data supporting a decreased risk of fragility fractures after surgery. Hypercalcemia is known to worsen renal function, and thus, a creatinine clearance <60 cc/min is a surgical indication. Lastly, hypercalciuria from PHPT leads to nephrolithiasis and nephrocalcinosis, so those with evidence of either of these entities should undergo parathyroidectomy. Furthermore, patients who present for workup of PHPT should undergo imaging to evaluate for nephrocalcinosis to determine if they should proceed with surgery. Parathyroidectomy is associated with a reduction in the development of nephrolithiasis and nephrocalcinosis [27].

While many patients with asymptomatic PHPT meet surgical criteria, many do not and these patients require monitoring to determine if they become surgical candidates. Per current guidelines, patients should have annual serum calcium levels, DXA should be performed every 1–2 years, X-ray or VFA of the spine should be ordered if height loss or back pain occurs, and renal function by eGFR and serum creatinine should be measured annually [3]. If nephrolithiasis is suspected, a 24-h urine stone profile in addition to renal imaging (X-ray, ultrasound, or CT) should be done [3]. The purpose of this laboratory and imaging testing is to find patients who become surgical candidates and to offer them a parathyroidectomy.

Despite meeting surgical criteria for a parathyroidectomy, some patients with PHPT are either not able to or do not wish to undergo surgery. These patients are therefore managed medically. Current guidelines recommend vitamin D repletion to above 20 ng/dL as hypovitaminosis D can lead to even higher PTH levels and more pronounced effects as described above. A goal vitamin D level >30 ng/dL is also reasonable as there are data to suggest that raising vitamin D levels to above 30 ng/dL can reduce PTH levels even further without an increase in hypercalcemia or hypercalciuria [19, 28]. Furthermore, increased lumbar spine bone mineral density was seen if a higher vitamin D goal was used.

Medications to consider for the treatment of PHPT include bisphosphonates and cinacalcet. The most studied bisphosphonate to date for the management of PHPT is alendronate. There is some evidence that alendronate can increase lumbar spine and hip BMD in nonsurgical patients with PHPT; however it is not clear there is an associated fracture risk reduction [29]. There is limited data examining zoledronic acid, pamidronate, or ibandronate therapy for nonsurgical PHPT treatment of low bone density. Women with PHPT who received 2 years of denosumab showed improvements in BMD compared to placebo [30].

The use of teriparatide and abaloparatide should be avoided in those with primary hyperparathyroidism. Based on the 2014 International Workshop guidelines for medical management of PHPT, bisphosphonate therapy is recommended if there is concern for low BMD [29]. The same guidelines suggest using cinacalcet (calcimimetic) if control of hypercalcemia is needed. Cinacalcet was approved by the FDA for the treatment of severe hypercalcemia in patients with PHPT who are not surgical candidates. Despite lowering of the serum calcium levels, it only has modest reduction on PTH and no effect on bone mineral density or urinary calcium excretion. Therefore, it is best used to treat symptoms of hypercalcemia in patients that are not surgical candidates for PHPT [29].

Conclusion

Our case demonstrates a particularly severe course of primary hyperparathyroidism presenting at a young age. Primary hyperparathyroidism is a common disorder that is diagnosed in primary care and endocrinology practices around the world. It is important to recognize the many clinical manifestations of this disorder, both common and rare, as well as establish how to make the diagnosis. Once the diagnosis is established, it is also important to be aware which individuals warrant consideration for genetic testing.

References

1. Wermers RA, Khosla S, Atkinson EJ, et al. Incidence of primary hyperparathyroidism in Rochester, Minnesota, 1993–2001: an update on the changing epidemiology of the disease. J Bone Miner Res. 2006;21(1):171–7.
2. Yeh MW, Ituarte PH, Zhou HC, et al. Incidence and prevalence of primary hyperparathyroidism in a racially mixed population. J Clin Endocrinol Metab. 2013;98(3):1122–9.
3. Bilezikian JP, Brandi ML, Eastell R, et al. Guidelines for the management of asymptomatic primary hyperparathyroidism: summary statement from the fourth international workshop. J Clin Endocrinol Metab. 2014;99(10):3561–9.
4. Castellano E, Attanasio R, Gianotti L, Cesario F, Tassone F, Borretta G. Forearm DXA increases the rate of patients with asymptomatic primary hyperparathyroidism meeting surgical criteria. J Clin Endocrinol Metab. 2016;101(7):2728–32.
5. De Geronimo S, Romagnoli E, Diacinti D, D'Erasmo E, Minisola S. The risk of fractures in postmenopausal women with primary hyperparathyroidism. Eur J Endocrinol. 2006;155(3):415–20.
6. Walker MD, Silverberg SJ. Primary hyperparathyroidism. Nat Rev Endocrinol. 2017.
7. Cipriani C, Abraham A, Silva BC, et al. Skeletal changes after restoration of the euparathyroid state in patients with hypoparathyroidism and primary hyperparathyroidism. Endocrine. 2017;55(2):591–8.

8. Misiorowski W, Czajka-Oraniec I, Kochman M, Zgliczyński W, Bilezikian JP. Osteitis fibrosa cystica-a forgotten radiological feature of primary hyperparathyroidism. Endocrine. 2017;58:380.
9. Silverberg S. Primary hyperparathyroidism. In: Rosen C, editor. Primer on the metabolic bone diseases and disorders of mineral metabolism. 8th ed. Hoboken: Wiley; 2013. p. 543–9.
10. Stein EM, Dempster DW, Udesky J, et al. Vitamin D deficiency influences histomorphometric features of bone in primary hyperparathyroidism. Bone. 2011;48(3):557–61.
11. Rejnmark L, Vestergaard P, Mosekilde L. Nephrolithiasis and renal calcifications in primary hyperparathyroidism. J Clin Endocrinol Metab. 2011;96(8):2377–85.
12. Espiritu RP, Kearns AE, Vickers KS, Grant C, Ryu E, Wermers RA. Depression in primary hyperparathyroidism: prevalence and benefit of surgery. J Clin Endocrinol Metab. 2011;96(11):E1737–45.
13. Walker MD, Rubin M, Silverberg SJ. Nontraditional manifestations of primary hyperparathyroidism. J Clin Densitom. 2013;16(1):40–7.
14. Ebert EC. The parathyroids and the gut. J Clin Gastroenterol. 2010;44(7):479–82.
15. Pepe J, Cipriani C, Sonato C, Raimo O, Biamonte F, Minisola S. Cardiovascular manifestations of primary hyperparathyroidism: a narrative review. Eur J Endocrinol. 2017;177(6):R297–308.
16. Persson A, Bollerslev J, Rosen T, et al. Effect of surgery on cardiac structure and function in mild primary hyperparathyroidism. Clin Endocrinol. 2011;74(2):174–80.
17. Silverberg SJ, Clarke BL, Peacock M, et al. Current issues in the presentation of asymptomatic primary hyperparathyroidism: proceedings of the fourth international workshop. J Clin Endocrinol Metab. 2014;99(10):3580–94.
18. Varghese J, Rich T, Jimenez C. Benign familial hypocalciuric hypercalcemia. Endocr Pract. 2011;17(Suppl 1):13–7.
19. Eastell R, Brandi ML, Costa AG, D'Amour P, Shoback DM, Thakker RV. Diagnosis of asymptomatic primary hyperparathyroidism: proceedings of the fourth international workshop. J Clin Endocrinol Metab. 2014;99(10):3570–9.
20. Wilhelm SM, Wang TS, Ruan DT, et al. The American association of endocrine surgeons guidelines for definitive management of primary hyperparathyroidism. JAMA Surg. 2016;151(10):959–68.
21. Newey PJ, Nesbit MA, Rimmer AJ, et al. Whole-exome sequencing studies of nonhereditary (sporadic) parathyroid adenomas. J Clin Endocrinol Metab. 2012;97(10):E1995–2005.
22. Costa-Guda J, Arnold A. Genetic and epigenetic changes in sporadic endocrine tumors: parathyroid tumors. Mol Cell Endocrinol. 2014;386(1–2):46–54.
23. Ibrahim Y, Mohamed SE, Deniwar A, Al-Qurayshi ZH, Kandil E. Lithium-associated hyperparathyroidism: a pooled analysis. ORL J Otorhinolaryngol Relat Spec. 2015;77(5):273–80.
24. Falchetti A, Marini F, Luzi E, et al. Multiple endocrine neoplasia type 1 (MEN1): not only inherited endocrine tumors. Genet Med. 2009;11(12):825–35.
25. Wasserman JD, Tomlinson GE, Druker H, et al. Multiple endocrine neoplasia and Hyperparathyroid-jaw tumor syndromes: clinical features, genetics, and surveillance recommendations in childhood. Clin Cancer Res. 2017;23(13):e123–32.
26. Rubin MR, Bilezikian JP, McMahon DJ, et al. The natural history of primary hyperparathyroidism with or without parathyroid surgery after 15 years. J Clin Endocrinol Metab. 2008;93(9):3462–70.
27. Mollerup CL, Vestergaard P, Frøkjaer VG, Mosekilde L, Christiansen P, Blichert-Toft M. Risk of renal stone events in primary hyperparathyroidism before and after parathyroid surgery: controlled retrospective follow up study. BMJ. 2002;325(7368):807.
28. Rolighed L, Rejnmark L, Sikjaer T, et al. Vitamin D treatment in primary hyperparathyroidism: a randomized placebo controlled trial. J Clin Endocrinol Metab. 2014;99(3):1072–80.
29. Marcocci C, Bollerslev J, Khan AA, Shoback DM. Medical management of primary hyperparathyroidism: proceedings of the fourth international workshop on the management of asymptomatic primary hyperparathyroidism. J Clin Endocrinol Metab. 2014;99(10):3607–18.
30. Eller-Vainicher C, Palmieri S, Cairoli E, et al. Protective effect of denosumab on bone in older women with primary hyperparathyroidism. J Am Geriatr Soc. 2018;66(3):518–24.

Chapter 3
Non-PTH-Mediated Hypercalcemia

Farah Meah, Gerald Charnogursky, Ruchita Patel, Namratha Reddy, and Lily Agrawal

Abbreviations

1-25D	1-25 dihydroxy vitamin D
24,25D	24, 25 dihydroxy vitamin D
25OHD	25-hydroxy vitamin D
GFR	Glomerular filtration rate
HHM	Hypercalcemia of malignancy
HPT	Hyperparathyroidism
MAS	Milk-alkali syndrome
PTH	Parathyroid hormone
PTHrp	Parathyroid hormone-related peptide

The original version of this chapter was revised. A correction to this chapter can be found at https://doi.org/10.1007/978-3-030-03694-2_16

F. Meah (✉) · L. Agrawal
Department of Medicine, Division of Endocrinology and Metabolism,
Edward Hines Jr. VA Hospital, Hines, Illinois, USA
e-mail: farah.meah@va.gov

G. Charnogursky · R. Patel
Department of Medicine, Division of Endocrinology and Metabolism,
Loyola University Medical Center, Maywood, Illinois, USA

N. Reddy
Department of Medicine, Loyola University Medical Center, Maywood, Illinois, USA

P. M. Camacho (ed.), *Metabolic Bone Diseases*,
https://doi.org/10.1007/978-3-030-03694-2_3

Case Presentation

A 55-year-old male smoker is brought to the emergency room by his wife for new-onset fatigue and weakness for the past 1–2 weeks. The wife states her husband has been very busy with work and rarely sees the doctor. He does not have time to eat and has lost nearly 30 lbs. in 6 months; however he has replaced meals with flavored Gatorade. Physical exam is notable for a cachectic male with sunken eyes and tenting of the skin. A left 2 cm hard, fixed neck mass along with left cervical lymphadenopathy is appreciated. Patient states he noticed the mass 2 months ago however was not concerned. Admission labs reveal a calcium level of 14.2 mg/dL, albumin 2.4 g/dL, undetectable PTH, and creatinine 2.5 mg/dl. CT neck confirms a left 2.5 cm infiltrating mass.

Introduction

Hypercalcemia is a heterogeneous group of disorders with nonspecific signs and symptoms related to the level of serum calcium, the rate of rise of calcium, and the underlying condition causing hypercalcemia. It can be due to increased influx of calcium into the circulation from the intestine, kidneys, or bones and the failure of renal excretion to compensate for it. Causes of hypercalcemia can be categorized into parathyroid-dependent (PTH-mediated) and parathyroid-independent (non-PTH-mediated) disorders as outlined in Fig. 3.1. Parathyroid-dependent causes include primary and tertiary hyperparathyroidism (HPT), familial hypocalciuric hypercalcemia, and lithium-induced hypercalcemia. Primary hyperparathyroidism and hypercalcemia of malignancy account for ~90% of hypercalcemia. The finding of high serum calcium with suppressed or low-normal PTH values should suggest the less common PTH-independent hypercalcemias. Parathyroid-independent hypercalcemia encompasses hypercalcemia of malignancy, granulomatous disorders, endocrinopathies, medications, and a few other disorders. In this chapter, we will focus on parathyroid-independent hypercalcemia.

Hypercalcemia of Malignancy

Nearly 80% of hypercalcemia of malignancy is mediated via production of parathyroid hormone-related protein (PTHrp) [1]. Fuller Albright initially discovered PTHrp in 1941 when he suspected that tumors might produce a PTH-like humor when trying to understand the pathophysiology behind hypercalcemia observed in malignancy. In the 1980–1990s, the syndrome of humoral hypercalcemia of malignancy (HHM) was identified. It was associated with the understanding that PTHrp and PTH were related molecules and both could stimulate the same type I PTH/PTHrp receptor (PTHR1) [2].

Low PTH				High PTH
Low Vitamin D		High Vitamin D (25OHD or 1-25D)		
Low PTHrp	High PTHrp	High 25OHD	High 1-25D	
Multiple myeloma Hyperthyroidism Pheochromocytoma Adrenal Insufficiency VIPoma Milk-alkali syndrome Vitamin A Intoxication Thiazide diuretics Lithium-mediated Hypercalcemia Immobilization Dehydration Jansen's metaphyseal chondrodysplasia Williams-Beuren syndrome Hypophosphatasia	Hypercalcemia of Malignancy Hypercalcemia of pregnancy	Vitamin D Intoxication	Hypercalcemia of malignancy Granulomatous disorders Acromegaly CYP24A1 mutation	Primary Hyperparathyroidism Familial Hypocalciuric Hypercalcemia Lithium -mediated Hypercalcemia

Fig. 3.1 Differential diagnosis of hypercalcemia

The human PTHrp gene is found on chromosome 12. PTHrp is found in many cell types and organs. It acts on the skeleton, mammary gland, placenta, smooth muscle, cardiovascular system, teeth, and pancreatic islets. At the level of the skeleton, PTHrp is involved with regulation of chondrocyte proliferation and differentiation. PTHrp leads to increased synthesis of receptor activator of nuclear factor-kappa B ligand (RANKL), leading to activation of osteoclasts and bone resorption, causing an elevation in plasma calcium. Additionally, PTHrp increases renal calcium reabsorption and renal phosphate excretion, similar to PTH. The malignancies most commonly associated with PTHrp-related hypercalcemia include squamous cell carcinomas (head and neck, esophageal, cervical, lung, and colon cancer) [3], urinary tract cancers (bladder and renal cell carcinoma), breast cancer, and ovarian cancer [4]. Hematologic malignancies associated with PTHrp-mediated hypercalcemia include multiple myeloma, lymphoma, and leukemia. Animal studies have shown that antibodies to PTHrp reverse hypercalcemia seen in allografts of human tumors [5].

Approximately 20% of malignancy-associated hypercalcemia arises from osteolytic metastases, with breast carcinoma and multiple myeloma being the two most common malignancies, causing excessive calcium release from the bone [1, 4]. In breast carcinoma, PTHrp has been shown to induce local osteolysis around bony metastases and contribute to its progression [5]. Transforming growth factor beta is a local growth factor, which produces PTHrp from metastatic breast cancer cells. The elevation in calcium further stimulates increased PTHrp release [4]. In multiple myeloma, bone remodeling leads to hypercalcemia after the local release of various cytokines, such as RANKL, interleukin-3, and interleukin-6, which lead to osteoclast activation [6]. Other humoral factors associated with increased remodeling and therefore hypercalcemia include tumor necrosis factor alpha, transforming growth factor alpha, interleukin-1, lymphotoxin, E-series prostaglandins, and macrophage inflammatory protein 1-alpha [3].

Vitamin D plays a major role in calcium homeostasis as seen in Fig. 3.2. With the help of sunlight, 7-dehydroxycholesterol is converted to D3 (cholecalciferol) in the skin; it is further hydroxylated to 25OHD in the liver by hepatic 25-hydroxylase. Vitamin D can also be obtained from diet through fatty fish (D3) or by UVB irradiation of the ergosterol in plants and fungi (D2, ergocalciferol). Subsequently, 25OHD is transported to the proximal tubules of the kidneys and is converted to the active form of vitamin D, 1-25D, by 1-α hydroxylase via stimulation by PTH. Although PTH and PTHrp act on the same receptors, PTHrp does not play a role in 1-25D production and thus does not increase intestinal absorption of calcium and phosphorous.

PTH-mediated causes of hypercalcemia seen in malignancy can occur through ectopic production of PTH by the tumor itself, although this is very rare, with a prevalence of less than 1% of cases [1].

Extrarenal production of 1-25D by tumor constitutes about 1% of cases of hypercalcemia in malignancy. This is most commonly seen in Hodgkin and non-Hodgkin lymphoma and ovarian dysgerminoma [3]. There have been a few reported cases of hypercalcemia in gastrointestinal stromal tumors with mechanism of overproduc-

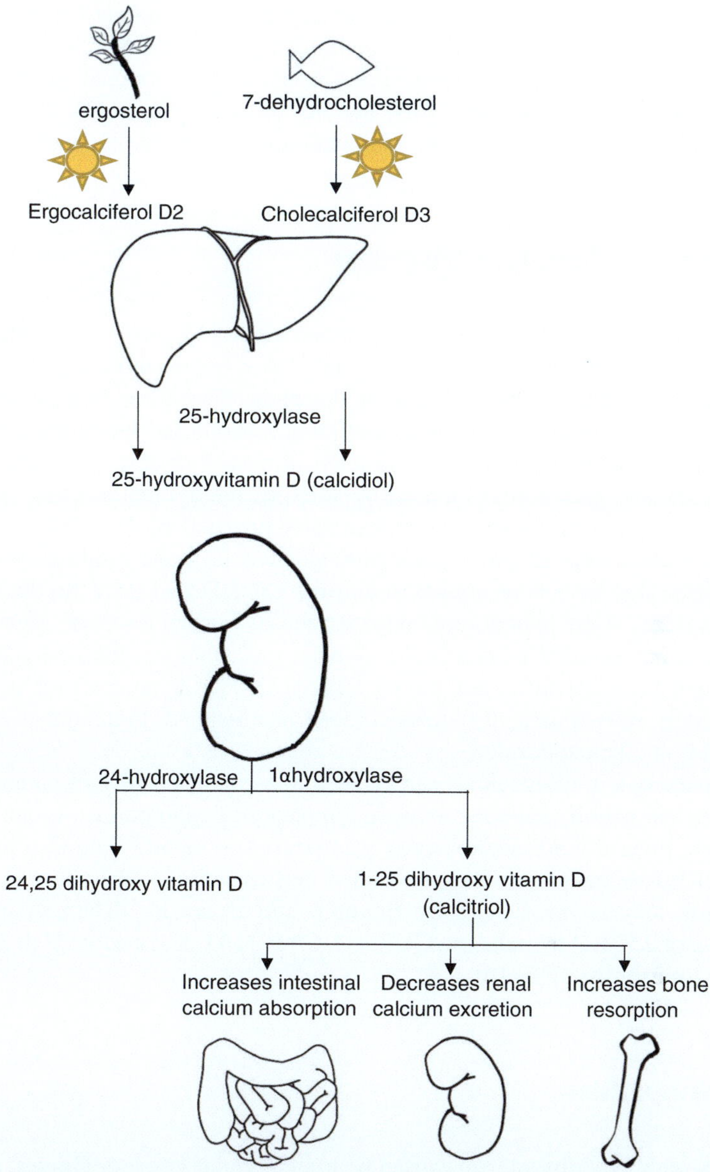

Fig. 3.2 Vitamin D Production. With the help of sunlight, 7-dehydroxycholesterol is converted to D3 (cholecalciferol) in the skin; it is further hydroxylated to 25OHD (calcidiol) in the liver by hepatic 25-hydroxylase. Vitamin D can also be obtained from diet through fatty fish (D3) or by UVB irradiation of the ergosterol in plants and fungi (D2, ergocalciferol). Subsequently, 25OHD is transported to the proximal tubules of the kidneys and is converted to the active form of vitamin D, 1-25D (calcitriol), by 1-α hydroxylase via stimulation by PTH. 1-25D acts that colon to increase intestinal calcium absorption, acts on the kidney to decrease renal calcium excretion, and acts on bone to increase bone resorption. 25OHD is also converted to 24,25D, an inactive form of vitamin D, by the enzyme 24-hydroxylase (CYP24A1)

tion of 1-25D, which was corrected with chemotherapy treatment [7]. It has been well described in the literature that nonmalignant granulomatous diseases such as sarcoidosis manifest with hypercalcemia secondary to extrarenal production of 1-25D via autonomous 1-αhydroxylase activity in macrophages [3]. Patients with HHM usually have clinically obvious malignant disease and have a poor prognosis.

Chronic Granulomatous Disorders

Granulomatous infections, including tuberculosis, leprosy, histoplasmosis, Pneumocystis jiroveci pneumonia, and many other fungal infections, have been associated with non-PTH-mediated hypercalcemia. These conditions, and other noninfectious granulomatous diseases including sarcoidosis, granulomatosis with polyangiitis (Wegener's granulomatosis) [8], Crohn's disease [9], infantile fat necrosis [10], and granulomas induced by silicone, methyl methacrylate, paraffin, and talc [11] have been associated with excessive production of 1-25D.

In sarcoidosis, sarcoid lymph node homogenates [12] and pulmonary alveolar macrophages [13] have been shown to convert 25OHD to 1-25D via the enzyme 1α-hydroxylase. These patients are characterized by normal levels of 25OHD, low PTH levels, and elevated 1-25D. In the alveolar macrophages, the 1α-hydroxylase is stimulated by γ-interferon and not by PTH [13]. This hypercalcemia is seen in approximately 10% of patients with sarcoidosis and responds to treatment with glucocorticoids and ketoconazole.

Hypercalcemia in tuberculosis can be seen in as many as 48% of patients [14]. 1α-hydroxylase activity has been found in lymphocytes, pulmonary alveolar macrophages, and pleural fluid macrophages. γ-interferon in pleural fluid also increases activity of 1α-hydroxylase. The prevalence and magnitude of hypercalcemia in tuberculosis may be modulated by rifampin and isoniazid. Rifampin increases breakdown of 25OHD by inducing CYP 384, CYP 24A1, and uridine 5′ diphosphoglucuronyltransferases [15, 16].

Endocrinopathies

In patients with hyperthyroidism caused by toxic nodular goiter or Graves' disease, 20% present with mild-moderate hypercalcemia [17]. PTH and 1-25D levels sometimes range from undetectable to low; however normal levels have also been reported [18, 19]. Phosphorus levels are typically normal which may be attributed to hypercalcemia in the setting of a low PTH. Alkaline phosphatase (ALP) levels may be elevated in up to 50% of individuals, and low bone mass can be attributed to thyrotoxicosis [17, 20]. The proposed mechanism is thyroid hormone stimulation of inflammatory mediators and markers of bone resorption. Patients with hyperthyroidism manifest higher levels of the inflammatory marker interleukin-6 (IL-6) [21].

IL-6 may encourage monocytic precursors to differentiate into osteoclasts [22, 23]. Increased osteoclast activity leads to hypercalcemia. The hypercalcemia typically resolves as hyperthyroidism is appropriately managed.

Pheochromocytomas are catecholamine-secreting tumors arising from the adrenal medulla that may occur sporadically or as part of the Multiple Endocrine Neoplasia 2 (MEN2) syndrome. Hypercalcemia can result from catecholamine stimulation of bone resorption or parathyroid gland PTH secretion [24, 25]. The tumor itself can produce ectopic PTH or PTHrp leading to hypercalcemia [24, 25]. Pheochromocytoma is most commonly treated with surgical resection.

Adrenal insufficiency is a clinical syndrome resulting from decreased adrenal glucocorticoid production of either a primary or secondary etiology. The most commonly proposed mechanism of hypercalcemia is volume depletion resulting in a reduced GFR leading to increased renal proximal tubule calcium reabsorption [26, 27].

VIPoma is a vasoactive intestinal peptide (VIP)-secreting neuroendocrine tumor characterized by watery diarrhea, hypokalemia, and achlorhydria. Hypercalcemia can result by VIP-mediated stimulation of parathyroid gland PTH secretion [28]. Similar to adrenal insufficiency, dehydration may also lead to a reduced GFR leading to increased renal proximal tubule calcium reabsorption.

Acromegaly is a clinical syndrome resulting from elevated growth hormone levels. Acromegaly can rarely be the etiology of 1-25D-mediated hypercalcemia of which the mechanism is unclear [29, 30].

PTHrp is produced in a variety of tissues including placenta. Hypercalcemia of pregnancy is mediated by placental production of PTHrp and typically resolves after delivery [31].

Medications

Milk-Alkali Syndrome (MAS)

MAS was originally described in the 1930s in association with the ingestion of large amounts of calcium (such as in milk), and absorbable alkali (such as sodium bicarbonate), known as Sippy's regimen for the treatment of peptic ulcer disease [32, 33]. It was more prevalent in males. Symptoms developed within several days to several weeks or months after the start of therapy and included nausea, vomiting, anorexia, headache, dizziness, vertigo, apathy, and confusion. Later muscle aches, psychosis, tremor, polyuria, polydipsia, pruritus, and abnormal calcifications (e.g., ocular keratopathy and calcium deposits in the conjunctiva, renal calcinosis, metastatic calcification in the periarticular tissue, subcutaneous tissue, central nervous system, liver, adrenal, bone, and lungs) were seen. Based on the chronicity of symptoms and prognosis, MAS was divided into two forms: Cope syndrome had a more acute presentation and an overall good prognosis [34]. The second form called Burnett syndrome was a chronic irreversible condition with band keratopathy in ~85% cases and nephrocalcinosis in ~ 60% cases; preexisting renal disease was seen in up to one-third of cases, and mortality due to chronic renal failure was common. Laboratory tests showed hypercalcemia, hyperphosphatemia, hypermagnesemia, azotemia, various degrees of renal failure, and metabolic alkalosis. With the introduction of histamine 2 blockers and proton pump inhibitors, the occurrence of MAS became rare in the 1970–1980s. However, a resurgence of MAS has occurred because of the increased use of calcium carbonate, the primary source of calcium and alkali. This is seen in postmenopausal women, patients receiving long-term corticosteroid therapy-mostly for osteoporosis prevention, and in dialysis patients who receive calcium carbonate as their principal phosphate binder. MAS is now considered the third most common cause of hypercalcemia, after primary HPT and HHM, with a prevalence of 9–12% among hospitalized patients with hypercalcemia [35]. Labs show hypercalcemia with appropriately low PTH and 1-25D, elevated serum bicarbonate, alkalosis, and variable degrees of renal impairment. Hyperphosphatemia is less common now since the etiology of MAS is often not due to consumption of large quantities of milk and dairy products, and due to the phosphate-binding properties of calcium carbonate. Contributing factors to the pathogenesis of MAS include excessive calcium intake and absorption, reduced renal calcium excretion due to increased tubular reabsorption induced by alkalosis, and failure to fully suppress 1-25D levels, despite high calcium intake and absorption from the gut. Treatment is supportive with hydration and withdrawal of the offending agents. Recovery from acute MAS usually occurs within 1–2 days, but in chronic forms, serum calcium levels can be elevated up to 6 months.

Vitamin D Intoxication (VDI)

Cholecalciferol (vitamin D3) is synthesized in the skin from 7-dehydrocholesterol by UV rays or taken as a nutrient or a supplement of vitamin D3 (cholecalciferol, from animal foods) or vitamin D2 (ergocalciferol, from plants) as seen in Fig. 3.2. After entering the blood, vitamins D2 and D3 from diet or the skin bind to vitamin D-binding protein and are carried to the liver, where they are hydroxylated to calcidiol [25OHD] which is the main storage form of vitamin D in the body. 25OHD (calcidiol) is then activated in the kidney by PTH-mediated 1α-hydroxylase, producing calcitriol [1-25D], the biologically active form of vitamin D3. Both 25OHD and 1-25D circulate bound to vitamin D-binding protein. Blood calcidiol levels are a direct assessment of the nutritional intake and skin conversion of vitamin D. Some clinical assays measure hydroxylated forms of both D2 and D3; others measure the total level of 25OHD (D2 + D3). Serum 25OHD levels >150 ng/ml are considered as VDI. Toxicity from high circulating levels of 25OHD may be due to displacement of 1-25D from vitamin D-binding protein, causing increase in free levels of 1-25D (despite normal total levels of calcitriol) [36]. At high concentrations, vitamin D metabolites such as 25OHD may compete for binding at vitamin D receptor sites, thereby producing effects similar to those of 1-25D by initiating translation of vitamin D receptor-responsive genes [37]. Hypervitaminosis D was a rare cause of hypercalcemia and renal impairment in the past. However, with increasing number of people using vitamin D supplements for bone health, and possibly for non-skeletal conditions, this may become more prevalent. High doses of vitamin D2 or vitamin D3 are often consumed either as prescription or over the counter, but are not common causes of hypercalcemia because 1α-hydroxylase activity is tightly regulated by calcium levels. Excessive administration of calcitriol or other active vitamin D analogs, such as paricalcitol or doxercalciferol, used as a treatment for hypoparathyroidism or in chronic kidney disease, bypasses the regulatory step at the level of the kidney and is more likely to lead to hypercalcemia. Excessive use of topical calcitriol has also been associated with hypercalcemia [38]. Laboratory tests show hypercalcemia, high serum 25OHD (usually >150 ng/mL), low serum PTH, normal or high serum phosphorus levels, normal or low levels of alkaline phosphatase, and high urine calcium/creatinine. Sometimes PTH may not be appropriately suppressed in response to hypercalcemia due to severe renal impairment induced by hypervitaminosis D [39]. Since vitamin D is lipophilic, the half-life of 25OHD is ~15 days and of 1-25D is ~15 h. Hypercalcemia due to excess 25OHD is usually prolonged and often requires therapy with corticosteroids and bisphosphonates, along with routine nonspecific measures. Calcitriol-induced hypercalcemia is short-lived because of its shorter half-life. Ensuring adequate hydration is usually enough.

Vitamin A Excess

Large doses of vitamins are being advocated and consumed for a multitude of health benefits without much scientific evidence. The term retinoids refers to vitamin A (retinol) and its metabolites and synthetic analogs (mainly retinal, retinyl esters, and retinoic acids). They are fat-soluble micronutrients mostly present in animal-derived diet, given as nutritional supplements containing pharmacologic doses of vitamin A to hemodialysis patients and also given as therapy for dermatological disorders, acute promyelocytic leukemia, and immunodeficiency treatment. Beta-carotene is plant derived. Vitamin A toxicity due to inadvertent intake of large doses or clinical utilization is a rare but well-documented cause of hypercalcemia, first recognized in the 1920s [40]. Symptoms include desquamative dermatitis, skeletal pain, hair loss, anorexia, pseudotumor cerebri, liver disease, and psychiatric complaints. The mechanism may be direct action on the bone to stimulate osteoclastic resorption and/or inhibit osteoblastic formation [41]. Treatment includes discontinuation of the medication, hydration, and administration of an anti-resorptive agent for the bones.

Thiazide Diuretics

Thiazides may produce hypercalcemia in the presence of abnormal calcium homeostasis. The exact mechanism is unknown, although "unmasking" of mild underlying primary hyperparathyroidism has been suggested. Other conditions that can predispose patients to thiazide-induced hypercalcemia are immobilization, Paget's disease, and high-dose vitamin D therapy. Thiazides decrease renal calcium excretion by inhibiting the thiazide-sensitive sodium chloride cotransporter and promote intravascular depletion and alkalemia [42].

Lithium

Patients on chronic lithium therapy may have hypercalcemia due to a defect in the calcium-sensing receptor, increasing the set point for inhibition of PTH release in parathyroid cells [43]. Long-term lithium exposure and the resulting parathyroid stimulation may trigger expression of parathyroid cell mutations and hyperplasia or adenoma formation, possibly because of loss of tumor suppression genes. The long-term sequela of mild lithium-induced hypercalcemia is not known. Bone density remains normal despite slightly higher levels of PTH, probably due to reduced urinary calcium excretion. After discontinuation of lithium, the hypercalcemia may not always resolve, and parathyroidectomy may be needed in some cases. Cinacalcet, a calcimimetic agent that lowers the threshold for activation of the calcium-sensing receptor by extracellular calcium resulting in decreased PTH secretion, can provide an alternative to surgery [44].

Teriparatide and Abaloparatide

Treatment of osteoporosis with teriparatide, recombinant human PTH analog (1-34), or abaloparatide (recombinant PTHrP 1-34 analog) are associated with improvement in bone density and fracture risk. Therapeutic use of these agents may lead to hypercalcemia via activation of bone remodeling, activation of the renal 1α-hydroxylase, and subsequent increase in 1-25D concentration resulting in increased intestinal calcium absorption or by increasing renal tubular reabsorption of filtered calcium [45]. It usually occurs within 1 month of treatment initiation but can occur any time during therapy. People who develop hypercalcemia or hypercalciuria had higher baseline calcium, 1-25D, and 24-h urinary calcium excretion [45]. Hypercalcemia is often mild and self limited.

Theophylline

Theophylline toxicity appears to cause hypercalcemia by mechanisms that are not clearly understood. It appears reversible with cessation of therapy. An adrenergic mechanism may be involved since calcium levels also fall after administration of a beta-blocker [46].

Estrogens and Antiestrogens

Hypercalcemia can be a potentially serious complication of tamoxifen therapy for breast cancer [47]. There are also case reports of hypercalcemia associated with the use of letrozole, an aromatase inhibitor, for breast cancer [48]. The mechanism is thought to be increased bone resorption due to longer life span of the osteoclasts mediated by estrogen deficiency. Hypercalcemia occurs within several days of starting therapy, it is generally short-lived and can be controlled with supportive measures, and serum calcium levels return to normal when the offending agent is withdrawn [47].

Aluminum Intoxication

In patients with ESRD, especially those on dialysis, excess aluminum accumulates in the body due to the use of aluminum-based phosphate binders, and aluminum found in the dialysate water [49]. This inhibits mineralization of osteoid. Available calcium can not be taken up by the bone, thereby causing hypercalcemia. Treatment consists of lowering calcium in the dialysis bath and stopping vitamin D. Sevelamer and lanthanum, synthetic non-aluminum and calcium-free phosphate binders, appear as effective as calcium-based binders in lowering phosphate but without the tendency to promote hypercalcemia [50].

Total Parenteral Nutrition (TPN)

Parenteral nutrition is a mixture of solutions containing dextrose, amino acids, electrolytes, vitamins, minerals, and trace elements tailored to the fluid and nutritional needs of a patient. Calcium gluconate is traditionally used since it is less likely to precipitate with the phosphorus. Modest intermittent hypercalcemia, hypercalciuria, low PTH, low 1-25D level, and osteomalacia have been reported [51]. Although the etiology and prevalence are unclear, the concentrations of calcium, phosphorous, and vitamin D in the TPN fluid may all play a role [52]. Hence early monitoring and treatment should be considered in all patients receiving TPN.

Other Diseases

Hypercalcemia of immobilization may be seen from a few days to several months after immobilization. It is mainly seen in people with rapid bone turnover such as children and adolescents. Immobilization can be associated with hypercalcemia in adults with underlying diseases associated with high bone turnover, such as Paget's disease and spinal cord injury, or in patients with end-stage renal disease. It occurs due to a relative change in bone turnover rate favoring resorption over bone formation. Lab findings include hypercalcemia with low PTH, low 1,25(OH)2 D level, normal serum 25(OH) D level, hypercalciuria, increased urinary hydroxyproline excretion, and marked osteopenia. Intravenous bisphosphonates [53] and denosumab [54] have been used successfully for treatment.

Hypercalcemia of dehydration/volume depletion: Since 50% of calcium is protein bound, dehydration may rarely result in pseudo-hypercalcemia due to hyperalbuminemia. Pseudo-hypercalcemia can also be seen with essential thrombocythemia and paraproteinemias [55]. To correct for an abnormal protein, the following formula can be used: corrected calcium (mg/dL) = measured total serum calcium (mg/dL) + [4.0- serum albumin (g/dL) X 0.8]; ionized calcium is normal in these patients.

Genetic disorders associated with short stature and hypercalcemia include Jansen's disease and Williams-Beuren syndrome. Jansen's metaphyseal chondrodysplasia is a rare form of dwarfism associated with hypercalcemia and hypophosphatemia with low PTH levels. This condition has been associated with activating mutations of the PTH and PTHrp receptors [56]. Williams-Beuren syndrome, caused by a deletion on chromosome 7q.11.23, occurs in approximately 1:10,000 live births and is associated with elfin facies, supravalvular aortic stenosis, and developmental delay with a friendly, social personality. Patients can also have structural abnormalities of the kidney and urinary tract and hypertension with an increased risk of renal artery stenosis. Most cases of hypercalcemia are mild and do not require specific therapy. Hypercalcemia has been attributed to several mechanisms including elevated 1-25D [57] and defective calcitonin production [58]. Hypophosphatasia is characterized by low levels of tissue nonspecific alkaline phosphatase (TNSALP) on osteoblasts and chondrocytes leading to impairment of bone mineralization. This rare metabolic bone disease is caused by mutations in the gene encoding TNSALP. The condition has variable degrees of severity depending on which of 200 known mutations is present. Laboratory testing reveals low levels of alkaline phosphatase and elevated levels of pyridoxal 5′ phosphate. Perinatal and infantile hypophosphatasia are the most severe forms. In the perinatal form, severe hypomineralization of bone and hypoplastic lungs cause respiratory failure and death soon after birth. Hypercalcemia and hypercalciuria, seen in infantile hypophosphatasia, may be caused by impaired mineralization with normal bone resorption [59]. The infantile form presents in the first year of life with mineralization defects in bony structures including skull and ribs, commonly leading to rib fractures and respiratory distress. The glycoprotein asfotase alfa contains the catalytic domain of TNSALP and can be used to treat this disorder.

Adynamic bone disease, a common form of renal osteodystrophy seen in patients on dialysis, is characterized by low bone formation and low bone turnover. This condition is characterized by over suppression of PTH due to the use of active vitamin D (e.g., calcitriol) and calcium-based phosphate binders to lower the hyperphosphatemia associated with chronic kidney disease. Hypercalcemia can occur in adynamic bone disease due to the use of these calcium-based phosphate binders coupled with reduced bone uptake of calcium [60]. Treatment of this form of renal osteodystrophy includes changing to non-calcium-based phosphate binders and reducing active vitamin D supplements to allow the PTH to rise.

Rhabdomyolysis-associated acute renal failure can be associated with hypocalcemia during the oliguric phase followed by hypercalcemia in up to 30% of patients in the diuretic phase [61]. Initial hypocalcemia reflects deposition of calcium in the injured muscles. This calcium is then mobilized in the diuretic phase in association with elevated levels of 25OHD and 1-25D leading to transient hypercalcemia. Patients developing hypercalcemia have low PTH in the diuretic phase. Authors suggest possible renal and extrarenal production of 1-25D as contributors to the hypercalcemia.

Hypercalcemia with suppressed PTH and low vitamin D levels can be seen in patients with advanced chronic liver disease in the absence of malignancy and other known causes of hypercalcemia [62–64]. While the etiology is not clear, increased bone resorption possibly mediated by factors including tumor necrosis factor, osteoclast-activating factor, interleukin-1, prostaglandins, and transforming growth factor may be contributing. This hypercalcemia can respond to calcitonin therapy.

Loss of function mutations in the CYP 24A1 gene causing impaired breakdown of 1-25D has been shown to produce a syndrome of hypercalcemia, hypercalciuria, nephrocalcinosis, and nephrolithiasis [15]. These mutations have been found in children previously described as idiopathic infantile hypercalcemia and in adults. Patients present with hypercalcemia, low PTH, and inappropriate 1-25D that is elevated or at the upper limits of normal. Hypercalcemia tends to be more severe in children and more modest in adults. Noting that calcitriol levels are commonly elevated in normal pregnancy, hypercalcemia during pregnancy has been seen in patients with this CYP24A1 mutation and can be the initial manifestation of this syndrome. Low levels of 24,25D are seen due to the decreased clearance of 1-25D.

Conclusion

Hypercalcemia is a common clinical problem. The evaluation of hypercalcemia involves understanding the hormones regulating mineral metabolism. Apart from PTH, various hormones and inflammatory mediators have effects on kidney, bone, and intestine resulting in hypercalcemia. In most cases, the etiology of hypercalcemia can be determined from the clinical setting and results of serum calcium, PTH, and vitamin D metabolites.

Case Management

The patient received aggressive hydration followed by one dose of denosumab. Additional laboratory studies revealed normal 25OHD; however PTHrp returned two times the upper limit of normal. Cervical lymph node biopsy was consistent with squamous cell carcinoma, and the patient was referred to oncology for further therapy.

References

1. Stewart AF. Clinical practice. Hypercalcemia associated with cancer. N Engl J Med. 2005;352(4):373–9.
2. Wysolmerski JJ. Parathyroid hormone-related protein: an update. J Clin Endocrinol Metab. 2012;97(9):2947–56.
3. Goldner W. Cancer-related hypercalcemia. J Oncol Pract. 2016;12(5):426–32.
4. Mirrakhimov AE. Hypercalcemia of malignancy: an update on pathogenesis and management. N Am J Med Sci. 2015;7(11):483–93.
5. Strewler GJ. The physiology of parathyroid hormone-related protein. N Engl J Med. 2000;342(3):177–85.
6. Roodman GD. Pathogenesis of myeloma bone disease. J Cell Biochem. 2010;109(2):283–91.
7. Barbaryan A, Bailuc S, Poddutoori P, Richardson A, Mirrakhimov AE. Gastrointestinal stromal tumor induced hypercalcemia. Case Rep Oncol Med. 2017;2017:4972017.
8. Edelson GW, Talpos GB, Bone HG 3rd. Hypercalcemia associated with Wegener's granulomatosis and hyperparathyroidism: etiology and management. Am J Nephrol. 1993;13(4):275–7.
9. Tuohy KA, Steinman TI. Hypercalcemia due to excess 1,25-dihydroxyvitamin D in Crohn's disease. Am J Kidney Dis. 2005;45(1):e3–6.
10. Shumer DE, Thaker V, Taylor GA, Wassner AJ. Severe hypercalcaemia due to subcutaneous fat necrosis: presentation, management and complications. Arch Dis Child Fetal Neonatal Ed. 2014;99(5):F419–21.
11. Woywodt A, Schneider W, Goebel U, Luft FC. Hypercalcemia due to talc granulomatosis. Chest. 2000;117(4):1195–6.
12. Mason RS, Frankel T, Chan YL, Lissner D, Posen S. Vitamin D conversion by sarcoid lymph node homogenate. Ann Intern Med. 1984;100(1):59–61.
13. Adams JS, Gacad MA, Singer FR, Sharma OP. Production of 1,25-dihydroxyvitamin D3 by pulmonary alveolar macrophages from patients with sarcoidosis. Ann N Y Acad Sci. 1986;465:587–94.
14. Lind L, Ljunghall S. Hypercalcemia in pulmonary tuberculosis. Ups J Med Sci. 1990;95(2):157–60.
15. Tebben PJ, Singh RJ, Kumar R. Vitamin D-mediated hypercalcemia: mechanisms, diagnosis, and treatment. Endocr Rev. 2016;37(5):521–47.
16. Wang Z, Lin YS, Dickmann LJ, Poulton EJ, Eaton DL, Lampe JW, et al. Enhancement of hepatic 4-hydroxylation of 25-hydroxyvitamin D3 through CYP3A4 induction in vitro and in vivo: implications for drug-induced osteomalacia. J Am Soc Bone Miner Res. 2013;28(5):1101–16.
17. Baxter JD, Bondy PK. Hypercalcemia of thyrotoxicosis. Ann Intern Med. 1966;65(3): 429–42.
18. Mosekilde L, Christensen MS. Decreased parathyroid function in hyperthyroidism: interrelationships between serum parathyroid hormone, calcium-phosphorus metabolism and thyroid function. Acta Endocrinol. 1977;84(3):566–75.
19. Bouillon R, Muls E, De Moor P. Influence of thyroid function on the serum concentration of 1,25-dihydroxyvitamin D3. J Clin Endocrinol Metab. 1980;51(4):793–7.
20. Iqbal AA, Burgess EH, Gallina DL, Nanes MS, Cook CB. Hypercalcemia in hyperthyroidism: patterns of serum calcium, parathyroid hormone, and 1,25-dihydroxyvitamin D3 levels during management of thyrotoxicosis. Endocr Pract. 2003;9(6):517–21.
21. Lakatos P, Foldes J, Horvath C, Kiss L, Tatrai A, Takacs I, et al. Serum interleukin-6 and bone metabolism in patients with thyroid function disorders. J Clin Endocrinol Metab. 1997;82(1):78–81.
22. Kurihara N, Bertolini D, Suda T, Akiyama Y, Roodman GD. IL-6 stimulates osteoclast-like multinucleated cell formation in long term human marrow cultures by inducing IL-1 release. J Immunol (Baltimore, MD: 1950). 1990;144(11):4226–30.
23. Cardoso LF, Maciel LM, Paula FJ. The multiple effects of thyroid disorders on bone and mineral metabolism. Arq Bras Endocrinol Metabol. 2014;58(5):452–63.

24. Kimura S, Nishimura Y, Yamaguchi K, Nagasaki K, Shimada K, Uchida H. A case of pheochromocytoma producing parathyroid hormone-related protein and presenting with hypercalcemia. J Clin Endocrinol Metab. 1990;70(6):1559–63.
25. Mune T, Katakami H, Kato Y, Yasuda K, Matsukura S, Miura K. Production and secretion of parathyroid hormone-related protein in pheochromocytoma: participation of an alpha-adrenergic mechanism. J Clin Endocrinol Metab. 1993;76(3):757–62.
26. Muls E, Bouillon R, Boelaert J, Lamberigts G, Van Imschoot S, Daneels R, et al. Etiology of hypercalcemia in a patient with Addison's disease. Calcif Tissue Int. 1982;34(6):523–6.
27. Montoli A, Colussi G, Minetti L. Hypercalcaemia in Addison's disease: calciotropic hormone profile and bone histology. J Intern Med. 1992;232(6):535–40.
28. Carroll R, Matfin G. Endocrine and metabolic emergencies: hypercalcaemia. Ther Adv Endocrinol Metabol. 2010;1(5):225–34.
29. Manroa P, Kannan S, Hatipoglu B, Licata A. Hypercalcemia and acromegaly – clarifying the connections. A case report and review of the literature. Endocr Pract. 2014;20(5):e86–90.
30. Shah R, Licata A, Oyesiku NM, Ioachimescu AG. Acromegaly as a cause of 1,25-dihydroxyvitamin D-dependent hypercalcemia: case reports and review of the literature. Pituitary. 2012;15(Suppl 1):S17–22.
31. Eller-Vainicher C, Ossola MW, Beck-Peccoz P, Chiodini I. PTHrP-associated hypercalcemia of pregnancy resolved after delivery: a case report. Eur J Endocrinol/Eur Fed Endocr Soc. 2012;166(4):753–6.
32. Cope C. Base changes in the alkalosis produced by the treatment of gastric ulcer with alkalies. Clin Sci. 1936;2:287–300.
33. Burnett CH, Commons RR, Albright F, Howard JE. Hypercalcemia without hypercalciuria or hypophosphatemia, calcinosis and renal insufficiency: a syndrome following prolonged intake of milk and alkali. N Engl J Med. 1949;240(20):787–94.
34. Medarov BI. Milk-Alkali syndrome. Mayo Clin Proc. 2009;84(3):261–7.
35. Picolos MK, Lavis VR, Orlander PR. Milk–alkali syndrome is a major cause of hypercalcaemia among non-end-stage renal disease (non-ESRD) inpatients. Clin Endocrinol. 2005;63(5):566–76.
36. Pettifor JM, Bikle DD, Cavaleros M, Zachen D, Kamdar MC, Ross FP. SErum levels of free 1,25-dihydroxyvitamin d in vitamin d toxicity. Ann Intern Med. 1995;122(7):511–3.
37. Haussler MR, Cordy PE. Metabolites and analogues of vitamin D: which for what? JAMA. 1982;247(6):841–4.
38. Hoeck HC, Laurberg G, Laurberg P. Hypercalcaemic crisis after excessive topical use of a vitamin D derivative. J Intern Med. 1994;235(3):281–2.
39. Bell D, Crooke M, Hay N, Glendenning P. Prolonged vitamin D intoxication: presentation, pathogenesis and progress. Intern Med J. 2013;43(10):1148–50.
40. Bhalla K, Ennis DM, Ennis ED. Hypercalcemia caused by iatrogenic hypervitaminosis A. J Am Diet Assoc. 2005;105(1):119–21.
41. Lippe B, Hensen L, Mendoza G, Finerman M, Welch M. Chronic vitamin a intoxication: a multisystem disease that could reach epidemic proportions. Am J Dis Child. 1981;135(7):634–6.
42. Nijenhuis T, Vallon V, van der Kemp AW, Loffing J, Hoenderop JG, Bindels RJ. Enhanced passive Ca 2+ reabsorption and reduced Mg 2+ channel abundance explains thiazide-induced hypocalciuria and hypomagnesemia. J Clin Invest. 2005;115(6):1651–8.
43. Haden ST, Stoll AL, McCormick S, Scott J, Fuleihan GE-H. Alterations in parathyroid dynamics in lithium-treated subjects. J Clin Endocrinol Metabol. 1997;82(9):2844–8.
44. Sloand JA, Shelly MA. Normalization of lithium-induced hypercalcemia and hyperparathyroidism with cinacalcet hydrochloride. Am J Kidney Dis. 2006;48(5):832–7.
45. Antoniucci DM, Sellmeyer DE, Bilezikian JP, Palermo L, Ensrud KE, Greenspan SL, et al. Elevations in serum and urinary calcium with parathyroid hormone (1–84) with and without alendronate for osteoporosis. J Clin Endocrinol Metab. 2007;92(3):942–7.
46. Mc PM, Prince SP, Atamer EP, Maxwell DB, Ross-Clunis H, Estep HL. Theophylline-induced hypercalcemia. Ann Intern Med. 1986;105(1):52–4.
47. Legha SS, Powell K, Buzdar AU, Blumenschein GR. Tamoxifen-induced hypercalcemia in breast cancer. Cancer. 1981;47(12):2803–6.

48. Ipekci SH, Baldane S, Ozturk E, Araz M, Korkmaz H, Colkesen F, et al. Letrozole induced hypercalcemia in a patient with breast cancer. Case Rep Oncol Med. 2014;2014:608585.
49. Visser W, Van de Vyver F. Aluminium-induced osteomalacia in severe chronic renal failure (SCRF). Clin Nephrol. 1984;24:S30–6.
50. Hutchison AJ. Oral phosphate binders. Kidney Int. 2009;75(9):906–14.
51. Shike M, Sturtridge WC, Tam CS, Harrison JE, Jones G, Murray TM, et al. A possible role of vitamin D in the genesis of parenteral-nutrition-induced metabolic bone disease. Ann Intern Med. 1981;95(5):560–8.
52. Hurley DL, McMahon MM. Long-term parenteral nutrition and metabolic bone disease. Endocrinol Metab Clin N Am. 1990;19(1):113–31.
53. Massagli TL, Cardenas DD. Immobilization hypercalcemia treatment with pamidronate disodium after spinal cord injury. Arch Phys Med Rehabil. 1999;80(9):998–1000.
54. de Beus E, Boer WH. Denosumab for treatment of immobilization-related hypercalcaemia in a patient with advanced renal failure. Clin Kidney J. 2012;5(6):566–71.
55. Jacobs TP, Bilezikian JP. Rare causes of hypercalcemia. J Clin Endocrinol Metabol. 2005;90(11):6316–22.
56. Schipani E, Langman CB, Parfitt AM, Jensen GS, Kikuchi S, Kooh SW, et al. Constitutively activated receptors for parathyroid hormone and parathyroid hormone-related peptide in Jansen's metaphyseal chondrodysplasia. N Engl J Med. 1996;335(10):708–14.
57. Garabedian M, Jacqz E, Guillozo H, Grimberg R, Guillot M, Gagnadoux MF, et al. Elevated plasma 1,25-dihydroxyvitamin D concentrations in infants with hypercalcemia and an elfin facies. N Engl J Med. 1985;312(15):948–52.
58. Culler FL, Jones KL, Deftos LJ. Impaired calcitonin secretion in patients with Williams syndrome. J Pediatr. 1985;107(5):720–3.
59. Barcia JP, Strife CF, Langman CB. Infantile hypophosphatasia: treatment options to control hypercalcemia, hypercalciuria, and chronic bone demineralization. J Pediatr. 1997;130(5):825–8.
60. Meric F, Yap P, Bia MJ. Etiology of hypercalcemia in hemodialysis patients on calcium carbonate therapy. Am J Kidney Dis. 1990;16(5):459–64.
61. Akmal M, Bishop JE, Telfer N, Norman AW, Massry SG. Hypocalcemia and hypercalcemia in patients with rhabdomyolysis with and without acute renal failure. J Clin Endocrinol Metab. 1986;63(1):137–42.
62. Gerhardt A, Greenberg A, Reilly JJ Jr, Van Thiel DH. Hypercalcemia. A complication of advanced chronic liver disease. Arch Intern Med. 1987;147(2):274–7.
63. Kuchay MS, Mishra SK, Farooqui KJ, Bansal B, Wasir JS, Mithal A. Hypercalcemia of advanced chronic liver disease: a forgotten clinical entity! Clin Cases Mineral Bone Metab. 2016;13(1):15–8.
64. Mateo RC, Apel J. Hypercalcemia induced by advanced chronic liver disease without malignancy. Endocrine Society's 97th Annual Meeting and Expo; San Diego, March 2015.

Chapter 4
Osteomalacia and Rickets

Sumeet Jain and Pauline M. Camacho

Abbreviations

$1,25(OH)_2D$	1,25-hydroxy vitamin D
25(OH)D	25-hydroxy vitamin D
mcg	Microgram
ng	Nanogram
pg	Picogram
PTH	Parathyroid hormone

Case

A 66-year-old woman presented to our clinic for multiple fractures and worsening bone density on bisphosphonate treatment. She recently had a pelvic fracture followed shortly by a Colles' fracture of her wrist after a fall. She had been taking risedronate 150 mg monthly for 4 years for presumed osteoporosis. She had chronic hip and leg pain for years. She had periodontal disease requiring multiple tooth extractions since she started bisphosphonate therapy. She had a history of uterine

S. Jain (✉)
Division of Endocrinology and Metabolism, Loyola University Medical Center, Maywood, IL, USA
e-mail: Sumeet.Jain@lumc.edu

P. M. Camacho
Division of Endocrinology and Metabolism, Loyola University Medical Center, Loyola University Osteoporosis and Metabolic Bone Disease Center, Maywood, IL, USA
e-mail: PCAMACH@lumc.edu

P. M. Camacho (ed.), *Metabolic Bone Diseases*,
https://doi.org/10.1007/978-3-030-03694-2_4

adenocarcinoma complicated by a small bowel obstruction that required a 20 cm resection of her distal ileum 10 years earlier. Her physical exam revealed varus deformities of her legs bilaterally. Her labs were significant for 25-hydroxy vitamin D of 8 ng/mL, parathyroid hormone of 174 pg/mL (reference range 10–65 pg/mL), bone alkaline phosphatase of 23.6 Ug/L (reference range in a postmenopausal woman 7–22.4 Ug/L), and 24-h urine calcium of 44 mg/24 h (reference range 50–400 mg/24 h).

She was diagnosed with osteomalacia based on her vitamin D deficiency, hypocalciuria, elevated bone alkaline phosphatase, and secondary hyperparathyroidism in the setting of bony pain and fractures. Her osteomalacia was thought to be related to malabsorption from her previous intestinal resection. Her risedronate was discontinued, and she was started on weekly ergocalciferol 50,000 IU with calcium citrate 1500 mg daily in divided dosing. Her bone alkaline phosphatase decreased to 18.8 in 5 months and decreased to 10.4 in 1 year. Her hip and leg pain dramatically improved in the next year.

Introduction

Osteomalacia and rickets are both caused by impaired mineralization. Osteomalacia is the softening of bone caused by impaired mineralization of the osteoid. Rickets is the impaired mineralization of the cartilaginous epiphyseal growth plate that occurs in children prior to growth plate closure. The osteoid is the organic matrix of collagen and glycosaminoglycans that is secreted by osteoblasts to form the unmineralized framework of bone. Mineralization involves incorporating calcium and phosphate hydroxyapatite crystals into the osteoid to provide the strength of bone. Defects or delays in mineralization result in rickets in children or osteomalacia in children and adults. Impaired mineralization may develop with deficiencies of calcium or phosphorous at the site of bone remodeling, abnormal collagen matrix, inhibitors of mineralization, or inadequate alkaline phosphatase activity.

Causes of Osteomalacia

Vitamin D and Calcium Deficiency

Due to vitamin D's importance in maintaining normal calcium and phosphorous levels, deficiency or abnormal metabolism of vitamin D is one of the most common causes of osteomalacia. Vitamin D deficiency can be caused most directly by inadequate dietary consumption or by lack of exposure to sunlight. Vitamin D deficiency due to malabsorption can be related to gluten enteropathy, small intestine disease or resection, bariatric surgery, pancreatic insufficiency, treatment with cholestyramines that bind dietary vitamin D, high phytic acid intake in vegetarian diets, or laxative abuse. Abnormal metabolism of vitamin D is seen in vitamin D-dependent rickets type I, vitamin D-resistant rickets type II, severe hepatic disease with decreased 1-hydroxylation, severe renal disease with decreased 25-hydroxylation, nephrotic syndrome with decreased vitamin D-binding protein, and with anti-epileptic use due to increased catabolism of vitamin D [19]. The same conditions that lead to vitamin D deficiency can also lead to calcium deficiency which leads to osteomalacia. Sometimes malabsorptive disorders such as celiac disease can lead to more pronounced deficiency in calcium than vitamin D.

Hypophosphatemia

Phosphorous deficiency results in osteomalacia due to its importance in bone mineralization. Hypophosphatemia may result from intracellular shifts of phosphorous, increased urination of phosphorous, or decreased intestinal absorption. Intracellular shifts of phosphorous are seen in refeeding syndrome, hungry bone syndrome, leukemia blast crisis, sepsis, and after glucose loads that increase insulin. Hypophosphatemia due to increased urinary excretion is caused by renal phosphate wasting disorders including X-linked hypophosphatemia and tumor-induced osteomalacia. X-linked hypophosphatemia presents with onset of symptoms in childhood with bowed legs, bony pain, pseudofractures, and elevated levels of the phosphaturic protein FGF23. An autosomal dominant form of the disease may present in adulthood with osteomalacia but without lower extremity deformities. The hyperphosphaturia in the autosomal dominant form may rarely self-resolve. Tumor-induced osteomalacia is a paraneoplastic syndrome caused by a mesenchymal tumor that secretes FGF23 or other phosphaturic agents [19].

Hyperphosphaturia is also seen in primary and secondary hyperparathyroidism, in diabetic ketoacidosis, and with certain medications: calcitonin, diuretics, glucocorticoids, and bicarbonates [19]. Other causes of hypophosphatemia are antacid-induced osteomalacia, chronic metabolic acidosis, treatment with saccharated ferric oxide, drug-induced Fanconi syndrome due to tenofovir, and cadmium toxicity [18].

Impaired Mineralization

Etidronate, an older bisphosphonate, can inhibit mineralization and result in osteomalacia. This effect is not seen significantly in newer bisphosphonates at the doses that are clinically used for osteoporosis. Fluoride, aluminum, and iron toxicity can all inhibit the process of bone mineralization resulting in osteomalacia. Treatment involves removing the inhibiting agent [18].

Hypophosphatasia

Deficient alkaline phosphatase activity seen in hypophosphatasia results in osteomalacia. Alkaline phosphatase helps break down phosphorous compounds that are inhibitory to mineralization and provides adequate elementary phosphorous levels to the site of mineralization in bone. Enzymatic replacement is now available with asfotase alfa.

Abnormal Collagen Matrix

Osteomalacia due to abnormal collagen is seen in fibrogenesis imperfecta ossium and axial osteomalacia.

Epidemiology

Population risk factors for osteomalacia are most often related to risk factors for vitamin D deficiency. They include advanced age, institutionalization, liver disease, kidney disease, bariatric surgery, inflammatory bowel disease, hospitalization, antiepileptic use, decreased sun exposure, and alcoholism [8]. The prevalence of vitamin D deficiency ranges from 25% to 57% in high-risk populations including medical inpatients, the elderly, and nursing home residents. The prevalence of vitamin D deficiency in noninstitutionalized outpatients is 9–14% depending on latitude per the NHANES III study [20]. The histological prevalence of osteomalacia from iliac crest biopsy in an autopsy study of 675 Northern German patients found a prevalence of osteomalacia as high as 25% [17]. Another study of elderly Europeans with hip fractures found an osteomalacia prevalence of only 2% on iliac crest biopsy [22]. Part of the difference between these two studies is explained by differing histologic definitions of osteomalacia.

Hypophosphatemia is observed in 5% of hospitalized patients. It is seen in 30–50% of patients with severe sepsis or alcoholism [9, 14]. X-linked hypophosphatemic rickets is the most common cause of hypophosphatemia-induced osteomalacia with incidence of 3–5 per 100,000 live births [19].

While the prevalence of rickets and osteomalacia decreased substantially in the western world after the mid-twentieth century following vitamin D supplementation public health campaigns, the prevalence has been increasing globally [21]. Global prevalence remains high in Asia, the Middle East, Africa, and in immigrants from these areas of the world. Contributing factors for increasing prevalence include traditional diets low in calcium and clothing that covers the majority of the body for cultural, religious, or climate-related reasons. Other global factors in developing countries that contribute to osteomalacia include depletion of nutrients in soil through intensive agriculture and exposure to industrial contaminants like arsenic, lead, and organophosphates [16].

Presentation

Patients with osteomalacia are at increased risk for fractures. They commonly have bone pain and hyperalgesia that is poorly localized. The pain is most often located in the lower back, pelvis, and legs. The pain is worse at night, worse with weight bearing, and worse with sudden movements. Patients develop symptoms of hypocalcemia like paresthesias, muscle cramps, and palpitations [6]. They develop clinical complications of hypocalcemia including seizures, tetany, and dilated cardiomyopathy. They develop symptoms of hypophosphatemia including myalgias and proximal muscle weakness [21]. In one review of 17 patients with osteomalacia in a GI malabsorptive disorder clinic, 16 out of 17 patients had bone pain or muscle weakness. Thirteen out of seventeen patients had a fracture. Only 2 out of 17 patients had cramps or muscle spasms [2].

Physical Exam

The most common physical exam sign associated with osteomalacia is bony tenderness to palpation. Fifteen out of 17 patients developed bony tenderness in the above study. Less commonly, 4 out of 17 patients developed a waddling gait. Due to hypocalcemia, 2 out of 17 patients had a positive Chvostek's sign [2]. Patients may exhibit Trousseau's sign of hypocalcemia. Proximal muscle weakness when present is symmetrical. Shoulder and pelvic girdle muscle weakness is most common. Patients may have difficulty standing up from a chair or climbing stairs. Muscle fasciculation may also be observed [6].

Labs

The pattern of lab abnormalities varies with the etiology of osteomalacia. Serum total and bone alkaline phosphatase are elevated in most causes of osteomalacia. Alkaline phosphatase is low when osteomalacia is due to hypophosphatasia. Parathyroid hormone may be elevated or normal when osteomalacia is related to low vitamin D, low phosphorous, or low calcium. In patients with osteomalacia due to vitamin D deficiency, hypocalcemia, hypophosphatemia, and elevated parathyroid hormone are often present. Twenty-four-hour urine calcium levels are low due to increased renal tubular resorption of calcium in patients with secondary hyperparathyroidism. $1,25(OH)_2D$ may be low due to severe 25(OH)D deficiency or may be elevated from increased conversion in secondary hyperparathyroidism [19].

In a case series of 21 patients with radiographic evidence of osteomalacia, 100% had PTH elevation, 95% had alkaline phosphatase elevation, 38% had hypophosphatemia, 38% had hypocalcemia, and 100% had vitamin D deficiency [3].

Following treatment of osteomalacia, alkaline phosphatase briefly increases prior to falling to normal levels within weeks to months. Hypocalcemia and hypophosphatemia normalize, PTH falls to normal levels, and urinary calcium increases to normal levels.

Histology

The gold standard diagnostic modality for the diagnosis of osteomalacia is iliac crest biopsy. When biopsy is required for ambiguous cases, the referring pathologist should be one who is familiar with the processing of undecalcified bone specimens and plastic embedding. The biopsy is analyzed with immunofluorescence images of tetracycline double labeling. In frank osteomalacia, double tetracycline labeling is not visible, but instead labeling may appear diffuse and of low intensity (Fig. 4.1). Bone resorption is generally increased with several Howship's lacunae and multinucleated osteoclasts due to concomitant hyperparathyroidism [19].

The diagnosis of osteomalacia histologically requires all three of the following [13]:

1. >10% osteoid in the cancellous bone area (normal <4%)
2. Osteoid width >15 μm or 4 lamellae (normal 4–12 μm)
3. Mineralization lag time >100 days (normal 9–20 days) (Fig. 4.2)

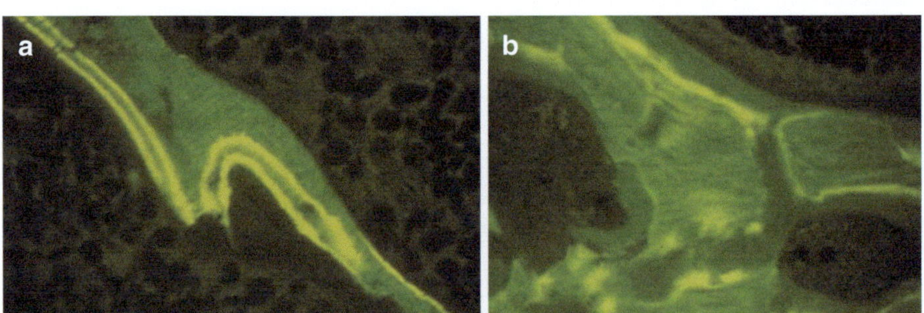

Fig. 4.1 Double tetracycline labeling fluorescence imaging. (**a**) Tetracycline double labeling discrete and widely spaced in normal mineralization. (**b**) Tetracycline labeling in osteomalacia appears diffuse and single despite two time-spaced doses of oral tetracycline [18]

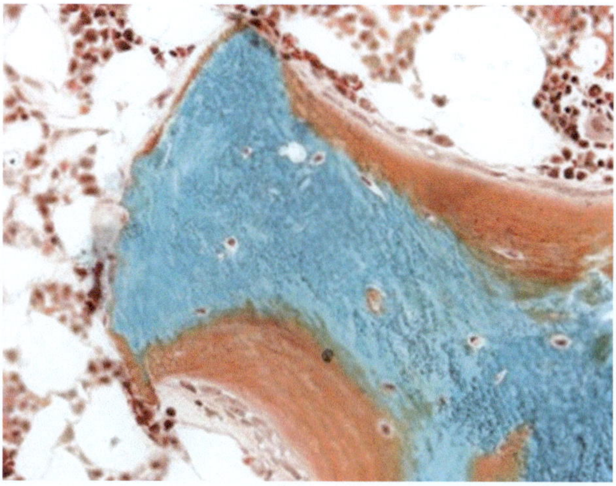

Fig. 4.2 Undecalcified bone biopsy shows abundant osteoid. Blue is normally mineralized bone. Red is unmineralized osteoid [18]

Imaging

Radiographs of bones in osteomalacia show less contrast and appear less sharp, as if the patient moved during the x-ray. A classic radiographic sign of osteomalacia is a pseudofracture, which is also called a Looser's zone or a Milkman's fracture. It is a radiolucent line through the cortical plate that is perpendicular to the periosteal surface. Looser's zones often have sclerosis at the margins (Fig. 4.3). They are seen most commonly in the ribs, pubic and ischial rami, femoral neck, metatarsals, or below the glenoid fossa on the outer border of the scapula [18]. Alternatively, radiographs in rickets show decreased mineralization around the epiphysis, less contrast, indistinct bone margins, and a decrease in ossification centers [18].

Looser's zones appear as hot spots on bone scintigraphy and may be confused as metastases [18]. Detection of Looser's zones is more sensitive with bone scintigraphy than on radiographs. Osteomalacia appears similar to hyperparathyroidism on scintigraphy with generalized increased uptake throughout the axial skeleton, a prominent calvarium and mandible, beading of costochondral junctions, and a "tie sternum" (Fig. 4.4) [5]. Osteomalacia and osteoporosis are generally indistinguishable on DEXA scans since both have decreased mineralized bone [19].

Treatment

Osteomalacia is treated by treating the underlying etiology causing osteomalacia. Treatment of osteomalacia often results in transient increases in alkaline phosphatase, bony pain, paresthesias, and hypocalcemia due to increased bone turnover with the initiation of therapy, so calcium levels should be followed closely at the start of treatment. Treatment results in rapid resolution of symptoms and normalization of

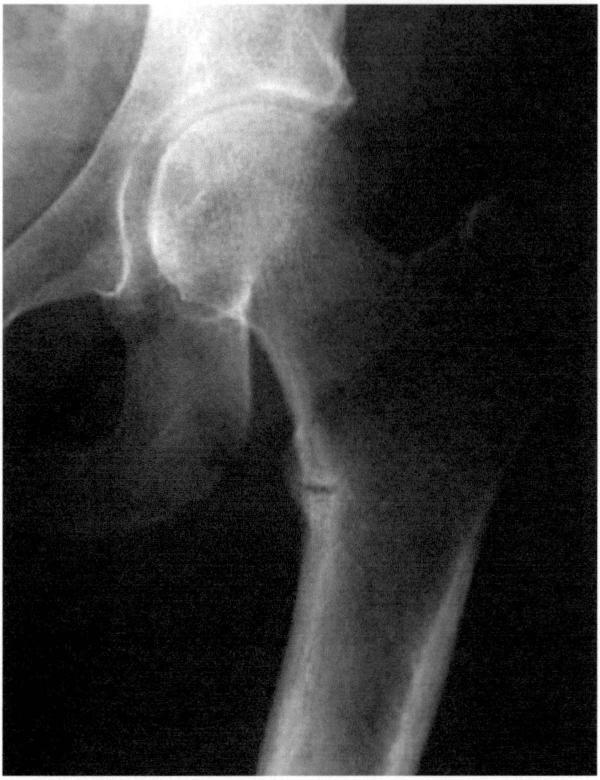

Fig. 4.3 Osteomalacia radiograph with pseudofracture [15]

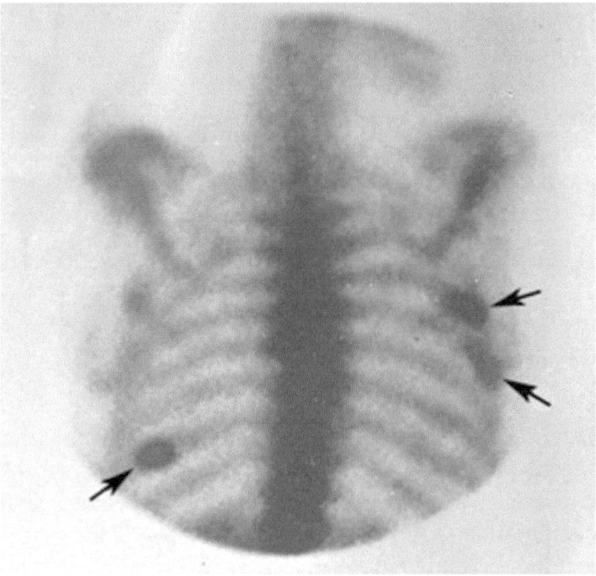

Fig. 4.4 Osteomalacia bone scan with increased uptake at areas of pseudofracture [18]

labwork. Healing of pseudofractures on imaging within months and increased ossification centers within weeks is seen in children. Healing of pseudofractures in adults may take up to 1 year [19]. Significant improvements in bone mineral density in the lumbar spine and the proximal femur occur after treatment of osteomalacia but are not seen at the radial diaphysis where patients may have had cortical osteoporotic bone loss related to secondary hyperparathyroidism [18]. Incorrect diagnosis as osteoporosis and treatment with bisphosphonates or other anti-resorptive agents prior to treatment of the underlying cause of osteomalacia may result in worsening osteomalacia symptoms.

Vitamin D and Calcium Deficiency

When osteomalacia develops due to 25(OH)D deficiency, treatment involves supplementation with cholecalciferol (D3) or ergocalciferol (D2). Symptoms of rickets and osteomalacia may resolve rapidly with very small daily amounts, 800–1200 IU, of vitamin D3 [19]. The optimal target vitamin D is an area of controversy. The Institute of Medicine recommends targeting 25(OH)D levels >20 ng/mL for the general population [12]. The AACE 2013 guidelines and the Endocrine Society 2011 guidelines recommend targeting 25(OH)D levels >30 ng/mL in bone disease [8, 11]. While the level at which low 25(OH)D results in hyperparathyroidism varies, there are studies that show for at least some patients PTH levels do not start decreasing until 25(OH)D is >31 ng/mL [4]. In a study evaluating what dose of vitamin D supplementation is required to reach goal levels, treatment with 100 IU vitamin D increased 25(OH)D by 0.7–1 ng/mL on average, though the dose response was four times larger when 25(OH)D was less than 20 ng/mL. Approximately 97.5% of people reached a 25(OH)D level of 30 ng/mL with 1600 IU of cholecalciferol per day over 6 months and 97.5% of people reached a 25(OH)D level of 20 ng/mL with 600 IU of cholecalciferol per day over 6 months. Increasing BMI is related to increasing resistance to vitamin D supplementation, and higher cholecalciferol doses are required to reach goals with BMI >30 [7]. When vitamin D deficiency is due to celiac disease or malabsorption, significantly higher doses of vitamin D may be required. Patients with celiac disease are also treated with strict avoidance of dietary gluten [19]. It is important to maintain age appropriate calcium intake in patients who are being treated with vitamin D (i.e., premenopausal women and men, 1000 mg, and postmenopausal women, 1200 mg of elemental calcium daily).

Vitamin D-Dependent Rickets Type I

Patients with osteomalacia due to autosomal recessive vitamin D-dependent rickets type I do not have 1-alpha-hydroxylase activity and cannot convert 25(OH)D to 1,25 $(OH)_2D$, so they are treated with lifelong calcitriol 0.5–1 mcg/day. If patients self-discontinue calcitriol, vitamin D deficiency redevelops within days. Calcium, creatinine, and 24-h urine calcium should be checked every 3–6 months due to risk of hypercalcemia with treatment [19].

Vitamin D-Resistant Rickets Type II

Patients with osteomalacia due to autosomal recessive vitamin D-resistant rickets type II have an abnormal vitamin D receptor and are unresponsive to $1,25(OH)_2D$. The only lab difference as compared to standard osteomalacia is an elevated $1,25(OH)_2D$ level. Treatment depends on the degree of vitamin D receptor unresponsiveness. If partially unresponsive, patients can be treated with calcitriol. If completely unresponsive, symptoms of osteomalacia, hypocalcemia, and hypophosphatemia can be prevented by IV calcium infusion or very high oral calcium and phosphorous loads [1]. Treatment with calcium and phosphorous has some efficacy at preventing osteomalacia because there is some passive intestinal absorption of calcium independent of vitamin D [10, 16].

Phosphate Disorders

Treatment of hypophosphatemia-induced osteomalacia requires balancing the increase of serum phosphate levels against the avoidance of secondary hyperparathyroidism or nephrocalcinosis. Treatment involves 1–2 g of phosphorous in three to four doses per day and 1–3 mcg of calcitriol to increase phosphorous absorption and prevent increases in parathyroid hormone. Phosphorous and calcitriol are titrated to treat symptoms and normalize alkaline phosphatase levels. To monitor treatment safely, serum and urine calcium, creatinine, and PTH should be monitored monthly at the beginning of treatment. If phosphorous-induced hyperparathyroidism develops, treatment becomes ineffective due to decreased phosphorous absorption and due to the negative effects of secondary hyperparathyroidism on bone health. Baseline and yearly kidney ultrasounds are required to evaluate for developing nephrocalcinosis during treatment.

A possible future treatment option for hypophosphatemia related to X-linked hypophosphatemia and other disorders that cause elevated FGF23 is an anti-FGF23 antibody, burosumab, which is currently FDA approved. Treatment of tumor-induced osteomalacia is with resection of the mesenchymal tumor [20].

References

1. Balsan S, et al. Long-term nocturnal calcium infusions can cure rickets and promote normal mineralization in hereditary resistance to 1,25-dihydroxyvitamin D. J Clin Investig. 1986;77(5):1661–7.
2. Basha B, et al. Osteomalacia due to vitamin D depletion: a neglected consequence of intestinal malabsorption. Am J Med. 2000;108(4):296–300.
3. Bhambri R, et al. Changes in bone mineral density following treatment of osteomalacia. J Clin Densitom. 2006;9(1):120–7.
4. Chapuy MC, et al. Prevalence of vitamin D insufficiency in an adult normal population. Osteoporos Int. 1997;7(5):439–43.
5. Fogelman I. The role of bone scanning in osteomalacia. J Nucl Med. 1978;19:245–8.
6. Francis RM, et al. National osteoporosis society practical clinical guideline on vitamin D and bone health. Maturitas. 2015;80(2):119–21. https://doi.org/10.1016/j.maturitas.2014.11.018.
7. Gallagher JC, et al. Dose response to vitamin D supplementation in postmenopausal women. Ann Intern Med. 2012;156(6):425–37.
8. Gonzalez-Campoy J, et al. Clinical practice guidelines for healthy eating for the prevention and treatment of metabolic and endocrine diseases in adults: cosponsored by the American Association of Clinical Endocrinologists/The American College of Endocrinology and The Obesity Society. Endocr Pract. 2013;19(Supplement 3):1–82.
9. Halevy J. Severe hypophosphatemia in hospitalized patients. Arch Intern Med. 1988;148(1):153–5.
10. Hogler W. Complications of vitamin D deficiency from the Foetus to the infant: one cause, one prevention, but who's responsibility? Best Pract Res Clin Endocrinol Metab. 2015;29(3):385–98.
11. Holick, et al. Evaluation, treatment, and prevention of vitamin D deficiency: an Endocrine Society Clinical Practice Guideline. J Clin Endocrinol Metab. 2011;96(7):1911–30.
12. IOM. Dietary reference intakes for calcium and vitamin D. Washington, DC: The National Academies Press; 2010.
13. Kulak CAM, Dempster DW. Bone Histomorphometry: a concise review for endocrinologists and clinicians. Arq Bras Endocrinol Metab. 2010;54(2):87–98.
14. Larsson L, et al. Severe hypophosphatemia-a hospital survey. Acta Med Scand. 1983;214(3):221–3.
15. Link TM, Adams JE. Metabolic and endocrine skeletal disease. In: Owens CM, Gillard JH, editors. Grainger & Allison's diagnostic radiology. Cambridge, UK: Elsevier; 2016.
16. Prentice A. Nutritional rickets around the world. J Steroid Biochem Mol Biol. 2013;136:201–6.
17. Priemel M, et al. Bone mineralization defects and vitamin D deficiency: histomorphometric analysis of iliac crest bone biopsies and circulating 25-hydroxyvitamin D in 675 patients. J Bone Miner Res. 2010;25(2):305–12.
18. Weinstein RS. Osteomalacia and rickets. In: Goldman L, Schafer AI, editors. Goldman-Cecil medicine. Philadelphia: Elsevier/Saunders; 2016. p. 1645–9.
19. Rosen C, et al. Primer on the metabolic bone diseases and disorders of mineral metabolism. Ames: Wiley; 2013.
20. Thomas MK, et al. Hypovitaminosis D in medical inpatients. N Engl J Med. 1998;338:777–83.
21. Uday S, Hogler W. Nutritional rickets and osteomalacia in the twenty-first century: revised concepts, public health, and prevention strategies. Curr Osteoporos Rep. 2017;15(4):293–302.
22. Wilton TJ, et al. Osteomalacia and femoral neck fractures in the elderly patient. J Bone Joint Surg Brit. 1987;69-B(3):388–90.

Chapter 5
Hypoparathyroidism

Susan Karam and Allison Hahr

Case Presentation

Our patient initially presented at the age of 20 with tetany and paresthesias. Her past medical history is significant for hypothyroidism and psoriasis. She has not had surgery or radiation to the head and neck. She has a sister with hyperthyroidism but no known family history of calcium abnormalities. Her only medication is levothyroxine. On the physical exam, she has positive Chvostek's and Trousseau's signs. On laboratory testing, she is found to have a calcium of 6.2 mg/dL (normal range 8.5–10.5 mg/dL) with albumin 4.0 mg/dL, magnesium 2.1 mg/dL, and phosphorus 6.7 mg/dL (normal range 2.5–5.0 mg/dL). Ionized calcium is 0.77 mmol/L (low) and PTH is low at 1 pg/mL. 25-hydroxyvitamin D was 24 ng/mL with reportedly normal levels of 1,25-hydroxyvitamin D (value not available). She was started on calcium carbonate 500 mg TID, calcitriol 0.25 mcg BID, as well as cholecalciferol. Hypocalcemia persisted even after repletion of vitamin D. She did not have features suggestive of the genetic syndromes which have a known association with hypoparathyroidism; thus a presumptive diagnosis of autoimmune hypoparathyroidism was made. She subsequently had testing of calcium-sensing receptor (CaSR) antibodies; however, the results were not clearly diagnostic of an activating mutation.

S. Karam · A. Hahr (✉)
Division of Endocrinology, Metabolism and Molecular Medicine, Northwestern University Feinberg School of Medicine, Chicago, IL, USA
e-mail: susan.karam@northwestern.edu; a-hahr@northwestern.edu

P. M. Camacho (ed.), *Metabolic Bone Diseases*,
https://doi.org/10.1007/978-3-030-03694-2_5

Introduction

Hypoparathyroidism is a disease characterized by hypocalcemia and hyperphosphatemia in the setting of absent or inappropriately low levels of parathyroid hormone (PTH) [1]. Hypoparathyroidism is considered a rare or "orphan" disease; the prevalence of hypoparathyroidism in the USA is estimated to be about 115,000 affected individuals [2]. PTH functions at the level of the bone to mobilize calcium, at the distal nephron to promote calcium reabsorption, and at the kidney to stimulate 1α-hydroxylase which converts 25-hydroxyvitamin D to 1,25-dihydroxyvitamin D for efficient intestinal absorption of calcium. Normal calcium levels are maintained by the interaction between PTH, vitamin D, and the calcium-sensing receptor (CaSR); alterations in any of these can result in the disruption of calcium homeostasis [3]. Hypocalcemia is identified by either low serum ionized calcium or albumin-corrected calcium and can have systemic effects. The symptoms of hypoparathyroidism are generally felt to be due to abnormal calcium levels; it is unclear if the deficiency of PTH itself also causes symptoms, although it has been proposed that it is possible as some symptoms do not resolve with normalization of calcium levels alone [4]. The presentation of hypoparathyroidism can differ between patients and is related to the duration, rate of development, and degree of hypocalcemia. Muscle symptoms are common and include tetany, paresthesias, muscle cramping, and spasms. More severe cases can present with bronchospasm, laryngospasm, seizures, heart failure, and prolonged QT interval. Persistent hypocalcemia and hyperphosphatemia promote development of cataracts, pseudotumor cerebri, and calcifications of intracranial structures including the basal ganglia [3, 5].

Diagnosis and Etiology

Determining the etiology of hypoparathyroidism is important as this can have implications for appropriate management. There are many possible causes of hypoparathyroidism including genetic and developmental defects, autoimmune processes, destruction from surgery, or, less commonly, radiation and severe magnesium deficiency or excess. Evaluation of hypocalcemia should include a thorough medical, surgical, and family history, physical exam, and measurement of ionized serum calcium, phosphorus, magnesium, PTH, and 25-hydroxyvitamin D. The need for further evaluation with genetic testing or referral to a geneticist, measurement of autoantibodies, and imaging should be patient-specific [1]. When evaluating hypocalcemia, it is essential to distinguish between hypoparathyroidism and pseudohypoparathyroidism, a group of conditions in which there is resistance to the action of PTH at target tissues. PTH levels are low or absent in hypoparathyroidism in contrast to pseudohypoparathyroidism in which they are elevated in an effort to overcome the target-tissue resistance [5]. Pseudohypoparathyroidism will be further discussed elsewhere in this book.

Destruction or Removal of Parathyroid Glands

Postsurgical hypoparathyroidism is the most common cause of hypoparathyroidism accounting for about 75% of all cases. It occurs as a result of either removal or devascularization causing damage to the glands during thyroid, parathyroid, or any other anterior neck surgery. Hypoparathyroidism may be transient following surgery although in some patients will become permanent [6]. Less commonly, hypoparathyroidism can develop because of damage from external radiation or neoplastic infiltration of the glands. Heavy metal deposition can also occur in the setting of hemochromatosis and Wilson's disease and has been observed in up to 14% of those with thalassemia and iron overload from frequent blood transfusions [5].

Genetic Disorders

After postsurgical hypoparathyroidism, autoimmune hypoparathyroidism (see below) and autosomal dominant hypocalcemic hypercalciuria (ADHH) due to activating mutations of the CaSR are the next most common causes of hypoparathyroidism. The CaSR is found at multiple sites including the parathyroid glands where it controls secretion of PTH and at the kidney where it promotes reabsorption of calcium. Over 70 gain-of-function mutations which lower the set point of the CaSR leading to inappropriate suppression of PTH relative to calcium levels have been identified. The hypocalcemia associated with ADHH is often mild, and patients may be asymptomatic; however, the hypercalciuria can be more pronounced. For this reason, treatment, if required, should be started cautiously because raising the serum calcium concentration can increase urinary calcium excretion leading to nephrocalcinosis [7, 8].

Less common forms of hypoparathyroidism can be inherited, either as an isolated entity or as part of a complex syndrome. Isolated hypoparathyroidism can be inherited in an autosomal dominant, autosomal recessive, or X-linked manner. Autosomal forms have been associated with PTH gene mutations while the X-linked form leads to agenesis of parathyroid glands [9]. DiGeorge syndrome is the result of developmental anomalies of the third and fourth branchial pouches leading to dysgenesis of the parathyroid glands and thymus. It also presents with congenital heart defects and deformities of the ear, nose, and mouth. Inheritance is usually sporadic, but autosomal dominant inheritance has been reported. It is the most common cause of persistent hypocalcemia in newborns but may resolve spontaneously in childhood. HDR presents with a phenotype similar to DiGeorge syndrome and includes *h*ypoparathyroidism, sensorineural *d*eafness, and *r*enal dysplasia and occurs due to haploinsufficiency of the GATA3 gene. Other syndromes associated with hypoparathyroidism include Kenny-Caffey (dwarfism, medullary stenosis of long bones, and eye abnormalities) and the hypoparathyroidism-retardation-dysmorphism (HRD) syndrome, also known as Sanjad-Sakati syndrome. Mitochondrial disorders such as

Kearns-Sayre syndrome, MELAS (mitochondrial encephalomyopathy, lactic acidosis, and stroke-like episodes), and mitochondrial trifunctional protein deficiency syndrome (MTPDS) have also been associated with hypoparathyroidism [9, 10].

Autoimmune Hypoparathyroidism

Autoimmune hypoparathyroidism may be either isolated or occur as part of a syndrome with other endocrine disorders. Autoimmune polyglandular syndrome 1 (APS1) is a complex of hypoparathyroidism, adrenal insufficiency, and mucocutaneous candidiasis. Inheritance can be either sporadic or autosomal recessive, and many different causative mutations in the AIRE-1 gene have been identified. APS1 is typically diagnosed during childhood with hypoparathyroidism and candidiasis in the first decade of life and adrenal insufficiency developing before age 15 [5]. When identified later in life, autoimmune hypoparathyroidism is often due to antibodies which activate the CaSR. These antibodies have been found both in those with isolated hypoparathyroidism and with APS1. Previously it was thought that autoimmune hypoparathyroidism resulted from destruction of parathyroid glands from circulating antibodies; however, it is now known that antibodies to the CaSR bind to and activate the receptor preventing PTH secretion [7].

Magnesium Deficiency or Excess

Both magnesium deficiency and excess have been demonstrated as reversible causes of hypoparathyroidism. Hypomagnesemia leads to impaired secretion of PTH as well as resistance to PTH action at the kidney and bone [11, 12]. Excess magnesium can also impair PTH secretion as demonstrated with the use of magnesium to treat preterm labor [13].

Treatment of Acute Hypocalcemia

Acute hypocalcemia may develop in the setting of neck surgery, medication noncompliance in those on chronic calcium and vitamin D replacement, or due to acute changes in calcium and vitamin D requirements often related to acute illness. Postsurgical hypoparathyroidism often develops within 1 day following surgery, and treatment is recommended if serum calcium levels fall below 7.5 mg/dL or if patients develop symptoms of hypocalcemia. Calcium can be given either orally or as an intravenous bolus infusion followed by continuous drip [14]. Calcium gluconate is preferred to calcium chloride which can cause skin necrosis if it extravasates from the IV and requires continuous cardiac monitoring. Vitamin D and magnesium are also often low in patients with postsurgical hypoparathyroidism and should be replaced with ergocalciferol and magnesium oxide, respectively, until replete [6].

Treatment of Chronic Hypocalcemia

The goal of chronic treatment of hypoparathyroidism is to maintain calcium levels in the low-normal range while avoiding symptoms associated with hypocalcemia which has historically been accomplished by supplementation of calcium and vitamin D or its analogs. Calcium supplementation is primarily limited by the degree of urinary calcium excretion as patients with hypoparathyroidism lose the ability to reabsorb calcium through the renal tubular system. This leads to an increased risk of hypercalciuria and nephrolithiasis when calcium levels are in the higher end of the normal range. Urinary calcium excretion should be monitored annually with goal of <300 mg/24 h [6, 14]. Thiazides can be used to increase calcium retention by the renal tubules if hypercalciuria is present. As in acute hypocalcemia, magnesium deficiency may be present and should be corrected.

Calcium Supplements

Calcium is given as either calcium carbonate or calcium citrate at typical doses of 1–2 g per day although there are some patients who require much higher doses. Doses should be divided throughout the day and taken with meals, particularly calcium carbonate which requires an acidic environment for absorption [15]. Calcium carbonate is the most common calcium salt used as it contains 40% elemental calcium compared to 20% found in calcium citrate. There are, however, certain circumstances in which calcium citrate is preferable to calcium carbonate. As calcium carbonate requires an acidic environment for proper absorption, calcium citrate should be given to those with achlorhydria [16] or those on a proton-pump inhibitor (PPI). It can also be used for those with severe constipation from calcium carbonate [14].

Vitamin D and Its Metabolites

In the absence of PTH and in the presence of hyperphosphatemia, renal conversion of 25-hydroxyvitamin D to its activated form 1,25-dihydroxyvitamin D by 1-α hydroxylase is impaired so treatment includes the activated form of vitamin D, calcitriol [5]. The required dose of active vitamin D needed to manage hypoparathyroidism varies between patients; however, typical doses range between 0.25 and 2.0 mcg daily. The parental forms of vitamin D, ergocalciferol (D2) and cholecalciferol (D3), are also often given as well [14].

Recombinant PTH

For many years, hypoparathyroidism was the only classic endocrine deficiency not treated by replacement of the missing hormone. Rather, it was primarily managed with calcium and vitamin D supplements given in multiple divided doses throughout the day which can be cumbersome to patients and lead to greater variability in calcium levels as well as side effects such as hypercalciuria, renal stones, impaired kidney function, and ectopic calcifications. In 2015, the FDA approved the use of recombinant human PTH (1–84) for the treatment of hypoparathyroidism [17]. Initial studies by Winer et al. on the use of rhPTH in the treatment of hypoparathyroidism used PTH (1–34) and demonstrated efficacy in maintaining calcium within the normal range with once daily dosing [18]. Her group later demonstrated that twice daily dosing was more effective than once daily dosing with less fluctuation of calcium levels and reduced total daily dose requirements [19]; this was proven to be a safe and effective strategy over a 3-year follow-up period [20].

Subsequent studies used PTH (1–84) as this is the full peptide missing in hypoparathyroidism. The pharmacokinetics are also such that PTH 1–84 can be administered once daily rather than twice daily or continuously in a pump as has been shown to be more effective with PTH (1–34) [19, 21]. The use of PTH (1–84) has been shown to be safe and effective in the management of hypoparathyroidism and is associated with substantial reduction of calcium and vitamin D supplementation requirements [22–24]. Treatment with PTH (1–84) has been recommended for patients who are not adequately controlled with traditional therapy, and guidelines outlining factors to consider when making this decision have been released [14]. Of note, PTH (1–84) was released with a black box warning for the risk of developing osteosarcoma as this was observed in rat models. The effect was dependent on both dose and treatment duration [17].

Clinical Course

The clinical course for patients with hypoparathyroidism can vary but for many is complicated by changing needs for calcium and vitamin D with subsequent hypocalcemia or hypercalcemia, decreased quality of life, and short- and long-term effects of calcium and vitamin D intake including effects on bone mineral density. A study which surveyed patients with hypoparathyroidism for varying reasons found that 79% of patients had emergency room visits or hospitalizations related to either symptoms or comorbidities of their condition illustrating the high burden of illness experienced by those with this condition [25]. Factors leading to inadequate control of calcium concentration include intercurrent illness, poor compliance, incomplete absorption, or intrinsic changes in requirements. Known complications of hypoparathyroidism include soft tissue calcification, renal stones, renal failure, and, less commonly, basal ganglia and diffuse brain calcifications [14].

Quality of Life

A common complaint among patients with hypoparathyroidism is reduced quality of life which has been demonstrated in studies quantifying mood and well-being. In these studies, patients have reported higher scores for depression, anxiety, and somatization and often complain of "brain fog." The normalization of calcium levels is not associated with the resolution of symptoms suggesting that the alteration of calcium-phosphorus homeostasis has some effect independent of absolute serum values [4, 26]. Patients have also demonstrated that the burden of illness is high and related to time-consuming monitoring and medication regimens; frequent and numerous symptoms which can be physical, cognitive, and emotional; and a limited ability to perform daily activities [25]. Fortunately, with the use of PTH (1–84), there has been documented improvement in quality of life in both mental and physical health [27]. This effect is seen early after treatment is started and persists over multiple years of treatment [28]. Another study did not demonstrate this benefit; however, larger fluctuations in calcium with frequent hypercalcemia were seen in the study indicating that maintaining more normal serum levels of calcium may play some role in the efficacy of the drug [29].

Effect on Bone

Bone remodeling is the process through which bone resorption and formation are balanced to maintain bone mineral density. PTH is an essential regulator of bone metabolism, and the absence or deficiency of PTH leads to a state of low bone turnover with measurable reduction in biochemical markers of resorption and formation [5]. Imaging with dual-energy x-ray absorptiometry (DXA) in patients with hypoparathyroidism shows an increase in bone mineral density (BMD) compared to age- and sex-matched controls in both trabecular and cortical bone with highest BMD at the lumbar spine [10, 30].

Further understanding of the unique properties of bone in those with hypoparathyroidism has been learned through advanced imaging with peripheral quantitative computed tomography (pQCT) as well as histomorphometric analysis of iliac crest bone biopsy. Chen et al. compared results of pQCT of the radius from 9 women with hypoparathyroidism to 36 women with hyperparathyroidism and to 100 matched controls. Compared to the women with hyperparathyroidism and the controls, those with hypoparathyroidism had increased cortical volumetric BMD at the cortical-enriched site at 20% of the midradius as well as significantly greater trabecular volumetric BMD in the trabecular-enriched 4% distal radius. Estimated bone strength was not found to be significantly different between the three groups [31]. Imaging with high-resolution pQCT has also shown increased cortical volumetric BMD at the radius and tibia in those with hypoparathyroidism and again did not show a significant difference in estimated bone strength [32]. A small study of iliac crest bone biopsies from 12 patients with hypoparathyroidism treated with vitamin D revealed a decreased resorption rate along with reduced bone formation and frequency of remodeling activation [33]. A later, larger study included 33 patients with hypoparathyroidism and again demonstrated decreased bone turnover with increase in cancellous bone volume and cortical bone width. Patients in both studies were treated with vitamin D, but even with repletion, skeletal abnormalities were seen [10]. Taken together, these studies indicate that PTH plays an important role in maintaining a normal skeleton, and the lack of PTH leads to low bone turnover and subsequent higher bone mass.

Fracture Risk

Although a deficiency in PTH clearly has effect on the structure of the bone, the risk of fracture in individuals with hypoparathyroidism is unclear. Two studies in Denmark have identified patients with hypoparathyroidism through a national registry and then determined the rate of fracture in this population. One study included 180 subjects diagnosed with nonsurgical hypoparathyroidism and found that the overall fracture risk was not different than age- and sex-matched controls but did find a significantly increased risk of fracture of the upper extremity [34]. Conversely, analysis of 866 subjects with postsurgical hypoparathyroidism found that the risk of fracture of the upper extremity was decreased with an overall fracture risk again similar to matched controls [35]. Evaluation of rates of vertebral fracture again revealed varying results with decreased incidence of vertebral deformity on radiograph shown in one study [36] and increased rates of morphometric vertebral fracture in another [37]. There does not appear to be a significant increase in fracture risk in hypoparathyroidism, but the exact risk remains unclear. Overall fracture risk is likely no different compared those with normal parathyroid function [38]

PTH (1–34)

With the increasing use of rhPTH to treat hypoparathyroidism, there has been interest in its effect on bone health, and this has been examined with the use of both PTH (1–34) and PTH (1–84). Studies using teriparatide (PTH (1–34)) compared a treatment group in which calcitriol was discontinued to those on standard therapy with calcitriol and calcium. In a 3-year study of adults aged 18–70 years treated with either twice daily PTH or standard therapy, it was demonstrated that each group had similar levels of serum calcium and phosphorus; however, those in the PTH treatment group had a significant increase in bone turnover markers. BMD was not significantly changed between the groups, but there was a downward trend in BMD at the distal one-third radius and a rise in BMD at the femoral neck in the PTH-treated group [20]. Similarly, a study of 12 children treated with PTH (1–34) or calcium and calcitriol for a 3-year period demonstrated a rise in bone turnover markers in the PTH-treated group as well as a significant downward trend in BMD at the distal radius with PTH treatment [39].

PTH (1–84)

The effect of PTH (1–84) has been demonstrated by open-label trials in which it was added to conventional therapy with calcium and calcitriol. After a period of 2 years of administration of PTH (1–84) at a dose of 100 mcg every other day, there was an observed increase in markers of bone formation and resorption. These levels peaked by 5–9 months with subsequent decline and stabilization over the duration of the study period. Histomorphometric studies revealed reduced trabecular thickness and increased trabecular number and cortical porosity in those treated with PTH as compared to controls [40]. Subsequent studies which reported results after 4 and 6 years of treatment with PTH (1–84) showed similar results with an initial rise in markers of bone turnover with subsequent gradual decline but overall higher levels as compared to baseline. Imaging in the cohort reported by Cusano et al. demonstrated an increase in BMD at the lumbar spine by year 2 with stable BMD at the femoral neck and total hip at the end of 4 years. BMD at the one-third radius declined by year 2 but then remained stable as compared to baseline by the end of the study period [22]. Results from the cohort followed for 6 years also showed an increase in lumbar spine BMD with a decrease in BMD at the one-third radius [41]. A study comparing hypoparathyroid patients treated with PTH (1–84) with subjects with primary hyperparathyroidism who had undergone parathyroidectomy showed significant increases in trabecular bone score, an indirect measure of bone microarchitecture, in the treated hypoparathyroid cohort [42]. Taken together, the available evidence does demonstrate the influence that rhPTH has on the abnormal bone remodeling seen in those with hypoparathyroidism although the long-term effect of treatment in regards to fracture risk is not yet known [38].

Conclusion

As has been reviewed here, the clinical course of hypoparathyroidism can vary between patients, but it can be very difficult to treat and can have a significant negative effect on quality of life. The patient presented in the vignette had great difficulty maintaining normal calcium levels and required escalating doses of supplemental calcium and calcitriol as well as ergocalciferol and cholecalciferol for over 15 years following diagnosis during which time she received care and close monitoring in our clinic. Even with 3000 mg of calcium carbonate divided between multiple daily doses and ergocalciferol, her calcium typically remained between 6.0 and 6.5 m/ dL. She was also hospitalized multiple times each year for acute worsening of hypocalcemia in the setting of viral illnesses or during her menstrual cycle which was observed to acutely increase her calcium and calcitriol requirements. For several months she required every other day calcium infusion via PICC line which was subsequently complicated by deep venous thrombosis (DVT) and infection. She also had multiple episodes of nephrolithiasis in the setting of high-dose calcium repletion. Unsurprisingly, she and her husband reported poor quality of life during this time with significant impairment in activity in both her professional and personal life due to frequent symptoms and hospitalizations as well as her complex medication regimen and frequent clinic visits and lab draws.

Given the difficulty in maintaining normal calcium levels and poor quality of life, she was enrolled in a clinical trial and started on PTH 1–84,100 mcg SQ daily when it became available. She was quickly able to decrease supplements to calcium carbonate 600 mg BID and calcitriol 0.25 mcg daily. The frequency of hospitalizations drastically declined, and calcium levels were maintained much more easily around 7.0 mg/dL. She and her husband reported significant improvement in their quality of life and overall sense of well-being.

Overall, hypoparathyroidism is a relatively uncommon disease where the lack of PTH leads to abnormalities in calcium and phosphate homeostasis with long-term consequences as reviewed here. The clinical course and severity can vary between patients, but it is highly associated with impaired quality of life and can be a complex disease to manage for both patients and providers. Bone structure and remodeling is abnormal in those with hypoparathyroidism even with replacement of calcium and vitamin D although the exact effect of bone quality on fracture risk is unclear. The relatively recent approval of rhPTH for the treatment of hypoparathyroidism has proven to be beneficial in the treatment of those with disease that is difficult to manage, leading to less fluctuation in levels of calcium and phosphate as well as overall improvement in quality of life. Improvement in bone turnover markers as well as abnormal bone structure has been demonstrated, but its exact role and long-term effect on bone remodeling are not yet known. While this is a promising new therapy, long-term studies are still needed to determine its role and safety in the chronic management of hypoparathyroidism.

References

1. Bilezikian JP, et al. Hypoparathyroidism in the adult: epidemiology, diagnosis, pathophysiology, target-organ involvement, treatment, and challenges for future research. J Bone Miner Res. 2011;26(10):2317–37.
2. Clarke BL, et al. Epidemiology and diagnosis of hypoparathyroidism. J Clin Endocrinol Metab. 2016;101(6):2284–99.
3. Shoback D. Clinical practice. Hypoparathyroidism. N Engl J Med. 2008;359(4):391–403.
4. Arlt W, et al. Well-being, mood and calcium homeostasis in patients with hypoparathyroidism receiving standard treatment with calcium and vitamin D. Eur J Endocrinol. 2002;146(2):215–22.
5. Rubin MR, Levine MA. Hypoparathyroidism and pseudohypoparathyroidism. In: Rosen CJ, editor. Primer on the metabolic bone diseases and disorders of mineral metabolism. Ames, Iowa : Wiley-Blackwell, 2013.

6. Khan MI, Waguespack SG, Hu MI. Medical management of postsurgical hypoparathyroidism. Endocr Pract. 2011;17(Suppl 1):18–25.
7. Hannan FM, Thakker RV. Calcium-sensing receptor (CaSR) mutations and disorders of calcium, electrolyte and water metabolism. Best Pract Res Clin Endocrinol Metab. 2013;27(3):359–71.
8. Marx SJ. Hyperparathyroid and hypoparathyroid disorders. N Engl J Med. 2000;343(25):1863–75.
9. Thakker RV. Genetics of endocrine and metabolic disorders: parathyroid. Rev Endocr Metab Disord. 2004;5(1):37–51.
10. Rubin MR, et al. Dynamic and structural properties of the skeleton in hypoparathyroidism. J Bone Miner Res. 2008;23(12):2018–24.
11. Rude RK, et al. Parathyroid hormone secretion in magnesium deficiency. J Clin Endocrinol Metab. 1978;47(4):800–6.
12. Tong GM, Rude RK. Magnesium deficiency in critical illness. J Intensive Care Med. 2005;20(1):3–17.
13. Cholst IN, et al. The influence of hypermagnesemia on serum calcium and parathyroid hormone levels in human subjects. N Engl J Med. 1984;310(19):1221–5.
14. Brandi ML, et al. Management of Hypoparathyroidism: summary statement and guidelines. J Clin Endocrinol Metab. 2016;101(6):2273–83.
15. Schafer AL, Shoback DM. Hypocalcemia: definition, etiology, pathogenesis, diagnosis, and management. In: Rosen CJ, editor. Primer on the metabolic bone diseases and disorders of mineral metabolism. Ames: Wiley; 2013.
16. Harvey JA, Zobitz MM, Pak CY. Dose dependency of calcium absorption: a comparison of calcium carbonate and calcium citrate. J Bone Miner Res. 1988;3(3):253–8.
17. Natpara (parathyroid hormone) [package insert]. NPS Pharmaceuticals, NJ; 2015. 2015.
18. Winer KK, Yanovski JA, Cutler GB Jr. Synthetic human parathyroid hormone 1-34 vs calcitriol and calcium in the treatment of hypoparathyroidism. JAMA. 1996;276(8):631–6.
19. Winer KK, et al. A randomized, cross-over trial of once-daily versus twice-daily parathyroid hormone 1-34 in treatment of hypoparathyroidism. J Clin Endocrinol Metab. 1998;83(10):3480–6.
20. Winer KK, et al. Long-term treatment of hypoparathyroidism: a randomized controlled study comparing parathyroid hormone-(1-34) versus calcitriol and calcium. J Clin Endocrinol Metab. 2003;88(9):4214–20.
21. Winer KK, et al. Synthetic human parathyroid hormone 1-34 replacement therapy: a randomized crossover trial comparing pump versus injections in the treatment of chronic hypoparathyroidism. J Clin Endocrinol Metab. 2012;97(2):391–9.
22. Cusano NE, et al. Therapy of hypoparathyroidism with PTH(1-84): a prospective four-year investigation of efficacy and safety. J Clin Endocrinol Metab. 2013;98(1):137–44.
23. Mannstadt M, et al. Efficacy and safety of recombinant human parathyroid hormone (1-84) in hypoparathyroidism (REPLACE): a double-blind, placebo-controlled, randomised, phase 3 study. Lancet Diabetes Endocrinol. 2013;1(4):275–83.
24. Sikjaer T, et al. The effect of adding PTH(1-84) to conventional treatment of hypoparathyroidism: a randomized, placebo-controlled study. J Bone Miner Res. 2011;26(10):2358–70.
25. Hadker N, et al. Understanding the burden of illness associated with hypoparathyroidism reported among patients in the PARADOX study. Endocr Pract. 2014;20(7):671–9.
26. Astor MC, et al. Epidemiology and health-related quality of life in hypoparathyroidism in Norway. J Clin Endocrinol Metab. 2016;101(8):3045–53.
27. Buttner M, Musholt TJ, Singer S. Quality of life in patients with hypoparathyroidism receiving standard treatment: a systematic review. Endocrine. 2017.
28. Cusano NE, et al. PTH(1-84) is associated with improved quality of life in hypoparathyroidism through 5 years of therapy. J Clin Endocrinol Metab. 2014;99(10):3694–9.
29. Sikjaer T, et al. Effects of PTH(1-84) therapy on muscle function and quality of life in hypoparathyroidism: results from a randomized controlled trial. Osteoporos Int. 2014;25(6):1717–26.
30. Duan Y, De Luca V, Seeman E. Parathyroid hormone deficiency and excess: similar effects on trabecular bone but differing effects on cortical bone. J Clin Endocrinol Metab. 1999;84(2):718–22.

31. Chen Q, et al. Effects of an excess and a deficiency of endogenous parathyroid hormone on volumetric bone mineral density and bone geometry determined by peripheral quantitative computed tomography in female subjects. J Clin Endocrinol Metab. 2003;88(10):4655–8.
32. Cusano NE, et al. Noninvasive assessment of skeletal microstructure and estimated bone strength in hypoparathyroidism. J Bone Miner Res. 2016;31(2):308–16.
33. Langdahl BL, et al. Bone histomorphometry in hypoparathyroid patients treated with vitamin D. Bone. 1996;18(2):103–8.
34. Underbjerg L, et al. The epidemiology of nonsurgical hypoparathyroidism in Denmark: a nationwide case finding study. J Bone Miner Res. 2015;30(9):1738–44.
35. Underbjerg L, et al. Postsurgical hypoparathyroidism – risk of fractures, psychiatric diseases, cancer, cataract, and infections. J Bone Miner Res. 2014;29(11):2504–10.
36. Fujiyama K, et al. Attenuation of postmenopausal high turnover bone loss in patients with hypoparathyroidism. J Clin Endocrinol Metab. 1995;80(7):2135–8.
37. Mendonca ML, et al. Increased vertebral morphometric fracture in patients with postsurgical hypoparathyroidism despite normal bone mineral density. BMC Endocr Disord. 2013;13:1.
38. Silva BC, et al. Bone imaging in hypoparathyroidism. Osteoporos Int. 2017;28(2):463–71.
39. Winer KK, et al. Long-term treatment of 12 children with chronic hypoparathyroidism: a randomized trial comparing synthetic human parathyroid hormone 1-34 versus calcitriol and calcium. J Clin Endocrinol Metab. 2010;95(6):2680–8.
40. Rubin MR, et al. PTH(1-84) administration reverses abnormal bone-remodeling dynamics and structure in hypoparathyroidism. J Bone Miner Res. 2011;26(11):2727–36.
41. Rubin MR, et al. Therapy of hypoparathyroidism with PTH(1-84): a prospective six year investigation of efficacy and safety. J Clin Endocrinol Metab. 2016;101(7):2742–50.
42. Cipriani C, et al. Skeletal changes after restoration of the euparathyroid state in patients with hypoparathyroidism and primary hyperparathyroidism. Endocrine. 2017;55(2):591–8.

Chapter 6
Pseudohypoparathyroidism

Bart L. Clarke

Case Description

A 38-year-old healthy female was referred for evaluation and management of hypocalcemia discovered incidentally during medical evaluation. She complained of intermittent mild tingling paresthesias and occasional muscle cramps in her legs. She had never had tetany, bronchospasm, laryngospasm, cardiac rhythm disturbances, seizures, or loss of consciousness. She had been advised by her primary care physician to take supplemental calcium carbonate with 500 mg elemental calcium once a day and calcitriol 0.25 mcg twice a day, but she did not take these supplements on a regular basis.

Her physical evaluation showed normal stature of 68 in, weight 140 lb, and BMI 21.3 kg/m^2. Her blood pressure was normal at 130/80 mm Hg, and her pulse was normal at 72 beats/min. Her physical exam showed a normal skeletal phenotype, without shortened fourth or fifth metacarpals or metatarsals or a dimple sign when she clenched her fists. She had no café au lait areas of macular hyperpigmentation, or subcutaneous calcifications, to suggest McCune-Albright syndrome.

Her initial serum calcium during evaluation was 7.5 mg/dL (normal, 8.9–10.1), with serum phosphorus upper normal at 4.5 mg/dL (normal, 2.5–4.5). Her serum creatinine was normal at 0.6 mg/dL (normal, 0.6–1.1). Her parathyroid hormone was increased at 540 pg/mL (normal, 15–65). Her serum 25-hydroxyvitamin D was optimal at 35 ng/mL (optimal, 20–50). Her serum magnesium was normal at 1.8 mg/dL (normal, 1.7–2.3).

B. L. Clarke (✉)
Mayo Clinic, Rochester, MN, USA
e-mail: clarke.bart@mayo.edu

P. M. Camacho (ed.), *Metabolic Bone Diseases*,
https://doi.org/10.1007/978-3-030-03694-2_6

Assessment for signs of hormone resistance other than to parathyroid hormone showed a normal sensitive TSH at 1.2 mIU/L (normal, 0.3–4.2). Her serum FSH was normal at 8.1 IU/L (normal, 1.8–22.5), with serum LH normal at 2.2 IU/L (normal, 1.2–100).

Her laboratory findings were consistent with pseudohypoparathyroidism. Because of her normal stature, lack of an apparent skeletal phenotype, or features of McCune-Albright syndrome, she was felt to most likely have pseudohypoparathyroidism type 1b and treated presumptively with calcium and calcitriol to try to lower her PTH level toward the normal range.

Introduction

Pseudohypoparathyroidism is a group of disorders characterized principally by proximal renal tubular resistance to parathyroid hormone (PTH) action [1]. These patients have impaired signaling by a number of hormones, particularly PTH, that activate cAMP-dependent pathways via Gsα proteins. Affected patients typically are characterized by hypocalcemia, hyperphosphatemia, and increased parathyroid hormone levels, with decreased serum 1,25-dihydroxyvitamin D levels. Patients with pseudohypoparathyroidism who are given exogenous biologically active PTH do not respond with an appropriate increase in urinary phosphate or cyclic adenosine monophosphate (cAMP). These patients do not demonstrate PTH resistance in other PTH target tissues, including the skeleton or thick ascending limb of the renal tubule [1].

Patients with pseudohypoparathyroidism usually develop neuromuscular irritability, manifesting as tingling paresthesias, muscle cramps, or seizures, unless treated with oral calcium supplementation and 1,25-dihydroxyvitamin D (calcitriol) [2]. Occasional patients are asymptomatic and have normal serum calcium and phosphate levels but maintain increased PTH levels. If these patients are not treated with calcium and/or calcitriol to lower their increased PTH secretion, they may develop significant bone disease over many years of chronic skeletal stimulation.

Pseudohypoparathyroidism was first described by Fuller Albright in 1942 as a disorder with target organ resistance to actions of PTH [3]. Since then a number of different variants have been described [4]. Patients with pseudohypoparathyroidism type 1 are characterized by unchanged serum cAMP and unchanged urinary phosphate and urinary cAMP after exogenous PTH injection. Patients with pseudohypoparathyroidism type 2 have increased plasma and urinary cAMP but unchanged urinary phosphate, after exogenous PTH injection.

This chapter will provide a broad overview of pseudohypoparathyroidism and discuss the clinical presentation, differential diagnosis, molecular pathophysiology, and treatment of the spectrum of disorders characterized by PTH resistance.

Epidemiology

Because of the rarity of pseudohypoparathyroidism, not much is known about the epidemiology of this disorder. Underbjerg et al. [5] identified all patients in Denmark with billing code diagnoses for pseudohypoparathyroidism through the Danish National Patient Registry and a prescription database. Billing code diagnoses were subsequently validated by records review. For each case, three age- (±2 years) and sex-matched controls were randomly selected from the general background population. A total of 60 cases of pseudohypoparathyroidism were identified, giving an estimated prevalence of 1.1 per 100,000 inhabitants. The average age at diagnosis in the cohort was 13 years (range, 1–62 years), and 42 of the patients were women. Only 14 patients had an identified mutation in their GNAS1 gene. Compared with controls, patients with pseudohypoparathyroidism had an increased risk of neuropsychiatric disorders ($P < 0.01$), infections ($P < 0.01$), seizures ($P < 0.01$), and cataracts ($P < 0.01$), whereas their risk of renal, cardiovascular, malignant disorders and fractures was comparable to the general background population. The same risks were found in a subgroup analysis in the 14 cases with genetically verified pseudohypoparathyroidism. The study concluded that patients with pseudohypoparathyroidism have an increased risk of neuropsychiatric disorders, infections, cataracts, and seizures, whereas mortality is comparable to that of the background population.

Clinical Presentation

Pseudohypoparathyroidism is typically defined by hypocalcemia, hyperphosphatemia, and increased PTH levels, associated with low-normal or decreased serum 1,25-dihydroxyvitamin D levels [1]. These biochemical abnormalities result from proximal renal tubular resistance to action of PTH. Physical symptoms have historically been attributed primarily to decreased ionized extracellular calcium, because studies have not demonstrated symptoms that correlated better with increased PTH levels than with low serum calcium.

Extracellular fluid hypocalcemia results in neuromuscular irritability, which may cause tingling paresthesias, muscle cramps, or tetany [6]. Patients may experience tingling sensations of their fingers, toes, lips, or tongue or nose tip and occasionally more diffuse tingling paresthesias over other facial areas. Symptoms can vary over time in the same patient, although many patients describe stereotypic symptoms that they learn to recognize as being due to low serum calcium. The level of serum calcium at which symptoms begin is quite variable between patients, but most patients describe symptoms with serum calcium below 7.5 mg/dL [7]. Some patients experience classical symptoms with serum calcium levels higher than this, and some seem to have few symptoms with serum calcium levels below 7.5 mg/dL.

Severe hypocalcemia usually presents in a more dramatic fashion, with seizures, bronchospasm, laryngospasm, cardiac rhythm disturbances, congestive heart failure, loss of consciousness, or, in extreme circumstances, sudden death.

Chvostek's sign is a characteristic of latent neuromuscular irritability, in which tapping the facial nerve in front of the ear causes ipsilateral twitching of the upper lip [8]. This sign is not pathognomonic of hypocalcemia, however, as about 10–15% of the general healthy population demonstrates this also [9]. Trousseau's sign is also characteristic of latent neuromuscular irritability, in which increasing pressure in a blood pressure cuff over the upper arm by 5 mm Hg above the systolic pressure will cause painful tetany in the arm below the blood pressure cuff within 3 min [10]. Trousseau's sign is also not pathognomonic of hypocalcemia, as about 1–2% of the general healthy population may have this sign [11].

Patients with chronic hypocalcemia may develop features such as pseudopapilledema, increased intracranial pressure, and dry rough skin [12]. Long-standing hypocalcemia and hyperphosphatemia associated with an increase in the calcium x phosphate product may cause cataracts or intracranial calcifications of the basal ganglia and other intracerebral structures [13]. Patients with extensive basal ganglia calcification may occasionally experience extrapyramidal dysfunction, but this is uncommon [14]. Spondyloarthropathy may occur rarely, causing significant joint pain and swelling and destruction [15]. Hypocalcemia may prolong the QT corrected interval on an electrocardiogram [16]. Congestive heart failure may occasionally develop due to prolonged severe hypocalcemia.

Patients with chronic mild to moderate hypocalcemia may adapt to their hypocalcemia fairly well and remain asymptomatic until low serum calcium is detected on routine blood testing.

Differential Diagnosis

Once other causes of hypocalcemia are ruled out, pseudohypoparathyroidism is usually easily diagnosed because of the classical biochemical changes. Patients with postsurgical or other forms of hypoparathyroidism have decreased serum calcium, upper-normal or increased serum phosphate, and lower PTH levels than expected for the simultaneously drawn serum calcium [17]. Patients with hypoparathyroidism demonstrate a significant increase in urinary phosphate and plasma and urinary cAMP after exogenous PTH administration [18]. In contrast, patients with pseudohypoparathyroidism type 1 have blunted increases in urinary phosphate and plasma and urinary cAMP after exogenous PTH, and patients with pseudohypoparathyroidism type 2 show increased plasma and urinary cAMP but blunted increases in urinary phosphate [19, 20] (Table 6.1).

Pseudohypoparathyroidism type 1 is caused by tissue deficiency of the alpha subunit of Gs (Gsα). Gsα is the signaling protein that couples stimulation of the PTH/PTH-rp receptor to stimulation of adenylyl cyclase [21]. Three forms of pseudohypoparathyroidism type 1 have been reported.

Table 6.1 Clinical characteristics of the types of pseudohypoparathyroidism and related disorders

Type (OMIM)	Gsα activity	AHO	PTH resistance	Urinary cAMP response	Multiple hormone resistance	Molecular defect
1a (103580)	Reduced	Yes	Yes	Reduced	PTH, TSH, Gn, GHRH	Heterozygous mutations in *GNAS*
PseudoPHP	Reduced	Yes	No	Normal	No	Heterozygous mutations in *GNAS*
1b (603233)	Normal	Yes	Kidney	Reduced	PTH, TSH	GNAS imprinting defect with *STX16* or *NESP55* deletions, paternal uniparental disomy 20q, sporadic cases
1c	Normal	No	No	Reduced	PTH, TSH, Gn	Heterozygous mutations in *GNAS*
POH	Normal	No	No	Normal	No	Heterozygous mutations in *GNAS*
2	Normal	No	Kidney	Normal	No	Unknown
Acrodysostosis type 1	Reduced	No	Yes	Reduced	Yes	*PRKAR1A* mutations
Acrodysostosis type 2	Reduce	No	Yes	Reduced	Yes	*PDE4D* mutations

AHO Albright's hereditary osteodystrophy, *cAMP* cyclic adenosine monophosphate, *GHRH* growth hormone-releasing hormone, *Gn* gonadotropins, *NESP55* neuroendocrine secretory protein-55, *PDE4D* phosphodiesterase 4D, *POH* progressive osseous heteroplasia, *PRKAR1A* protein kinase cAMP-dependent type 1 regulatory subunit alpha, *PTH* parathyroid hormone, *PseudoPHP* pseudopseudohypoparathyroidism, *STX16* syntaxin-16, *TSH* thyroid-stimulating hormone

Pseudohypoparathyroidism type 1a (OMIM 103580) is the result of generalized deficiency of Gsα due to mutations within *GNAS* exons 1–13 [1]. Pseudohypoparathyroidism type 1b (OMIM 603233) is caused by more restricted deficiency of Gsα due to mutations affecting GNAS imprinting [22]. Patients with pseudohypoparathyroidism type 1a typically have resistance to multiple hormones and certain somatic features not seen in pseudohypoparathyroidism type 1b. Pseudohypoparathyroidism type 1c is thought to be a variant of type 1a in which resistance to multiple hormones is present without a defect in Gsα [23].

Pseudohypoparathyroidism type 1a is the most frequent type of pseudohypoparathyroidism and usually more easily identified than other types because of associated physical features. Patients with pseudohypoparathyroidism type 1a have Albright's hereditary osteodystrophy (AHO), characterized by variable short stature, round facies, dental abnormalities, shortened fourth and fifth metacarpals and metatarsals, mild to moderate mental retardation, and subcutaneous calcifications [24]. Many of these patients have early-onset obesity, and some have sensory neuropathy, and they appear to have GNAS mutations causing abnormal Gsα signaling in the hypothalamus and central nervous system [25]. The obesity appears to be due to decreased expression of Gαs in imprinted regions of the hypothalamus [26], thereby leading to reduced energy expenditure rather than increased caloric intake.

Pseudohypoparathyroidism type 1a is caused by heterozygous mutations of the maternal allele of the imprinted *GNAS* gene on chromosome 20q13.2-q13.3, causing decreased expression or function of the Gsα protein. The requirement of normal expression of Gsα protein for signal transduction by many hormones and neurotransmitters leads to hormone resistance in patients with pseudohypoparathyroidism type 1a to not just PTH but also thyroid-stimulating hormone (TSH), luteinizing hormone (LH), follicle-stimulating hormone (FSH), calcitonin, and growth hormone-releasing hormone (GHRH) [27, 28], in tissues that express the maternal *GNAS* allele. Hormone resistance is not present in patients with pseudohypoparathyroidism type 1a in tissues where *GNAS* is not imprinted and both parental alleles are expressed. Because of this, response to adrenocorticotropic hormone (ACTH) and vasopressin is normal in these patients.

Patients with paternally inherited *GNAS* mutations have physical features of AHO but no evidence of resistance to PTH or other hormones. This disorder was first described in 1952 [29] and is known as pseudopseudohypoparathyroidism [30]. Kindreds with pseudopseudohypoparathyroidism without hormone resistance often have family members with pseudohypoparathyroidism with hormone resistance, with the variation in expression depending on the parental origin of the *GNAS* mutation.

Molecular Causes of Pseudohypoparathyroidism

The *GNAS* gene maintains flexible expression in different tissues by using alternative first exons upstream of exon 1, alternative splicing of downstream exons, antisense mRNA transcripts, or reciprocal imprinting (Fig. 6.1). Gsα is encoded by exons 1–13 of the *GNAS* gene, with inclusion or exclusion of exon 3 leading to expression of either 52 kDa or 45 kDa proteins. These two Gsα isoforms both appear to function normally in signal transduction.

Different Gsα mRNA transcripts are produced by three alternative first exons upstream of exon 1, each splicing to exons 2–13. The first alternative exon XL is expressed only by the paternal allele and generates an mRNA transcript with overlapping open reading frames that encode XLsα [31] and ALEX. Both proteins are able to interact with each other and are expressed specifically in neuroendocrine cells. XLsα measures about 78 kDa and therefore is much larger than Gsα, which is either 52 or 45 kDa. XLsα interacts with PTH/PTH-rp receptors and other receptors in cell systems, but it is not yet clear whether this protein can interact with these receptors in the whole organism.

The second alternative first exon is encoded only by the maternal allele and generates a secretory protein called neuroendocrine secretory peptide 55 (NESP55) [32]. This protein has no sequence homology with Gsα.

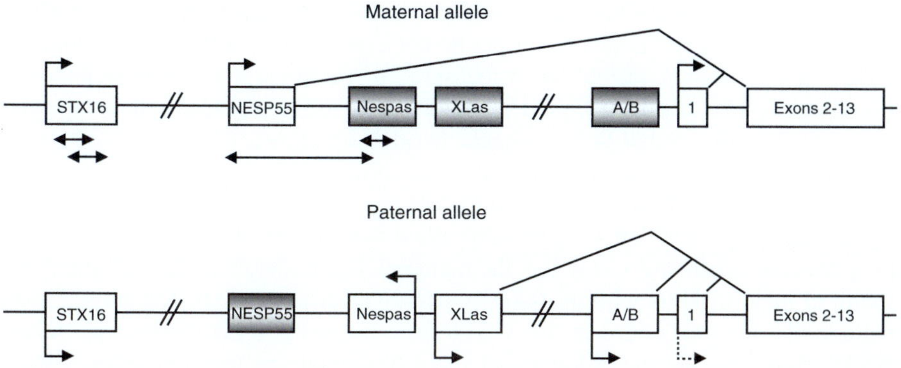

Fig. 6.1 General organization and imprinting of *GNAS*. The maternal and paternal alleles of *GNAS* are shown. Methylated regions are indicated in *gray*, and active promoters are indicated by *arrows in the direction of transcription*. The alternative first exons and common exon 2 are shown as *rectangles* with exon 1 being the first coding exon for Gsα. The *dashed line at the paternal Gsα promoter* indicates tissue-specific imprinting of the gene. For clarity only the first exon for Nespas is shown, and the localization of DMR (differentially methylated regions) has been omitted in the figure. The figure also shows representation of the maternally derived deletions (*double-headed arrows*) found to cause familial PHP-Ib. The diagram is not drawn to scale. (Used with permission from Mantovani [1])

The third alternative first exon 1A or A/B (associated first exon) is encoded only by the paternal allele. Transcripts from this alternative first exon may be translated from an initiator codon in the second exon and produce an N-terminal truncated protein that competitively inhibits Gsα [33].

These three alternative first exons for Gsα are associated with differentially methylated promotor regions. Methylation results in silencing of the affected allele. Unlike the three alternative first exons, the promotor for exon 1 is within a CpG island and remains unmethylated on both alleles in all tissues. Cis-acting elements that control tissue-specific paternal imprinting of Gsα are thought to be located within the primary imprint region in exon 1A [34].

Multiple kindreds with pseudohypoparathyroidism type 1a have four-base deletions in exon 7, and because the missense mutation A366S has been found in exon 13 in two unrelated boys, it is possible that exons 7 and 13 may represent sites of frequent *GNAS* mutations. About 80% of patients with AHO have been identified as having small deletions or point mutations in *GNAS*, whereas other cases have been reported to have larger rearrangements or uniparental disomy, where both *GNAS* alleles are inherited from the mother.

Patients with pseudohypoparathyroidism type 1b may have postzygotic somatic mutations in *GNAS* that increase the expression of the Gsα protein, with constitutive activation of adenylyl cyclase, resulting in proliferation and autonomous increased function of hormonally responsive tissues [35]. Activating mutations of the *GNAS* maternal allele expressed in imprinted tissues may lead to clinically significant effects. Variable Gsα activity in different tissues may help determine hormone action in the different tissues.

Patients with pseudohypoparathyroidism type 1b may have shortened fourth or fifth metacarpal or metatarsal bones but do not express most of the other features of AHO. Gsα activity is normal when measured in various tissues of these patients. Pseudohypoparathyroidism type 1b patients have PTH resistance and, in some cases, TSH resistance but lack resistance to other hormones. Changes in bone density over time in these patients correlate with serum PTH levels [36]. Patients with sporadic or inherited pseudohypoparathyroidism type 1b have switched their pattern of maternal methylation of the Gsα allele to a pattern of paternal methylation [37]. Mutations causing a switch in the maternal to paternal methylation pattern are found in most patients with pseudohypoparathyroidism type 1b. These mutations include two microdeletions in the *STX16* gene located 220 kB centromeric to the *GNAS* exon 1A [38] and deletions of the differentially methylated region of the NESP55 exon and exons 3 and 4 of the antisense mRNA transcript. Inheritance of the mutation from the mother, or a spontaneous mutation of a maternally derived allele, negates the maternal *GNAS* methylation pattern. Patients with pseudohypoparathyroidism type 1b have not been reported to have small mutations, but uniparental disomy has been reported, where both *GNAS* alleles were inherited from the father. It is believed that conversion of the maternal GNAS allele epigenotype to the paternal GNAS allele epigenotype, or inheritance of two paternal GNAS alleles, results in transcriptional silencing of the Gsα promoter in imprinted tissues by both alleles, with resultant limited or absent expression of Gsα in these tissues.

Patients with pseudohypoparathyroidism type 1c have AHO features with resistance to multiple hormones, without evidence of Gsα or Giα signaling transduction abnormalities. These patients may have *GNAS* mutations resulting in functional defects in Gsα [39].

The heterotopic ossifications of AHO are a unique feature of this disorder [40]. These ossifications are not mature calcifications and not related to serum calcium or phosphorus levels or the calcium x phosphate product. These ossifications are areas of intramembranous bone that seem to develop without prior inflammation or trauma. It is thought that Gsα deficiency leads to expression of ectopic Cbfa1/Runx2 in mesenchymal stem cells in the skin, causing these cells to differentiate into osteoblasts that cause new bone to form in the skin.

Osteoma cutis and progressive osseous heteroplasia (POH) are two forms of AHO in which abnormal bone formation is the only feature present [41]. In osteoma cutis, abnormal bone formation occurs only in the skin, whereas in POH, abnormal bone formation occurs in the skin, subcutaneous tissues, muscles, tendons, and ligaments. Progressive osseous heteroplasia may result in limitation of joint or limb movement due to widespread calcification of the skin during childhood, followed by gradual conversion of skeletal muscles and deeper connective tissues into the bone. Bony nodules and strands of heterotopic bone may extend from the skin and superficial connective tissues into the subcutaneous fat and deeper connective tissues.

Patients with osteoma cutis and POH may have paternally inherited inactivating heterozygous *GNAS* mutations. These patients lack other features of AHO or pseudohypoparathyroidism.

Pseudohypoparathyroidism type 2 is thought to result from normal PTH/PTH-rp receptor-Gsα-adenylyl cyclase complex function but reduced action of the generated cAMP on downstream intracellular targets, such as sodium-phosphate cotransporters that mediate renal tubular phosphate reabsorption. Pseudohypoparathyroidism type 2 currently lacks a defined genetic or familial inheritance, with the clinical and biochemical presentation similar to severe vitamin D deficiency or vitamin D resistance. It is possible that cases of pseudohypoparathyroidism type 2 may result from unsuspected vitamin D deficiency [42].

Acrodysostosis is a form of pseudohypoparathyroidism type 2 characterized by increased basal and PTH-stimulated urinary cAMP excretion but lack of PTH-induced phosphate excretion [43]. This disorder has several forms, with type 1 due to mutations in protein kinase A regulatory subunit 1A and type 2 due to mutations in phosphodiesterase 4D.

Transient pseudohypoparathyroidism of the newborn may occur in infants within 5–7 days of birth [44]. Most infants developing hypocalcemia at this age have decreased PTH levels causing hypoparathyroidism, but as many as 25% may have increased PTH levels. These infants may have delayed development of the post-cAMP signaling pathway limited to the proximal renal tubule. Affected infants seem to recover from this delay in post-receptor signaling maturation within 6 months of birth.

Patients with pseudohypoparathyroidism type 1 commonly have an apparent dissociation between circulating bioactive PTH and serum immunoreactive PTH. Plasma from these patients may have reduced biological activity in in vitro cytochemical bioassays, implying inhibition of PTH action. A potential explanation for this inhibition may be accumulated fragments of PTH 7–84 and other fragments that inhibit the hypercalcemic and hypophosphatemic effects of PTH 1–84. PTH 7–84 fragments are often increased in patients with pseudohypoparathyroidism types 1a and 1b, with the proportion of these fragments increased compared to biologically active PTH 1–84. These and other fragments could accumulate in patients with pseudohypoparathyroidism type 1 due to the duration of their long-standing hyperparathyroidism and may not play a significant role in the pathogenesis of the disorder.

Hypomagnesemia and severe vitamin D deficiency may both cause biochemical findings of PTH resistance, so it is important to measure serum magnesium and 25-hydroxyvitamin D before confirming a suspected diagnosis of pseudohypoparathyroidism.

The AHO features seen in pseudohypoparathyroidism type 1a may be also seen in other genetic disorders such as Prader-Willi syndrome or Ullrich-Turner syndrome. Patients with small terminal deletions of chromosome 2q37 may appear to have AHO, but they have normal hormone function and normal Gsα activity.

The classical test for pseudohypoparathyroidism, the Ellsworth-Howard test, was later modified by Chase, Melson, and Aurbach [45, 46]. This test required intravenous infusion of 200–300 USP units of purified bovine PTH or parathyroid extract. Since purified bovine PTH is no longer available, this protocol has been modified to use teriparatide (human recombinant parathyroid hormone 1–34) either by intravenous infusion or subcutaneous injection. One version of this modified protocol [47] recommends having patients drink 250 mL of water each hour from 6 a.m. to 12 p.m. Two 30-min control urine collections are obtained before 9 a.m. Teriparatide is given at 9 a.m. at 0.625 mcg/kg body weight to a maximum of 25 mcg by intravenous infusion over 15 min or to a maximum of 40 mcg by subcutaneous injection. Thirty-minute urine collections are started at 9 a.m. and 9:30 a.m., and 1-h urine collections are started at 10 a.m. and 11 a.m. Serum phosphate and creatinine are drawn at 9 a.m. and 11 a.m. The urine samples from the different time points are measured for cAMP, phosphorus, and creatinine. Cyclic AMP results are expressed as nmol cAMP per 100 mL glomerular filtrate and renal tubular phosphate reabsorption as TmP/GFR. Normal healthy subjects typically demonstrate a 10–20-fold increase in urinary cAMP excretion and 20–30% decrease in TmP/GFR. Patients with pseudohypoparathyroidism types 1a and 1b show markedly blunted responses no matter how low their serum calcium.

Genetic testing may help in the diagnosis of pseudohypoparathyroidism type 1a but is not helpful in making a diagnosis of pseudohypoparathyroidism type 1b or other types of pseudohypoparathyroidism.

A new classification schema has recently been established by the EuroPHP network to cover all disorders of the PTH receptor and its signaling pathway [48, 49]. Inactivating PTH/PTH-related protein signaling disorder (iPPSD) is the new name proposed for these disorders. These disorders are divided into subtypes iPPSD1 through iPPSD6. PTH receptor inactivation mutations leading to Eiken and Blomstrand dysplasia are classified as iPPSD1. Inactivating Gsα mutations causing pseudohypoparathyroidism type 1a, pseudohypoparathyroidism type 1c, and pseudopseudohypoparathyroidism are classified as iPPSD2. Mutations leading to loss of methylation of GNAS disease-modifying regions leading to pseudohypoparathyroidism type 1b are classified as iPPSD3. Mutations of protein kinase A regulatory subunit 1A (PRKAR1A) leading to acrodysostosis type 1 are classified as iPPSD4. Mutations of phosphodiesterase 4D (PDE4D) leading to acrodysostosis type 2 are classified as iPPSD5. Mutations of phosphodiesterase 3A (PDE3A) causing autosomal dominant hypertension with brachydactyly are classified as iPPSD6. iPPSDx is the designation given for unknown molecular defects, and iPPSDn+1 is the term used for new molecular defects not yet described.

Treatment

Treatment of pseudohypoparathyroidism is focused on correcting the biochemical abnormalities of low serum calcium, high serum phosphorus, and associated hyperparathyroidism [50]. These goals include improving serum calcium to as close to the normal range as possible, thereby helping suppress PTH secretion as much as possible toward normal. The target PTH level is as close to the upper limit of normal as possible to minimize increased bone resorption leading to osteitis fibrosa cystica.

Because the distal renal tubular effects of PTH in patients with pseudohypoparathyroidism remain intact, calcium reabsorption from the glomerular filtrate occurs normally. This minimizes the amount of calcium supplement required to keep serum calcium normal and to suppress PTH secretion.

Because proximal renal tubular production of 1,25-dihydroxyvitamin D from 25-hydroxyvitamin D via 1α-hydroxylase is limited in pseudohypoparathyroidism, calcitriol supplementation is typically required [51]. Combination therapy with calcium and calcitriol usually does not increase urinary calcium because the distal renal tubular mechanisms for reabsorption of calcium from glomerular filtrate remain intact. Urinary calcium excretion may increase before serum calcium normalizes. The best way to prevent significant hypercalciuria in this situation is to target serum calcium in the low-normal range.

Low-phosphate diets or phosphate binders are sometimes necessary to reduce increased serum phosphate levels.

Calcium supplementation with 1–2 g elemental calcium each day is usually sufficient to increase serum calcium levels into the low-normal range, as well as to block intestinal phosphate absorption to limit hyperphosphatemia. Calcium supplements should be taken with meals to reduce intestinal phosphate absorption.

Calcitriol has a short half-life of 2–3 h and is usually given at starting doses of 0.25–0.50 mcg at least twice daily. Alfacalcidol is not approved for use in the USA but is available in Europe and much of the rest of the world. Alfacalcidol has a longer half-life and is usually given at starting doses of 0.50–1.00 mcg once daily. Vitamin D2 or D3 may be given in age-appropriate doses for skeletal health as per the Institute of Medicine 2011 dietary reference intakes [52] but should not be given in very large doses as in the past, as these very high doses may lead to markedly increased serum 25-hydroxyvitamin D levels that may become toxic and cause significant hypercalcemia and kidney dysfunction. Vitamin D2 or D3 toxicity may take weeks to months to resolve after vitamin D2 or D3 are stopped, during which renal dysfunction may worsen or become permanent.

Thiazide-type diuretics limit urinary calcium loss, and these may be helpful in stabilizing or improving serum calcium levels in pseudohypoparathyroidism. Because thiazide-type diuretics cause urinary potassium loss, potassium supplementation may be necessary to prevent hypokalemia with long-term thiazide-type diuretic use.

Cinacalcet has been used as adjunctive therapy to reduce very high levels of PTH secretion in at least one pediatric patient and one young man with pseudohypoparathyroidism type 1b when calcium and activated vitamin D supplementation in combination were not sufficient to control the hyperparathyroidism [53, 54].

Recombinant human growth hormone has been used to treat short stature in eight prepubertal children with pseudohypoparathyroidism type 1a for 3–8 years, with reported results similar to children with idiopathic growth hormone deficiency [55].

PTH treatment is not recommended for pseudohypoparathyroidism because serum PTH levels are significantly increased already. Tissue resistance to endogenous PTH secretion makes it difficult for exogenous PTH administration to have a significant beneficial effect.

Summary and Conclusions

Pseudohypoparathyroidism is a rare disorder that results from proximal renal tubular resistance to parathyroid hormone. This tissue resistance results in hyperparathyroidism associated with decreased serum calcium, increased serum phosphate, and decreased 1,25-dihydroxyvitamin D. A variety of forms of pseudohypoparathyroidism have been described. Pseudohypoparathyroidism type 1 results in inability of exogenous PTH to stimulate urinary cAMP and phosphate excretion. Pseudohypoparathyroidism type 2 is associated with increased urinary cAMP excretion but normal urinary phosphate excretion after administration of exogenous PTH. PTH resistance occurs in the proximal renal tubule but not in other PTH target tissues. Most patients develop symptoms of hypocalcemia, including tingling paresthesias, muscle cramps, tetany, or seizures without adequate supplementation. Calcium and calcitriol supplementation is recommended for all patients with pseudohypoparathyroidism to prevent sustained hyperparathyroidism and resultant bone disease.

References

1. Mantovani G. Clinical review: pseudohypoparathyroidism: diagnosis and treatment. J Clin Endocrinol Metab. 2011;96:3020–30.
2. Singla M, Garg G, Gupta A. Pseudohypoparathyroidism type 1a. QJM. 2018;111:331–3.
3. Albright F, Burnett CH, Smith PH, Parson W. Pseudohypoparathyroidism – an example of "Seabright-Bantam syndrome". Endocrinology. 1942;39:922–32.
4. Cianferotti L, Brandi ML. Pseudohypoparathyroidism. Minerva Endocrinol. 2018;43:156–67.
5. Underbjerg L, Sikjaer T, Mosekilde L, Rejnmark L. Pseudohypoparathyroidism – epidemiology, mortality and risk of complications. Clin Endocrinol. 2016;84:904–11.
6. Tafaj O, Jüppner H. Pseudohypoparathyroidism: one gene, several syndromes. J Endocrinol Invest. 2017;40:347–56.
7. Mantovani G, Spada A, Elli FM. Pseudohypoparathyroidism and Gsα-cAMP-linked disorders: current view and open issues. Nat Rev Endocrinol. 2016;12:347–56.
8. Athappan G, Ariyamuthu VK. Images in clinical medicine. Chvostek's sign and carpopedal spasm. N Engl J Med. 2009;360:e24.
9. Kotowicz J. Occurrence of Chvostek's sign in healthy people and its significance. Pol Med J. 1969;8:440–3.
10. Meininger ME, Kendler JS. Images in clinical medicine. Trousseau's sign. N Engl J Med. 2000;343:1855.
11. van Bussel BC, Koopmans RP. Trousseau's sign at the emergency department. BMJ Case Rep. 2016;2016.
12. Kuzel AR, Lodhi MU, Rahim M. Classic and non-classic features in pseudohypoparathyroidism: case study and brief literature review. Cureus. 2017;9:e1878.
13. Kobayashi Y, Tsuyuzaki J, Koizumi Y. Pseudohypoparathyroidism causing multiple brain calcifications. Intern Med. 2018;57:153–4.
14. Song CY, Zhao ZX, Li W, Sun CC, Liu YM. Pseudohypoparathyroidism with basal ganglia calcification: a case report of rare cause of reversible parkinsonism. Medicine (Baltimore). 2017;96:e6312.

15. Sharma M, Nolkha N, Sharma A, Bhadu D, Dhakad U, Singh R, Das SK. Spondyloarthropathy-like findings and diffuse osteosclerosis as the presenting feature of pseudohypoparathyroidism. J Clin Rheumatol. 2016;22:102–4.
16. Heemskerk CPM, Pereboom M, van Stralen K, Berger FA, van den Bemt PMLA, Kuijper AFM, van der Hoeven RTM, Mantel-Teeuwisse AK, Becker ML. Risk factors for QTc interval prolongation. Eur J Clin Pharmacol. 2018;74:183–91.
17. Bilezikian JP, Khan AA, Potts JT Jr, Brandi ML, Clarke BL, Shoback D, Jüppner H, D'Amour P, Fox J, Rejnmark L, Mosekilde L, Rubin MR, Dempster D, Gafni R, Collins MT, Sliney J, Sanders J. Hypoparathyroidism in the adult: epidemiology, diagnosis, pathophysiology, target-organ involvement, treatment, and challenges for future research. J Bone Miner Res. 2011;26:2317–37.
18. Shoback D. Clinical practice. Hypoparathyroidism. N Engl J Med. 2008;359:391–403.
19. Chase LR, Melson GL, Aurbach. Pseudohypoparathyroidism: defective excretion of 3′,5′-AMP in response to parathyroid hormone. J Clin Invest. 1969;48:1832–44.
20. Drezner M, Neelon FA, Lebovitz HE. Pseudohypoparathyroidism type II: a possible defect in the reception of the cyclic AMP signal. N Engl J Med. 1973;289:1056–60.
21. Weinstein LS, Yu S, Warner DR, Liu J. Endocrine manifestations of stimulatory g protein alpha-subunit mutations and the role of genomic imprinting. Endocr Rev. 2001;22:675–705.
22. Mantovani G, Elli FM. Pseudohypoparathyroidism type Ib in 2015. Ann Endocrinol (Paris). 2015;76:101–4.
23. Brix B, Werner R, Staedt P, Struve D, Hiort O, Thiele S. Different pattern of epigenetic changes of the GNAS gene locus in patients with pseudohypoparathyroidism type Ic confirm the heterogeneity of underlying pathomechanisms in this subgroup of pseudohypoparathyroidism and the demand for a new classification of GNAS-related disorders. J Clin Endocrinol Metab. 2014;99:E1564–70.
24. Salemi P, Skalamera Olson JM, Dickson LE, Germain-Lee EL. Ossifications in Albright hereditary osteodystrophy: role of genotype, inheritance, sex, age, hormonal status, and BMI. J Clin Endocrinol Metab. 2018;103:158–68.
25. Grüters-Kieslich A, Reyes M, Sharma A, Demirci C, DeClue TJ, Lankes E, Tiosano D, Schnabel D, Jüppner H. Early-onset obesity: unrecognized first evidence for GNAS mutations and methylation changes. J Clin Endocrinol Metab. 2017;102:2670–7.
26. Chen M, Shrestha YB, Podyma B, Cui Z, Naglieri B, Sun H, Ho T, Wilson EA, Li YQ, Gavrilova O, Weinstein LS. Gsα deficiency in the dorsomedial hypothalamus underlies obesity associated with Gsα mutations. J Clin Invest. 2017;127:500–10.
27. Mantovani G, Maghnie M, Weber G, De Menis E, Brunelli V, Cappa M, Loli P, Beck-Peccoz P, Spada A. Growth hormone releasing hormone resistance in pseudohypoparathyroidism type ia: new evidence for imprinting of the Gs alpha gene. J Clin Endocrinol Metab. 2003;88:4070–4.
28. Germain-Lee EL, Groman J, Crane JL, Jan de Beur SM, Levine MA. Growth hormone deficiency in pseudohypoparathyroidism type 1a: another manifestation of multihormone resistance. J Clin Endocrinol Metab. 2003;88:4059–69.
29. Albright F, Forbes AP, Henneman PH. Pseudopseudohypoparathyroidism. Trans Assoc Am Phys. 1952;65:337–50.
30. Thiele S, Werner R, Grötzinger J, Brix B, Staedt P, Struve D, Reiz B, Farida J, Hiort O. A positive genotype-phenotype correlation in a large cohort of patients with Pseudohypoparathyroidism type Ia and pseudo-pseudohypoparathyroidism and 33 newly identified mutations in the GNAS gene. Mol Genet Genom Med. 2015;3:111–20.
31. Kehlenbach RH, Matthey J, Huttner WB. XLαs is a new type of G protein. Nature. 1995;372:804–9.
32. Ischia R, Lovisetti-Scamihorn P, Hogue-Angeletti R, Wolkersdorfer M, Winkler H, Fischer-Colbrie R. Molecular cloning and characterization of NESP55, a novel chromogranin-like precursor of a peptide with 5HT1B receptor agonist activity. J Biol Chem. 1997;272:11657–62.
33. Basteppe M, Pincus JE, Sugimoto T, Tojo K, Kanatami M, Azuma Y, Kruse K, Rosenbloom AL, Koshiyama H. Positional dissociation between the genetic mutation responsible for pseu-

dohypoparathyroidism type Ib and the associated methylation defect at exon A/B: evidence for a long-range regulatory element within the imprinted GNAS1 locus. Hum Mol Genet. 2001;10:1231–41.
34. Williamson CM, Ball ST, Nottingham WE, Skinner A, Plagge A, Turner MD, Powles N, Hough T, Papworth D, Fraser WD, et al. A cis-acting control region is required exclusively for the tissue imprinting of Gnas. Nat Genet. 2004;36:894–9.
35. Elli FM, Bordogna P, Arosio M, Spada A, Mantovani G. Mosaicism for GNAS methylation defects associated with pseudohypoparathyroidism type 1B arose in early post-zygotic phases. Clin Epigenetics. 2018;10:16.
36. Chu X, Zhu Y, Wang O, Nie M, Quan T, Xue Y, Wang W, Jiang Y, Li M, Xia W, Xing X. Bone mineral density and its serial changes are associated with PTH levels in pseudohypoparathyroidism type 1b patients. J Bone Miner Res. 2018;33:743–52.
37. Bastepe M, Frolich LF, Hendy GN, Indridason OS, Josse RG, Koshiyama H, Korkko J, Nakamoto JM, Rosenbloom AL, Slyper AH, et al. Autosomal dominant pseudohypoparathyroidism type 1b is associated with a heterozygous microdeletion that likely disrupts a putative imprinting control element of GNAS. J Clin Invest. 2003;112:1255–63.
38. Linglart A, Gensure RC, Olney RC, Juppner H, Bastepe M. A novel STX16 deletion in autosomal dominant pseudohypoparathyroidism type 1b redefines the boundaries of a cis-acting imprinting control element of GNAS. Am J Hum Genet. 2005;76:804–14.
39. Thiele S, de Sanctis L, Werner R, Grotzinger J, Aydin C, Juppner H, Bastepe M, Hiort O. Functional characterization of GNAS mutations found in patients with pseudohypoparathyroidism type 1c defines a new subgroup of pseudohypoparathyroidism affecting selectively Gsalpha-receptor interaction. Hum Mutat. 2011;32:653–60.
40. Bastepe M. GNAS mutations and heterotopic ossification. Bone. 2018;109:80–5.
41. Kaplan FS, Shore EM. Progressive osseous heteroplasia. J Bone Miner Res. 2000;15:2084–94.
42. Shriraam M, Bhansali A, Velayutham P. Vitamin D deficiency masquerading as pseudohypoparathyroidism type 2. J Assoc Physicians India. 2003;51:619–20.
43. Silve C. Acrodysostosis: a new form of pseudohypoparathyroidism? Ann Endocrinol (Paris). 2015;76:110–2.
44. Lee CT, Tsai WY, Tung YC, Tsau YK. Transient pseudohypoparathyroidism as a cause of late-onset hypocalcemia in neonates and infants. J Formos Med Assoc. 2008;107:806–10.
45. Chase LR, Melson GL. Aurbach GD Pseudohypoparathyroidism: defective excretion of 3′,5′-AMP in response to parathyroid hormone. J Clin Invest. 1969;48:1832–44.
46. Sohn HE, Furukawa Y, Yumita S, Miura R, Unakami H, Yoshinaga K. Effect of synthetic 1-34 fragment of human parathyroid hormone on plasma adenosine 3′,5′-monophosphate (cAMP) concentrations and the diagnostic criteria based on the plasma cAMP response in Ellsworth-Howard test. Endocrinol Jpn. 1984;31:33–40.
47. Rubin MR, Levine MA. Hypoparathyroidism and pseudohypoparathyroidism. In: Rosen CJ editor. Primer on the metabolic bone diseases and disorders of mineral metabolism. 8th ed. Wiley; 2013. p. 579–89.
48. Thiele S, Mantovani G, Barlier A, Boldrin V, Bordogna P, De Sanctis L, Elli FM, Freson K, Garin I, Grybek V, Hanna P, Izzi B, Hiort O, Lecumberri B, Pereda A, Saraff V, Silve C, Turan S, Usardi A, Werner R, de Nanclares GP, Linglart A. From pseudohypoparathyroidism to inactivating PTH/PTHrP signaling disorder (iPPSD), a novel classification proposed by the EuroPHP network. Eur J Endocrinol. 2016;175:P1–P17.
49. Turan S. Current nomenclature of pseudohypoparathyroidism: inactivating parathyroid hormone/parathyroid hormone-related protein signaling disorder. J Clin Res Pediatr Endocrinol. 2017;9(Suppl 2):58–68.
50. Lopes MP, Kliemann BS, Bini IB, Kulchetscki R, Borsani V, Savi L, Borba VZ, Moreira CA. Hypoparathyroidism and pseudohypoparathyroidism: etiology, laboratory features and complications. Arch Endocrinol Metab. 2016;60:532–6.
51. Ishii A, Imanishi Y, Kurajoh M, Nagata Y, Kobayashi K, Miki T, Inaba M, Nishizawa Y. The administration of an active vitamin D(3) analogue reduced the serum concentrations of 1-84

and truncated parathyroid hormone in pseudohypoparathyroidism type Ib patients. Endocr J. 2010;57:609–14.

52. IOM (Institute of Medicine). Dietary reference intakes for calcium and vitamin D. Washington, DC: The National Academies Press; 2011.
53. Srivastava T, Krudys J, Mardis NJ, Sebestyen-VanSickle J, Alon US. Cinacalcet as adjunctive therapy in pseudohypoparathyroidism type 1b. Pediatr Nephrol. 2016;31:795–800.
54. Koch M, Kohnle M. Successful off-label use of cinacalcet HCl after standard therapy failure in a young man with pseudohypoparathyroidism type 1b and vitamin D intoxication sequelae. Clin Nephrol. 2008;70:439–44.
55. Mantovani G, Ferrante E, Giavoli C, Linglart A, Cappa M, Cisternino M, Maghnie M, Ghizzoni L, de Sanctis L, Lania AG, Beck-Peccoz P, Spada A. Recombinant human GH replacement therapy in children with pseudohypoparathyroidism type Ia: first study on the effect on growth. J Clin Endocrinol Metab. 2010;95:5011–7.

Chapter 7
Phosphorus Disorders: Hypophosphatemic Rickets

Bart L. Clarke

Case Description

A 22-year-old female was referred for evaluation and management of hypophosphatemia first diagnosed during a general medical evaluation. She complained of intermittent muscle weakness and pain, bone and joint pain, and decreased energy level. She had previously been noted to have mild bowing of her legs, with several lower extremity stress fractures affecting her metatarsal bones, but not had other fractures. She had not had kidney stones previously. She has had multiple abscessed teeth over the years. She had not been previously advised to take phosphorus or vitamin D supplements. She thinks she may have taken a liquid form of phosphorus in childhood for several years but stopped this by the time she was in kindergarten. She has been advised by her primary care physician to take a supplemental multivitamin for general health. Her family history was significant for multiple family members with short stature and bowing of the legs.

Her physical evaluation showed short stature of 58 inches, weight 110 lb, and BMI 23.0 kg/m^2. Her blood pressure was normal at 110/70 mm Hg, and her pulse was normal at 68 beats/min. Her physical exam showed short stature, with mild lateral bowing of her tibiae, without other significant abnormalities.

Her fasting serum phosphorus was decreased at 1.8 mg/dL (normal, 2.5–4.5), with serum calcium normal at 9.2 mg/dL (normal, 8.9–10.1). Her serum creatinine was normal at 0.8 mg/dL (normal, 0.6–1.1). Her serum total alkaline phosphatase was increased at 180 units/L (normal, 45–115). Her parathyroid hormone was normal at 35 pg/mL (normal, 15–65). Her serum 25-hydroxyvitamin D was optimal at

B. L. Clarke (✉)
Mayo Clinic, Rochester, MN, USA
e-mail: clarke.bart@mayo.edu

P. M. Camacho (ed.), *Metabolic Bone Diseases*,
https://doi.org/10.1007/978-3-030-03694-2_7

25 ng/mL (optimal, 20–50), but her serum 1,25-dihydroxyvitamin D was decreased at 16 pg/mL (normal, 18–78). Her serum magnesium was normal at 2.1 mg/dL (normal, 1.7–2.3).

Her clinical and laboratory findings were felt to be compatible with childhood-onset hypophosphatemic rickets, most likely X-linked based on her family history with multiple male and female family members affected. Because of her decreased serum phosphorus level and history of lower extremity stress fractures, she was treated with potassium phosphate 250 mg elemental phosphorus one packet twice daily and calcitriol 0.25 mcg twice a day. She was advised to maintain dietary calcium intake at 1000 mg elemental calcium and to continue her multivitamin containing vitamin D3 400 international units per tablet.

Compliance with potassium phosphate supplementation was difficult for her over the next 2 years due to stomach distress and intermittent diarrhea, and she was variably compliant with therapy, but did not have further lower extremity stress fractures or dental abscesses.

Introduction

Phosphorus is a critical element for skeletal development and maturation, as well as bone mineralization, cell membrane structure, nucleotide formation, and intracellular signaling. Phosphorus forms complexes with oxygen in living tissues to form anionic phosphate. Phosphate homeostasis in humans is largely maintained by the balance between parathyroid hormone (PTH), 1,25-dihydroxyvitamin D, and fibroblast growth factor-23 (FGF-23). Serum phosphorus is influenced by these hormones, as well as by dietary intake, acid-based changes in the blood, renal function, skeletal metabolism, and intestinal absorption.

Low serum phosphorus is seen in up to 5% of hospitalized patients [1, 2]. Hypophosphatemia is more common in patients who abuse alcohol or who develop sepsis, where it may be seen in as many as 30–50% of patients.

Clinical findings related to hypophosphatemia are variable, depending on the severity of the low serum phosphorus and how long it has been present. Chronic long-standing hypophosphatemia may cause fewer symptoms in patients than acute hypophosphatemia. Severe hypophosphatemia may be seen in chronic alcoholism, during repletion of nutrition in patients with poor nutrition, treatment of diabetic ketoacidosis, or severe illness in patients in critical care settings.

Symptoms of hypophosphatemia are usually attributed to the direct effects of decreased intracellular phosphorus. Intracellular phosphorus depletion results in tissue hypoxia caused by reduced 2,3-diphosphoglycerate (2,3-DPG) in erythrocytes, which increases the affinity of hemoglobin for oxygen. This deprives the tissues of oxygen delivery by the blood. Cells that are depleted of phosphorus make insufficient adenosine 3′,5′-triphosphate (ATP) to maintain energy metabolism, with resulting suboptimal cellular function.

This chapter will provide a review of hypophosphatemic rickets and discuss the differential diagnosis of hypophosphatemia, focusing on different genetic and acquired disorders causing renal tubular loss of phosphorus, with an emphasis on X-linked hypophosphatemic rickets.

Differential Diagnosis of Hypophosphatemia

The three most common causes of hypophosphatemia are intestinal malabsorption of phosphorus, redistribution of tissue fluid phosphorus into cells, and increased renal tubular loss of phosphorus. Many patients with hypophosphatemia can be diagnosed based on their medical history, but some cannot. Serum and 24-h urine phosphorus should be measured in most patients to document levels to confirm the diagnosis. Fractional excretion of filtered phosphate on a random urine specimen may be helpful in patients unable to complete a 24-h urine collection. Fractional excretion of filtered phosphate is calculated from the formula $FEPO_4 = (UPO_4 \times PCr)/(PPO_4 \times UCr)$, where U and P represent urine and plasma, PO_4 is phosphate concentration, and Cr is creatinine. In patients with hypophosphatemia, fractional excretion of phosphate greater than 5%, or 24-h urinary phosphorus greater than 100 mg, is indicative of increased renal tubular phosphate loss.

Table 7.1 shows the differential diagnosis of hypophosphatemia. Reduced intestinal absorption may be due to many different causes, whereas intracellular shifts of phosphorus are caused by a smaller number of disparate causes. The differential diagnosis of hypophosphatemia due to renal tubular losses is wide and includes primary renal tubular transport defects, hyperparathyroidism, increased FGF-23 levels, and increased expression of KLOTHO or other phosphaturic proteins. These causes are listed in Table 7.2.

Epidemiology of Hypophosphatemic Rickets

Because of the relative rarity of hypophosphatemic rickets, prevalence and incidence estimates for this group of disorders have not been published in most countries. Previous studies have reported that X-linked hypophosphatemic rickets occurs in 3.9–5.0 per 100,000 live births.

Beck-Nielson et al. [3] estimated the incidence of nutritional rickets and incidence and prevalence of hereditary rickets in Southern Denmark in a population-based retrospective cohort study based on a review of medical records. Patients aged 0–14.9 years referred to or discharged from hospitals in Southern Denmark from 1985 to 2005 with a diagnosis of rickets were identified by register search, and their medical records were retrieved. Patients fulfilling the diagnostic criteria of primary rickets were included. A total of 112 patients were identified with nutritional rickets,

Table 7.1 Differential diagnosis of hypophosphatemia

Intracellular shifts
Hyperinsulinemia due to insulin treatment, treatment of diabetic ketoacidosis, or refeeding
Hungry bone syndrome
Acute respiratory alkalosis
Tumor cell uptake in leukemia blast crisis, lymphoma
Sepsis
Dietary intake of glucose, fructose, or glycerol
Recovery from metabolic acidosis
Decreased intestinal absorption
Vitamin D deficiency or resistance due to
Nutritional deficiency
Low sunlight exposure
Low dietary intake
Malabsorption
Celiac or Crohn's disease
Previous gastrectomy, small intestinal resection, intestinal bypass surgery
Pancreatitis
Chronic diarrhea of any cause
Chronic liver disease
Chronic kidney disease
Increased catabolism due to anticonvulsant therapy
Vitamin D receptor defects: vitamin D-dependent rickets, type 2
Vitamin D synthetic defects
Vitamin D-dependent rickets, type 1 (CYP27B1)
CYP27A1
Nutritional deficiencies: alcoholism, anorexia nervosa, starvation
Antacids containing aluminum or magnesium
Increased renal tubular loss
Renal tubular phosphate loss disorders
Primary and secondary hyperparathyroidism
Diabetic acidosis with osmotic diuresis
Medications: calcitonin, diuretics, glucocorticoids, bicarbonate
Acute volume expansion

of which 74% were immigrants. From 1995 to 2005, the average incidence of nutritional rickets in children aged 0–14.9 and 0–2.9 years was 2.9 and 5.8 per 100,000 per year, respectively. Among immigrant children born in Denmark, the average incidence was 60 (0–14.9 years) per 100,000 per year. Ethnic Danish children were only diagnosed in early childhood, and the average incidence in the age group 0–2.9 years declined from 5.0 to 2.0 per 100,000 per year during 1985–1994 to

Table 7.2 Disorders causing renal phosphate loss

Disease (OMIM)	Defect	Pathogenesis
TIO	Mesenchymal tumor	Ectopic unregulated production of FGF-23, sFRP4, MEPE, FGF-7
XLH (307800)	PHEX mutation	Inappropriate FGF-23 synthesis in the bone
ADHR (193100)	FGF-23 mutation	Increased circulating intact FGF-23 due to mutations making it resistant to cleavage
HHRH (241530)	SLC34A3 mutation	Loss-of-function NaPi-IIc mutations that cause renal phosphate wasting without a defect in 1,25-D synthesis
ARHR1 (241520)	DMP1 mutation	Loss of DMP1 causes impaired osteocyte differentiation and increased FGF-23 production
ARHR2 (613312)	ENPP1 mutation	Increased FGF-23 production
HR and HPT (612089)	α-KLOTHO translocation	Increased KLOTHO, FGF-23, and downstream FGF-23 signaling
Fibrous dysplasia (139320)	GNAS mutation	Increased FGF-23 production from dysplastic bone
Linear nevus sebaceous syndrome	Excess FGF-23 production	Increase FGF-23 production from dysplastic bone and nevi
Osteoglophonic dysplasia (166250)	FGFR1 mutation	Increased FGF-23 production from dysplastic bone
NPHLOP1 (612286)	SLC34A1 mutation	Renal phosphate wasting without a defect in 1,25-D synthesis
NPHLOP2 (612287)	SLC9A3R1 mutation	Renal phosphate wasting through potentiation of PTH-mediated cAMP production
FRTS2 (613388)	SLC34A1 mutation	Renal phosphate wasting without a defect in 1,25-D synthesis

1995–2005. Sixteen cases of hereditary rickets were diagnosed during the study period giving an average incidence of 4.3 per 100,000 (0–0.9 years) per year. The prevalence of hypophosphatemic rickets and vitamin D-dependent rickets type 1 was 4.8 and 0.4 per 100,000 (0–14.9 years), respectively. The study concluded that nutritional rickets is rare in Southern Denmark and largely restricted to immigrants, but the incidence among ethnic Danish children was unexpectedly high. Hereditary rickets was the most common cause of rickets in ethnic Danish children, but nutritional rickets was most frequent among all young children.

Clinical Presentation of Genetically Inherited Renal Tubular Phosphate-Wasting Disorders

X-Linked Hypophosphatemic (XLH) Rickets

This is the most common genetic cause of renal tubular phosphate wasting. XLH was first described by Fuller Albright in 1939 [4]. Patients with XLH most often have short stature, rachitic and osteomalacic bone disease, and dental abscesses, similar to the case presented above. The X-linked inheritance of this form of rickets was first established in 1958 [5]. X-linked inheritance means that males with an appropriate mutation on their X chromosome will express the disorder and that females with appropriate mutations on both X chromosomes will have the condition but that females with an appropriate mutation on only one X chromosome will not express the disorder.

It took many years to work out the genetic basis for this disorder. Mutations in the *PHEX* gene on the X chromosome were eventually reported in the 1990s to cause XLH, with up to 285 mutations reported to date in the *PHEX* database at www.PHEXdb@mcgill.ca. *PHEX* is an acronym for *p*hosphate-regulating gene with *h*omologies to *e*ndopeptidases on the *X* chromosome [6]. This gene transcribes a protein with as-yet-unknown function that is a member of the M13 family of membrane-bound metalloproteinases and present in osteoblasts, osteocytes, and odontoblasts, but not in renal tubular cells [7].

Patients with XLH usually have no symptoms or recognized skeletal phenotype before they start to walk. Most new patients come from families known to have this disorder. When starting to walk, children develop bowing of their lower extremities due to weight bearing on weakened bones due to their rickets. Height gain usually decreases around this time, and bone and/or joint pain begins. Tooth abnormalities, including dental abscesses in the teeth without cavities, enamel defects, enlarged pulp spaces, and taurodontism, may develop. Taurodontism is a condition found in human molar teeth in which the body of the tooth and pulp chamber is enlarged vertically at the expense of the roots. As a result, the floor of the pulp chamber and the furcation of the tooth are moved apically down the root. Skull abnormalities, including frontal bossing and increased anteroposterior skull length, may be noted. As patients mature into adulthood, the presentation of XLH often changes to more diffuse bone and joint pain due to osteomalacia, with pseudofractures and enthesopathy in the spine characterizing the radiographic findings.

Laboratory abnormalities are classically decreased serum phosphorus, normal serum calcium, increased urinary phosphorus, increased serum total and bone alkaline phosphatase, normal serum PTH, and low or inappropriately normal serum 1,25-dihydroxyvitamin D for the level of serum phosphorus. Children may have normal serum phosphorus initially, but this decreases later during the first several years of life. These changes suggest that serum phosphate regulators other than PTH and 1,25-dihydroxyvitamin D may play a role in XLH. Serum FGF-23 secreted by osteocytes and osteoblasts seems to play a role in the pathogenesis of this disorder also. Serum FGF-23 levels are either increased or inappropriately normal, even though PHEX does not cleave FGF-23 directly. FGF-23 is known to increase throughout life in the bones of *hyp* mice lacking PHEX, an animal model of XLH [8–13]. It appears that PHEX is involved in the downregulation and control of FGF-23, but the precise mechanism has not yet been elucidated.

The diagnosis of XLH is based on the clinical presentation, physical examination, radiologic rachitic changes or evidence of osteomalacia, appropriate biochemical findings, and family history consistent with multiple generational or sporadic appearance of XLH. PHEX gene mutational analysis is available, but mutations are only found in 50–70% of suspected individuals when testing is done [14].

Treatment of XLH in children requires high-dose oral phosphate supplementation three to five times a day and high-dose calcitriol several times a day. Phosphate treatment should normally be started at low doses to minimize gastrointestinal irritation and diarrhea. Doses are then titrated upward to achieve a weight-based dose of phosphate three to five times a day given at peak doses of 20–40 mg/kg/day and calcitriol given at peak doses of 20–30 ng/kg/day several times a day [13]. When initiating therapy, some physicians prefer high-dose calcitriol therapy for the first year, given with phosphate as described above, with calcitriol 50–70 ng/kg/day up to a maximum of 3.0 mcg/day [13]. No comparison trials have evaluated the two strategies for treatment efficacy.

Treatment with phosphate and calcitriol in childhood leads to marked improvement in radiologic signs of rickets, as well as improvement in, but not normalization of, growth. Studies have shown that age and height at initiation of treatment, and possibly the sex of the patient, influence the peak height attained. Patients not responding to phosphate and calcitriol supplementation may eventually require orthopedic surgical intervention to correct lower extremity bony deformities.

Adult patients with XLH have low bone turnover and have had early closure of their epiphyses, such that phosphate and calcitriol requirements are often significantly less than in children. The role for therapy in adults remains unclear. Patients may be treated with no therapy, low-dose phosphate alone, low-dose calcitriol alone, or low-dose phosphate and calcitriol. It is not yet clear which adult patients require long-term treatment and which patients can safely discontinue therapy. Adult patients who are symptomatic likely will benefit from the treatment to improve their symptoms and bone architecture and to cure osteomalacia that may be present. Treatment should be given to patients with spontaneous insufficiency fractures, upcoming orthopedic surgical procedures, biochemical evidence of osteomalacia, or significant skeletal pain [13].

Clinical extension trials evaluating a monthly subcutaneously injectable monoclonal antibody to FGF-23 called burosumab (KRN23) in patients with XLH were completed and the drug is now FDA approved [15–17]. These trials have shown an increase in bone density at the spine, but this may have been due to increased calcific enthesopathy rather than increased bone strength, and it is unclear yet whether burosumab reduces fracture risk. Serum FGF-23 levels have been shown to increase with phosphate and calcitriol supplementation, but the clinical significance of this is not yet known [18]. A small trial with subcutaneously injected calcitonin showed a transient increase in serum phosphate and a decrease in FGF-23 levels [19]. Further clinical trials are needed to demonstrate whether any of these agents are efficacious for the treatment of XLH.

Autosomal-Dominant Hypophosphatemic Rickets (ADHR)

This rare form of hypophosphatemic rickets is similar in many ways to XLH. Early reports described a renal tubular phosphate-wasting disorder characterized by male to male transmission, indicating this form of rickets was distinct from XLH [20, 21].

Evaluation of kindreds with this condition showed incomplete penetrance in family members, another feature quite different from XLH. Extensive efforts using positional mapping, cloning, and sequence analysis eventually showed that the cause of ADHR was mutations in FGF-23 [22, 23]. Missense mutations in one or two arginine residues at positions 176 or 179 of FGF-23 have been identified in affected members of ADHR families. These mutated residues are located in the consensus proprotein convertase cleavage RXXR motif of the protein, preventing cleavage of the protein and thereby preventing its inactivation. As a result, serum FGF-23 levels are increased, causing increased or prolonged FGF-23 activity in the circulation [24].

Patients with ADHR have clinical and biochemical features similar to XLH. Other features that distinguish this disorder from XLH may include delayed onset until the late 20s and apparent complete spontaneous resolution of previously recognized renal tubular phosphate loss [24]. Serum FGF-23 levels vary with disease status [24]. Kindreds with ADHR may have two distinct presentations within the same family. One group with childhood onset usually has clinical and biochemical features similar to XLH, whereas the other group with late onset does not have lower extremity bowing deformities, presumably because the onset of the disorder occurred after fusion of the epiphyses. Iron deficiency may mimic late-onset ADHR, and lower serum iron levels are associated with increased FGF-23 levels [25].

Patients with childhood-onset ADHR are treated with phosphate and calcitriol supplementation similar to patients with XLH. Those who do not respond to supplementation may require orthopedic surgery to straighten bowed limbs eventually. Adult-onset patients may or may not require phosphate or calcitriol supplementation.

Hereditary Hypophosphatemic Rickets with Hypercalciuria (HHRH)

This rare form of hypophosphatemic rickets is characterized by hypophosphatemia, increased renal tubular phosphate loss, and increased serum 1,25-dihydroxyvitamin D in response to hypophosphatemia. The appropriate increase in serum 1,25-dihydroxyvitamin D in response to low serum phosphorus causes increased intestinal calcium absorption and consequent hypercalciuria and kidney stones. The genetic cause for this disorder is loss-of-function mutations in *SLC34A3*, leading to reduced renal tubular expression of the sodium-phosphate cotransporter IIc [26, 27]. This is one of the three sodium-phosphate cotransporters responsible for reabsorption of calcium from the renal tubule. Mutations may be homozygous or heterozygous [28].

The clinical presentation is similar to that of tumor-induced osteomalacia, but patients with HHRH have increased rather than decreased 1,25-dihydroxyvitamin D levels and hypercalciuria rather than normal or decreased urinary calcium.

Patients with HHRH are treated with phosphate supplementation alone, and not given calcitriol because their serum 1,25-dihydroxyvitamin D levels are appropriately increased already.

Autosomal Recessive Hypophosphatemic Rickets Type 1 (ARHR1)

This rare disorder is caused by loss-of-function mutations in dentin matrix protein-1 (DMP-1). DMP-1 is a matrix protein related to matrix extracellular phosphoglycoprotein (MEPE) and belongs to the small integrin-binding ligand N-linked glycoprotein (SIBLING) family of matrix proteins [29, 30]. The DMP-1 protein apparently has two functions. Early during osteocyte proliferation, it migrates to the nucleus and regulates gene transcription. Later during osteocyte differentiation, it becomes phosphorylated and is transported outside the osteocyte in response to calcium fluxes, where it facilitates matrix mineralization by hydroxyapatite after the full-length protein is cleaved. Loss of DMP-1 function in ARHR results in variably modestly increased serum FGF-23 levels, markedly increased bone FGF-23, defects in osteocyte differentiation, and impaired skeletal mineralization. Immature osteocytes may overproduce FGF-23, causing the kidneys to lose phosphorus in the urine and reduce production of 1,25-dihydroxyvitamin D. Treatment requires high-dose phosphate and calcitriol supplementation, similar to XLH.

Autosomal Recessive Hypophosphatemic Rickets Type 2 (ARHR2)

This rare disorder is caused by inactivating mutations in ectonucleotide pyrophosphatase/phosphodiesterase-1 (ENPP-1). This gene is associated with generalized arterial calcification of infancy. It normally regulates extracellular pyrophosphate and is critical for bone mineralization with phosphate. Five families with ARHR2 have been reported with loss-of-function mutations [31, 32]. Treatment requires high-dose phosphate and calcitriol supplementation, similar to XLH.

Other Rare Causes of Hypophosphatemic Rickets

Hyperphosphatemic rickets with hyperparathyroidism has been reported previously in one patient [33]. This patient was characterized by renal tubular phosphate loss, inappropriately normal serum 1,25-dihydroxyvitamin D, and hyperparathyroidism due to a genetic translocation causing increased α-KLOTHO levels. Alpha-KLOTHO is the cofactor required for binding of FGF-23 to its FGFR1 receptor. Serum FGF-23 levels are increased in this disorder also, implicating α-KLOTHO in the regulation of serum phosphate, FGF-23 expression, and parathyroid gland function.

Fibrous dysplasia is caused by activating mutations in the *GNAS* gene. These mutations cause constitutive activation of Gsα protein signaling. Fibrous dysplasia is associated with replacement of the medullary bone with undermineralized bone, and normal bone marrow with fibrotic bone marrow. Gsα mutations in dysplastic bone may help differentiate fibrous dysplasia, where they are present, from benign fibrous osseous lesions, where they are absent [34]. McCune-Albright syndrome is characterized by precocious puberty, café au lait hyperpigmented skin lesions, and fibrous dysplasia. Phosphate wasting may be associated with this syndrome, with increased serum FGF-23 levels in some cases. The serum FGF-23 level correlates generally with the extent of skeletal involvement with fibrous dysplasia. The hypophosphatemia in this disorder is not associated with classical rickets, so there is debate as to whether this should be treated with high-dose phosphate or calcitriol [35].

Linear nevus sebaceous syndrome, or epidermal nevus syndrome, is a rare form of hypophosphatemic rickets. Patients with this disorder are characterized by multiple cutaneous nevi and fibrous dysplasia and often have severe hypophosphatemic rickets caused by increased serum FGF-23 [36]. Treatment is usually given with high-dose phosphate and calcitriol.

Osteoglophonic dysplasia is a rare dominantly inherited form of dwarfism associated with renal tubular phosphate wasting and inappropriately low serum 1,25-dihydroxyvitamin D levels. This disorder is caused by activating mutations in the FGF receptor 1 (FGFR1) [37]. Not all patients with this disorder have renal tubular phosphate loss, with the mechanism of the phosphate loss thought to be FGF-23 overproduction by a high burden of non-ossifying bony lesions seen in many of these patients. Serum FGF-23 and renal tubular phosphate loss generally correlate with the burden of skeletal disease.

Hypophosphatemic nephrolithiasis/osteoporosis type 1 (NPHLOP1) is a rare disorder associated with renal tubular phosphate loss and osteopenia or nephrolithiasis. Two patients have been reported with this condition, both with heterozygous dominant-negative mutations in the renal sodium-phosphate cotransporter type 2a gene SLC34A1 [38]. Neither of these patients had bone pain or muscle weakness.

Hypophosphatemic nephrolithiasis/osteoporosis type 2 (NPHLOP2) is a rare disorder associated with renal tubular phosphate loss and nephrolithiasis and low bone mineral density. This disorder has been associated with mutations in the gene for the sodium/hydrogen exchanger regulatory factor 1 SLC9A3R1 [39].

Fanconi renotubular syndrome 2 (FRTS2) is a rare disorder associated with renal tubular phosphate loss. This condition is due to in-frame duplication of the SLC34A1 gene [40]. Two patients presenting with fractures, bone deformities, and severe short stature were reported to have these mutations causing autosomal recessive renal Fanconi's syndrome and hypophosphatemic rickets. Similar to *NPHLOP1*, in which SLC34A1 loss-of-function mutations have also been reported, these patients had hypercalciuria and increased serum 1,25-dihydroxyvitamin D levels.

In conclusion, it appears that renal tubular phosphate loss in these rare genetic syndromes is due either to mutations in the sodium-phosphate cotransporters, damage to the proximal renal tubule, or abnormal regulation of FGF-23.

Tumor-Induced Osteomalacia

Tumor-induced osteomalacia (TIO), or oncogenic osteomalacia, is a rare acquired disorder first described in 1947 [41], in which tumors produce factors called phosphatonins that cause renal tubular phosphate loss and decreased production of 1,25-dihydroxyvitamin D [42]. This condition is an acquired paraneoplastic syndrome in which the majority of tumors oversecrete FGF-23 but may also oversecrete secreted frizzled-related protein 4 (sFRP4), MEPE, FGF7, or other as-yet-unknown phosphatonins. The clinical presentation and biochemistries of TIO are similar to what is seen in the genetic forms of hypophosphatemic rickets, with long-standing bone, joint, and muscle pain, stress fractures, fractures, and low serum phosphate, increased urinary phosphate loss, low serum 1,25-dihydroxyvitamin D levels, and increased total and bone alkaline phosphatase. Patients frequently have increased serum FGF-23 levels. Adult patients presenting for the first time with hypophosphatemic osteomalacia must be suspected of having this disorder, as they are highly unlikely to have a genetic form of hypophosphatemic rickets, unless they have late-onset ADHR.

Patients with TIO usually present for the first time in their 50s or 60s, but this condition may occur at any age in life. Children with TIO usually develop rickets with waddling gait, slowing of growth, and skeletal deformities. Because of the rarity of this condition and the occult nature of the tumor causing the syndrome, the average time from symptom onset until correct diagnosis is often longer than 2.5 years [43]. Once TIO is recognized, it takes an average of 5 years to localize the tumor [44]. Documentation of previously normal serum phosphorus in an adult supports a diagnosis of TIO, but in patients where this is not available, genetic testing to rule out genetic hypophosphatemic rickets may be necessary. This involves performing gene mutation analysis of the *PHEX*, *FGF23*, *DMP1*, and *ENPP1* genes.

Patients with TIO present with biochemistries similar to many of the genetic forms of hypophosphatemic rickets described above. Serum calcium and PTH are usually normal. Bone biopsies, if done, show severe osteomalacia with increased osteoid and prolonged mineralization lag time.

Tumors causing TIO are usually slow-growing phosphaturic mesenchymal tumors of the mixed connective tissue type [45], occurring either in soft tissues or in the bone. Most are benign, but some may be cancerous. These tumors overexpress and secrete FGF-23 and other phosphatonin proteins, which increase renal tubular loss of phosphorus by causing internalization of the sodium-phosphate cotransporters NaPi-IIa and NaPi-IIc from the renal brush-border membrane [46], while also decreasing serum 1,25-dihydroxyvitamin D levels by decreasing expression of renal tubular 1α-hydroxylase that synthesizes 1,25-dihydroxyvitamin D and increasing expression of renal tubular 24-hydroxylase that breaks down 1,25-dihydroxyvitamin D [47]. Serum FGF-23 levels are often increased in patients with TIO [48].

These tumors are often difficult to localize, even when they are suspected, and serum FGF-23 levels are increased. They may occur in the long bones, vertebrae, periarticular locations in the distal extremities, the nasopharynx, sinuses, and groin. Palpable lesions in the subcutaneous tissues may be detected by a thorough skin exam. Because mesenchymal tumors often express somatostatin receptors, ^{111}indium-pentetreotide (octreotide) scanning is often done first [49]. If this is negative, whole-body sestamibi scans, DOTATATE PET/CT scans, whole-body MRI scans, and venous sampling have been employed with variable success.

Removal of the causative tumor usually allows TIO to completely resolve, with rapid improvement in low serum phosphorus, reduction in urine phosphorus, and normalization in serum 1,25-dihydroxyvitamin D levels, within minutes to days of tumor resection. Osteomalacia typically takes several weeks to completely resolve. If the tumor cannot be completely resected, radiofrequency or cryotherapy ablation of the tumor has been reported to improve serum FGF-23 oversecretion also.

Patients with TIO where the tumor cannot yet be localized, or can only be incompletely resected, are usually treated with high-dose phosphate and calcitriol supplementation to reverse the biochemical changes and heal the osteomalacia. Phosphate supplementation with 1–2 g/day in 3–4 divided doses, and calcitriol 1–3 mcg/day in 2–3 divided doses, is usually given. The monoclonal antibody burosumab (KRN23) was recently approved by the FDA to treat TIO [50]. Patients who develop severe hyperparathyroidism in response to long-term high-dose phosphate supplementation may eventually require parathyroidectomy or cinacalcet therapy [51]. Octreotide therapy has been used in severe cases that are refractory to high-dose phosphate and calcitriol.

Treatment

Treatment of hypophosphatemic rickets is targeted to correcting the biochemical abnormalities resulting from low serum phosphorus and low serum 1,25-dihydroxyvitamin D levels. Treatment goals include increasing both serum phosphorus and 1,25-dihydroxyvitamin D as close to the normal range as possible, with the intent that this will help heal skeletal osteomalacia or rickets that is present.

Patients with XLH should be treated as described above with high-dose phosphate and calcitriol supplementation. Adult patients require lower supplement doses than children. The monoclonal antibody burosumab (KRN23) has been approved by the FDA to treat XLH. Those who do not respond to medical therapy may require orthopedic surgery to straighten bowed limbs eventually.

Patients with childhood-onset ADHR are treated with phosphate and calcitriol supplementation, similar to patients with XLH. Those who do not respond to supplementation may require orthopedic surgery.

Patients with HHRH are treated with phosphate supplementation alone, and not given calcitriol because their serum 1,25-dihydroxyvitamin D levels are increased already.

For all the other forms of genetically inherited hypophosphatemic rickets, patients are treated with high-dose phosphate and calcitriol as appropriate.

Patients with nonlocalizable or unresectable TIO are usually treated with high-dose phosphate and calcitriol supplementation. Patients with TIO refractory to these treatments may occasionally be treated with cinacalcet, octreotide, or radiofrequency or cryotherapy ablation. Parathyroidectomy is sometimes recommended to control hyperparathyroidism. The monoclonal antibody burosumab (KRN23) is also being used to treat TIO in current clinical trials.

Summary and Conclusions

Hypophosphatemic rickets occurs due to a wide range of causes. Typically the cause of hypophosphatemia falls into one of the three categories, including decreased intestinal absorption, intracellular shifts, or increased urinary losses. Patients with increased urinary loss of phosphorus typically have uncommon or rare genetic disorders or acquired tumor-induced osteomalacia. Patients with disorders causing renal tubular loss of phosphorus typically have low serum phosphorus, increased urinary phosphorus, inappropriately normal or low serum 1,25-dihydroxyvitamin D, and increased total or bone alkaline phosphatase. Diagnosis is dependent on the clinical presentation, biochemistries, radiologic phenotype, and family history. Genetic mutational analysis of the PHEX, FGF23, DMP1, and ENPP1 genes may be done for diagnostic purposes in some settings. Treatment in most cases involves high-dose phosphate and calcitriol supplementation. Burosumab is now available for the treatment of XLH.

References

1. Halevy J, Bulvik S. Severe hypophosphatemia in hospitalized patients. Arch Intern Med. 1988;148:153–5.
2. Larsson L, Rebel K, Sorbo B. Severe hypophosphatemia – a hospital survey. Acta Med Scand. 1983;214:221–3.
3. Beck-Nielsen SS, Brock-Jacobsen B, Gram J, Brixen K, Jensen TK. Incidence and prevalence of nutritional and hereditary rickets in southern Denmark. Eur J Endocrinol. 2009;160:491–7.
4. Albright F, Butler A, Bloomberg E. Rickets resistance to vitamin D therapy. Am J Dis Child. 1939;54:529–47.
5. Winters RW, Graham JB, Williams TF, McFalls VW, Burnett CH. A genetic study of familial hypophosphatemia and vitamin D resistant rickets with a review of the literature. Medicine (Baltimore). 1958;37:97–142.
6. The Hyp Consortium. A gene (PEX) with homologies to endopeptidases is mutated in patients with X-linked hypophosphatemic rickets. Nat Genet. 1995;11:130–6.

7. Beck L, Soumounou Y, Martel J, Krishnamurthy G, Gauthier C, Goodyer CG, Tenenhouse HS. Pex/PEX tissue distribution and evidence for a deletion in the 3′ region of the Pex gene in X-linked hypophosphatemic mice. J Clin Invest. 1997;99:1200–9.
8. Jonsson KB, Zahradnik R, Larsson T, White KE, Sugimoto T, Imanishi Y, Yamamoto T, Hampson G, Koshiyama H, Ljunggren O, Oba K, Yang IM, Miyauchi A, Econs MJ, Lavigne J, Jüppner H. Fibroblast growth factor 23 in oncogenic osteomalacia and X-linked hypophosphatemia. N Engl J Med. 2003;348:1656–63.
9. Weber TJ, Liu S, Indridason OS, Quarles LD. Serum FGF23 levels in normal and disordered phosphorus homeostasis. J Bone Miner Res. 2003;18:1227–34.
10. Yamazaki Y, Okazaki R, Shibata M, Hasegawa Y, Satoh K, Tajima T, Takekuchi Y, Fujita T, Nakahara K, Yamashita T, Fukumoto S. Increased circulatory level of biologically active full-length FGF-23 in patients with hypophosphatemic rickets/osteomalacia. J Clin Endocrinol Metab. 2002;87:4957–60.
11. Liu S, Tang W, Fang J, Ren J, Li H, Xiao Z, Quarles LD. Novel regulators of Fgf23 expression and mineralization in Hyp bone. Mol Endocrinol. 2009;23:1505–18.
12. Ruppe MD, Brosnan PG, Au KS, Tran PX, Dominguez BW, Northrup H. Mutational analysis of PHEX, FGF23, and DMP1 in a cohort of patients with hypophosphatemic rickets. Clin Endocrinol. 2011;74:313–8.
13. Carpenter TO, Imel EA, Holm IA, Jan de Beur SM, Insogna KL. A clinician's guide to X-linked hypophosphatemia. J Bone Miner Res. 2011;26:1381–8.
14. Sabbagh Y, Tenenhouse HS, Econs MJ. The online metabolic and molecular bases of inherited disease. In: Valle D, editor. Mendelian hypophosphatemias. New York: McGraw-Hill Companies.
15. Carpenter TO, Imel EA, Ruppe MD, Weber TJ, Klausner MA, Wooddell MM, Kawakami T, Ito T, Zhang X, Humphrey J, Insogna KL, Peacock M. Randomized trial of the anti-FGF23 antibody KRN23 in X-linked hypophosphatemia. J Clin Invest. 2014;124:1587–97.
16. Imel EA, Zhang X, Ruppe MD, Weber TJ, Klausner MA, Ito T, Vergeire M, Humphrey JS, Glorieux FH, Portale AA, Insogna K, Peacock M, Carpenter TO. Prolonged correction of serum phosphorus in adults with X-linked hypophosphatemia using monthly doses of KRN23. J Clin Endocrinol Metab. 2015;100:2565–73.
17. Ruppe MD, Zhang X, Imel EA, Weber TJ, Klausner MA, Ito T, Vergeire M, Humphrey JS, Glorieux FH, Portale AA, Insogna K, Peacock M, Carpenter TO. Effect of four monthly doses of a human monoclonal anti-FGF23 antibody (KRN23) on quality of life in X-linked hypophosphatemia. Bone Rep. 2016;5:158–62.
18. Imel EA, DiMeglio LA, Hui SL, Carpenter TO, Econs MJ. Treatment of X-linked hypophosphatemia with calcitriol and phosphate increases circulating fibroblast growth factor 23 concentrations. J Clin Endocrinol Metab. 2010;95:1846–50.
19. Liu ES, Carpenter TO, Gundberg CM, Simpson CA, Insogna KL. Calcitonin administration in X-linked hypophosphatemia. N Engl J Med. 2011;364:1678–80.
20. Econs MJ, McEnery PT, Lennon F, Speer MC. Autosomal dominant hypophosphatemic rickets is linked to chromosome 12p13. J Clin Invest. 1997;100:2653–7.
21. ADHR Consortium. Autosomal dominant hypophosphatemic rickets is associated with mutations in FGF23. Nat Genet. 2000;26:345–8.
22. Shimada T, Muto T, Urakawa I, Yoneya T, Yamazaki Y, Okawa K, Takeuchi Y, Fujita T, Fukumoto S, Yamashita T. Mutant FGF-23 responsible for autosomal dominant hypophosphatemic rickets is resistant to proteolytic cleavage and causes hypophosphatemia in vivo. Endocrinology. 2002;143:3179–82.
23. Econs MJ, McEnery PT. Autosomal dominant hypophosphatemic rickets/osteomalacia: clinical characterization of a novel renal phosphate-wasting disorder. J Clin Endocrinol Metab. 1997;82:674–81.
24. Imel EA, Hui SL, Econs MJ. FGF23 concentrations vary with disease status in autosomal dominant hypophosphatemic rickets. J Bone Miner Res. 2007;22:520–6.
25. Imel EA, Peacock M, Gray AR, Padgett LR, Hui SL, Econs MJ. Iron modifies plasma FGF23 differently in autosomal dominant hypophosphatemic rickets and healthy humans. J Clin Endocrinol Metab. 2011;96:3541–9.

26. Bergwitz C, Roslin NM, Tieder M, Loredo-Osti JC, Bastepe M, Abu-Zahra H, Frappier D, Burkett K, Carpenter TO, Anderson D, Garabedian M, Sermet I, Fujiwara TM, Morgan K, Tenenhouse HS, Juppner H. SLC34A3 mutations in patients with hereditary hypophosphatemic rickets with hypercalciuria predict a key role for the sodium-phosphate cotransporter NaPi-IIc in maintaining phosphate homeostasis. Am J Hum Genet. 2006;78:179–92.
27. Lorenz-Depiereux B, Benet-Pages A, Eckstein G, Tenenbaum-Rakover Y, Wagenstaller J, Tiosano D, Gershoni-Baruch R, Albers N, Lichtner P, Schnabel D, Hochberg Z, Strom TM. Hereditary hypophosphatemic rickets with hypercalciuria is caused by mutations in the sodium-phosphate cotransporter gene SLC34A3. Am J Hum Genet. 2006;78:193–201.
28. Tencza AL, Ichikawa S, Dang A, Kenagy D, McCarthy E, Econs MJ, Levine MA. Hypophosphatemic rickets with hypercalciuria due to mutation in SLC34A3/type IIc sodium-phosphate cotransporter: presentation as hypercalciuria and nephrolithiasis. J Clin Endocrinol Metab. 2009;94:4433–8.
29. Lorenz-Depiereux B, Bastepe M, Benet-Pagès A, Amyere M, Wagenstaller J, Müller-Barth U, Badenhoop K, Kaiser SM, Rittmaster RS, Shlossberg AH, Olivares JL, Loris C, Ramos FJ, Glorieux F, Vikkula M, Jüppner H, Strom TM. DMP1 mutations in autosomal recessive hypophosphatemia implicate a bone matrix protein in the regulation of phosphate homeostasis. Nat Genet. 2006;38:1248–50.
30. Feng JQ, Ward LM, Liu S, Lu Y, Xie Y, Yuan B, Yu X, Rauch F, Davis SI, Zhang S, Rios H, Drezner MK, Quarles LD, Bonewald LF, White KE. Loss of DMP1 causes rickets and osteomalacia and identifies a role for osteocytes in mineral metabolism. Nat Genet. 2006;38:1310–5.
31. Levy-Litan V, Hershkovitz E, Avizov L, Leventhal N, Bercovich D, Chalifa-Caspi V, Manor E, Buriakovsky S, Hadad Y, Goding J, Pavari R. Autosomal-recessive hypophosphatemic rickets is associated with an inactivation mutation in the ENPP1 gene. Am J Hum Genet. 2010;86:273–8.
32. Lorenz-Depiereux B, Schnabel D, Tiosano D, Hausler G, Strom TM. Loss-of-function ENPP1 mutations cause both generalized arterial calcification of infancy and autosomal-recessive hypophosphatemic rickets. Am J Hum Genet. 2010;86:267–72.
33. Brownstein CA, Adler F, Nelson-Williams C, Iijima J, Li P, Imura A, Nabeshima Y, Reyes-Mugica M, Carpenter TO, Lifton RP. A translocation causing increased alpha-klotho level results in hypophosphatemic rickets and hyperparathyroidism. Proc Natl Acad Sci U S A. 2008;105:3455–60.
34. Liang Q, Wei M, Hodge L, Fanburg-Smith JC, Nelson A, Miettenen M, Foss RD, Wang G. Quantitative analysis of activating alpha subunit of the G protein (Gsalpha) mutation by pyrosequencing in fibrous dysplasia and other bone lesions. J Mol Diagn. 2011;13:137–42.
35. Dumitrescu CE, Collins MT. McCune-Albright syndrome. Orphanet J Rare Dis. 2008;3:12.
36. Hoffman WH, Jueppner HW, Deyoung BR, O'Dorisio MS, Given KS. Elevated fibroblast growth factor 23 in hypophosphatemic linear nevus sebaceous syndrome. Am J Med Genet A. 2005;134:233–6.
37. White KE, Cabral JM, Davis SI, Fishburn T, Evans WE, Ichikawa S, Fields J, Yu, Shaw NJ, McLellan NJ, McKeown C, Fitzpatrick D, Yu K, Ornitz DM, Econs MJ. Mutations that cause osteoglophonic dysplasia define novel roles for FGFR1 in bone elongation. Am J Hum Genet. 2005;76:361–7.
38. Prie D, Huart V, Bakouh N, Planelles G, Dellis O, Gerard B, Hulin P, Benque-Blanchet F, Silve C, Grandchamp B, Friedlander G. Nephrolithiasis and osteoporosis associated with hypophosphatemia caused by mutations in the type 2a sodium-phosphate cotransporter. N Engl J Med. 2002;347:983–91.
39. Karim Z, Gera B 3rd, Bakouh N, Alili R, Leroy C, Beck L, Silve C, Planelles G, Urena-Torres P, Grandchamp B, Friedlander G, Prie D. NHERF1 mutations and responsiveness of renal parathyroid hormone. N Engl J Med. 2008;359:1128–35.
40. Magen D, Berger L, Coady MJ, Ilivitzky A, Militianu D, Tieder M, Selig S, Lapointe JY, Zelikovic I, Skorecki K. A loss-of-function mutation in NaPi-IIa and renal Fanconi's syndrome. N Engl J Med. 2010;362:1102–9.

41. McCance R. Osteomalacia with Looser's nodes (Milkman's syndrome) due to a raised resistance to vitamin D acquired about the age of 15 years. Q J Med. 1947;16:33–46.
42. Minisola S, Peacock M, Fukumoto S, Cipriani C, Pepe J, Tella SH, Collins MT. Tumour-induced osteomalacia. Nat Rev Dis Primers. 2017;3:17044.
43. Ruppe MD, Jan de Beur SM. Disorders of phosphate homeostasis. In: Rosen CJ, editor. Primer on the metabolic bone diseases and disorders of mineral metabolism. 8th ed. Ames: Wiley-Blackwell; 2013. p. 601–12.
44. Jan de Beur SM. Tumor-induced osteomalacia. JAMA. 2005;294:1260–7.
45. Folpe AL, Fanburg-Smith JC, Billings SD, Bisceglia M, Bertoni F, Cho JY, Econs MJ, Inwards CY, Jan de Beur SM, Mentzel T, Montgomery E, Michal M, Miettinen M, Mills SE, Reith JD, O'Connell JX, Rosenberg AE, Rubin BP, Sweet DE, Vinh TN, Wold LE, Wehrli BM, White KE, Zaino RJ, Weiss SW. Most osteomalacia-associated mesenchymal tumors are a single histopathologic entity: an analysis of 32 cases and a comprehensive review of the literature. Am J Surg Pathol. 2004;28:1–30.
46. Gattineni J, Bates C, Twombley K, Dwarakanath V, Robinson ML, Goetz R, Mohammadi M, Baum M. FGF23 decreases renal NaPi-2a and NaPi-2c expression and induces hypophosphatemia in vivo predominantly via FGF receptor 1. Am J Physiol Ren Physiol. 2009;297:F282–91.
47. Shimada T, Hasegawa H, Yamazaki Y, Muto T, Hino R, Takeuchi Y, Fujita T, Nakahara K, Fukumoto S, Yamashita T. FGF-2 is a potent regulator of vitamin D metabolism and phosphate homeostasis. J Bone Miner Res. 2004;19:429–35.
48. Jonsson KB, Zahradnik R, Larsson T, White KE, Sugimoto T, Imanishi Y, Yamamoto T, Hampson G, Koshiyama H, Ljunggren O, Oba K, Yang IM, Miyauchi A, Econs MJ, Lavigne J, Juppner H. Fibroblast growth factor 23 in oncogenic osteomalacia and X-linked hypophosphatemia. N Engl J Med. 2003;348:1656–63.
49. Jan de Beur SM, Steeten EA, Civelek AC, McCarthy EF, Uribe L, Marx SJ, Onobrakpeya O, Raisz LG, Watts NB, Sharon M, Levine MA. Localisation of mesenchymal tumours by somatostatin receptor imaging. Lancet. 2002;359:761–3.
50. Kinoshita Y, Fukumoto S. X-linked hypophosphatemia and FGF23-related hypophosphatemic diseases -Prospect for new treatment. Endocr Rev. 2018;39:274–91.
51. Geller JL, Khosravi A, Kelly MH, Riminucci M, Adams JS, Collins MT. Cinacalcet in the management of tumor-induced osteomalacia. J Bone Miner Res. 2007;22:931–7.

Chapter 8
Paget's Disease of Bone

Alaleh Mazhari, Vinita Singh, Nicholas Emanuele, and Mary Ann Emanuele

Case Presentation

A 71-year-old man presents with a 3-year history of low back pain that is getting worse. On specific questioning, he admits that his head is enlarging and that he has lost hearing over the last 2 years. On physical examination, the head is larger especially in the frontal area when compared to a photograph taken 5 years ago. The neurologic examination is unremarkable except for hearing loss.

Spine x-rays show coarsening of the trabecular pattern in several lumbar vertebrae and expansion of several lumbar vertebral bodies. The total serum alkaline phosphatase level is four times the upper limit of normal. Other liver function tests and routine laboratory tests are normal.

Epidemiology, Pathogenesis, Genetics, and Histology

Historically, Paget's disease of bone can be traced to the skull of a Neanderthal man demonstrating changes consistent with this disease [1]. It was first described by Sir James Paget's in 1876 and was initially known as osteitis deformans and believed to be an age-related focal disorder of bone metabolism. The hallmark feature of Paget's

A. Mazhari · V. Singh · M. A. Emanuele
Department of Medicine, Division of Endocrinology and Metabolism, Loyola University Medical Center, Maywood, IL, USA

N. Emanuele (✉)
Endocrinology Section, Hines VA Hospital, Loyola University of Chicago Stritch School of Medicine, Hines, IL, USA
e-mail: amazhari@lumc.edu

P. M. Camacho (ed.), *Metabolic Bone Diseases*,
https://doi.org/10.1007/978-3-030-03694-2_8

is an accelerated rate of bone remodeling, resulting in overgrowth of the bone at single or multiple sites resulting in compromised integrity of affected bone. The most frequently involved sites are the skull, spine, pelvis, and long bones of the lower extremities.

Epidemiology

Paget's disease of the bone is the second most common bone disease and is most often seen in older women and men, typically after age 55, with prevalence estimates ranging from 2.3% to 9% in geographic areas most affected [2]. These areas include Central Europe, the United Kingdom, parts of Canada, the United States, and Australia [3–7]. The recognition of both geographic and familial clusters of the disease led to a search for both environmental and genetic causes [8–10].

In the older literature, the prevalence has been reported at 3–3.7% [1, 11]. More recent data [12] demonstrate that Paget's disease is rare under age of 55 years but increases in prevalence thereafter. Paget's disease has been shown to affect 5% of women and 8% of men by the eighth decade of life in some countries. Individuals of European descent are predominantly affected, while it is rare in Africans, Asians, and individuals from the Indian subcontinent. Paget's is speculated to have originated in Northwestern Europe through one or more genetic mutations. However epidemiologic data investigating the prevalence of Paget's can be misleading, as some studies have relied on abdominal imaging to detect involvement in the proximal femur, pelvis, and lumbar spine without examining the skull and other potentially involved areas. Elevations in bone turnover markers have also been the basis for prevalence in epidemiological studies, specifically alkaline phosphatase [13]. Interestingly, the prevalence appears to be decreasing and the degree of skeletal involvement declining [10, 14]. This decrease may be due to changes in environmental factors that affect the tendency to disease, including improved nutrition, reduced exposure to infections, and a more sedentary lifestyle with decreased mechanical loading and skeletal injuries [10, 14].

Pathogenesis and Genetics

Paget's disease of the bone is characterized by an accelerated rate of bone remodeling resulting in overgrowth of bone at selected sites and impaired integrity of affected bone. It is believed to be a disease of the osteoclast based on the abnormal appearance of the osteoclasts, which contain excessive nucleoli and intranuclear inclusion bodies. The increase in bone resorption is coupled with aberrant bone formation over years. Osteoblastic activity can result in sclerosis and deformation of the bone. The antiresorptive agents used in treating Paget's largely inhibit osteoclastic activity and normalize bone remodeling. Osteoclasts from pagetic bone also demonstrate hypersensitivity to vitamin D [15, 16].

Genetic and environmental causes are both suspected to contribute to the pathogenesis of the disease [17]. Many individuals with Paget's, up to 40% [8], have a family history of the disease with an autosomal dominant pattern of inheritance but with incomplete penetrance. Individuals with familial Paget's disease may differ from those with sporadic Paget's disease by having an earlier onset, more skeletal involvement, deformity, and fracture [18–21].

Mutations in SQSTM1 (which encodes sequestosome-1, also known as ubiquitin-binding protein p62) appear to account for the susceptibility to develop Paget's disease in some families, and involvement of other genes is currently under investigation. Candidate gene analyses have identified 15 genetic loci associated with Paget's [22–24]. Most of these risk loci identify proteins known to affect bone physiology. Several directly affect RANK-RANKL pathway activity, such as the *TNFRSF11A* locus that encodes RANKL. A germline mutation in the gene for OPG, the decoy receptor for receptor activator for NFkB ligand (RANKL), leading to a deficiency of OPG, has been reported. Juvenile Paget's disease (or hyperphosphatasia), is an autosomal recessive bone dysplasia with childhood onset that is unrelated to Paget's disease in adults.

In addition to a genetic cause, environmental factors have been proposed to have a role in the pathogenesis of Paget's disease. There are data that infection contributes to the disease based on the observation of intranuclear inclusion bodies resembling paramyxovirus nucleocapsids in pagetic osteoclasts. Although other evidence has been presented for measles virus as an etiologic factor, some studies have not confirmed its involvement. The decreasing incidence of Paget's disease could be attributed to measles vaccination [25]. While measles remains a problem worldwide where vaccinations are not available, Paget's disease of the bone has not been described as more prevalent in these populations [6]. Also immunohistochemical and molecular approaches to confirming the presence of virus in bone biopsies from individuals with Paget's have generated conflicting findings [25–27]. Outside of the cellular responses to measles virus nucleocapsid protein and an interferon-gamma connection, the exact role of the immune system in Paget's disease of the bone is not well understood. The increased levels of cytokines including IL-6 and interferon-gamma noted in Paget's are similar to those seen in other osteo-immunological disorders. As a potential osteo-immunological disorder, the future treatment of Paget's disease of the bone may include targeted immune modulator therapy, particularly the receptor activator of nuclear factor kappa-B ligand and IL-6 signaling inhibition.

There are no consistent correlates found between the occurrence of Paget's disease and other environmental exposures including lead, dog ownership, urban versus rural living, heavy metals, milk ingestion, or family size [25].

Histology

The osteoclasts in patients with Paget's disease of the bone are multinucleated, numerous, and unusual in appearance. The accelerated bone turnover results in lamellar bone being deposited interspersed with woven bone, resulting in increased bone volume and a chaotic appearance. The trabeculae are enlarged and contain numerous osteoblasts. A mosaic pattern is characteristic of the disease, which is attributed to disorganized units of lamellar bone surrounded by irregular cement borders. Normal marrow is replaced by highly vascular stromal tissue.

Clinical Presentation

Changing Presentation

The various modes of presentation are clear and related to the bone, nervous system, and, cardiovascular system. However, the frequency of discrete systemic involvement is difficult to determine for various reasons. First, studies tend to come from specialty referral sites where it is likely that more difficult patients are sent. These patients may not reflect the general population. Second, there is a very large variation in clinical presentation over time. Third, there is regional variation as well [13, 28].

Skeletal and Rheumatic Aspects

The lumbar spine and sacrum are the most commonly involved skeletal sites [29]. There are enlarged, sclerotic vertebrae, and there can be compression fractures and consequent kyphosis [29]. The femur and tibia can undergo plastic deformation resulting in bowing [30]. Repeated loading on these weakened bones can accelerate degenerative disease of the hip and/or knee and cause gait disturbance and ultimately fractures [30]. Fractures in long bones are seen usually in the lower extremities, more often the femur than the tibia and typically transverse in nature [29, 30]. The humerus can sometimes be affected by Paget's, and this may lead to severe degenerative disease in the shoulder and occasionally in a humeral fracture if there is extensive involvement coupled with a fall [30]. Involvement of the skull with greater enlargement over the frontal and occipital areas can lead to hearing loss, tinnitus, and rarely hydrocephalus [29, 31]. If the jaw is affected, there can be malocclusion and migration and loss of teeth [29].

Bone pain can result from fractures or associated osteoarthritis. Less commonly, nerve root or spinal cord compression, pseudo-fractures, or increased bone turnover can account for pain [13, 29, 32].

Franck et al. did a careful study of 55 patients with Paget's disease to better define the pain syndromes [32]. They found a high frequency of rheumatic complaints distinct from Paget's bone disease or degenerative arthritis. These included gouty arthritis, calcific periarthritis, rheumatoid arthritis and its variants, and low back pain syndromes. Six of the patients had classic podagra. Twenty of 55 patients had periarticular calcifications identified on x-ray, mainly involving shoulder joints, and acute inflammatory episodes occurred at 14 sites. Eight patients had rheumatoid arthritis and its variants. Six patients appeared to have ankylosing spondylitis or a clinical syndrome very close to ankylosing spondylitis. Six patients who had low back pain had spinal cord or nerve root compression demonstrated on myelogram. Although the frequency in this report might not reflect the general population, since these were patients referred to a specialty care center, all of these various causes of pain need to be considered.

Neurologic Aspects

Up to 76% of patients with Paget's disease may have some neurologic complication [33]. About 90% of these have more than one affected bone. Reported prevalence data for neurologic complications vary widely [33].

Hearing Loss

Hearing loss is the most common complications, seen in up to 76%, but prevalence estimates are from 2% to 76% [33]. It is generally seen when the temporal bone is involved [13, 30], though there may be difficulty in distinguishing Paget's-related hearing loss from presbycusis. The mechanism of hearing loss has been speculated to be multifactorial involving compression or stretching of the auditory nerve, loss of hair cells or ganglion cells, vascular shunts, or epitympanic spurs, among other things [30]. Not all of these potential mechanisms have been verified. In a CT study of 37 patients with Paget's of the skull compared to 20 controls, there was no compression or stretching of the auditory nerve, and auditory brain stem responses gave no evidence of auditory nerve dysfunction [34]. However, high-resolution QCT uncovered a strong correlation between high-frequency pure tone hearing loss and decreased bone mineral density of the cochlear capsule associated with invasion by pagetic bone [34].

Skull Involvement

In most cases when the skull is involved in Paget's disease, the effects are largely cosmetic [30]. However, in extreme situations, there may be platybasia or even syringomyelia as well as brainstem compression [33]. Rarely, this may result in acute tonsillar herniation and death. There may be no pain or disabling headaches. Optic atrophy and papilledema have been described and attributed to narrowing of the optic foramen but could also be caused by hydrocephalus and attendant increased intracranial pressure [13, 30]. Hearing loss in Paget's disease is well known (see above), but patients may also have ophthalmoplegia, anosmia, trigeminal neuralgia, and facial and bulbar palsy [30, 33]. The prevalence of cranial nerve lesions (other than hearing loss) varies from 0.2% to 41% [33].

Dementia even in the absence of hydrocephalus has been attributed to direct compression of the cerebral hemispheres [33]. A rare syndrome of inclusion body myopathy and frontotemporal dementia in Paget's patients has been reported [33]. The dementia is characterized by personality change and language dysfunction and has a rapid progression.

Intracranial expansion of tumors, most often sarcomas, can cause intense headaches, exophthalmos, and the expected localizing neurologic signs depending on location [33]. These tumors are rare (<1% of Paget's patients), and only about 10% occur in the cranium. Rapid neurologic deterioration may indicate hemorrhage into such tumors.

Pagetic change in the maxilla and ethmoids results in facial deformity, either bilateral or strikingly asymmetric, and nasal obstruction [35]. The nasal obstruction may generate anosmia, but there may be nerve compression as well. Thickening of the alveolar ridges leads to loosening and drifting of teeth [35].

Vertebral Involvement

Neck or back pain has been reported in 10–54% of patients and evidence of spinal cord or nerve root damage in 4–34%, again illustrating the wide range of prevalence of various symptoms and signs of Paget's disease [33].

Whether back pain is due to pagetic bone involvement or associated osteoarthritis can always be debated in a particular patent, and both etiologies must be kept in mind.

When the vertebrae are involved in the pagetic process, there can be impingement on the spinal cord and alteration of blood flow resulting in pain as well as quadriparesis or paraparesis depending on the level of the significant lesion [30]. Blood flow to pagetic bone can be quite high, and it has been hypothesized that when this occurs in a vertebral body, a "steal" of blood flow from the adjacent spinal cord may occur, causing reversible spinal cord ischemia [30, 33]. Symptoms are slowly progressive, but new symptoms or rapid progression of the neck or neck symptoms should suggest fracture, hematoma, or sarcoma [33].

Peripheral Nerve Involvement

Peripheral nerve involvement is relatively rare (2–5% prevalence) and is usually due to nerve entrapment syndromes such as those of the ulnar, sciatic, medial, and posterior tibial nerves [33].

Cardiovascular Aspects

High-output congestive heart failure occurs in about 3% of patients with very active Paget's disease with very high blood flow to the bone, muscle, and overlying skin [29, 30, 36, 37]. It is of interest that, in one small study, most of the increased extremity blood flow in patients with active Paget's disease was to the skin [38]. Nonetheless, increased blood flow may cause shunting and lower peripheral vascular resistance. Significant bony involvement (usually defined as >15%) may then lead to heart failure [39]. Echocardiographic data compared those with very active Paget's disease (15–22% skeletal involvement) to those with less active disease (<15% 15–22% skeletal involvement) and control non-pagetic subjects [39]. Cardiomegaly was more frequent and left ventricular mass greater in those with very active Paget's disease compared to those with less active disease and controls.

Vascular calcification has been seen in patients with Paget's disease as well. After adjustment for a variety of cardiovascular risk factors, the frequency of arterial calcification was not greater in Paget's disease patient than controls, but the calcifications were longer and thicker in Paget's [40]. The prevalence of calcified aortic valves is higher in Paget's disease than in control subjects [41]. Furthermore, the clinical severity of the Paget's was associated with higher frequency of aortic valvular disease. Whether there is an increased risk for mitral calcification is not clear [39, 41].

Neoplasms

The frequency of giant cell tumors is low, <1%. Though low, this is a 30 times higher risk than the general population [31]. There is data from the United Kingdom that these tumors are becoming more rare [42]. Most, about 85%, are osteosarcomas, but there are rare fibrosarcomas and chondrosarcomas [29]. Acute bone pain, either recent in onset, or an increase in pre-existing pain may be the signal that sarcomatous degeneration has occurred. In fact, in the published UK series, 58% of 32 patients with osteosarcomas had the tumor as a presenting manifestation of Paget's disease [42]. Median survival was 8 months from diagnosis, and only four patients (12.5%) lived more than 2 years from diagnosis. Tumors can also metastasize to pagetic bone, probably when there is active disease with high blood flow [29].

Diagnosis and Differential Diagnosis

The diagnosis of Paget's disease can be achieved by combination of clinical signs and symptoms with imaging and biochemical testing. Since many, if not most of the patients are asymptomatic, clinicians mainly rely on imaging and biochemical testing to confirm the diagnosis of Paget's disease.

Imaging

The diagnosis of Paget's disease is mostly radiological [43]. The most commonly affected bones are the pelvis (70% of cases), femur (55%), lumbar spine (53%), skull (42%), and tibia (32%).

The initial test is a plain x-ray of the involved bone, which can show osteolytic lesions, overgrowth, deformity, or fractures if present. An early radiological stage of Paget's disease is the osteolytic lesion, which has been observed to progress in a long bone at an average rate of about 8 mm/year [44]. The second stage of the disease is increase in osteoblastic activity with mixed osteolytic-osteosclerotic appearance on the x-ray, disturbing the normal trabecular architecture of the bone. In the third stage, the sclerotic lesion predominates which might cause bony overgrowth [45]. It can also depict cortical thickening and bone expansion. Untreated patients might have an increase in size of the bone thereby leading to bony deformity mostly in the form of bowing of long bones. X-rays can also help to diagnose "fissure fractures" which are linear transverse radiolucencies mostly seen in convex aspect of long bones [44].

Paget's disease of the bone can be polyostotic or monostotic [46]. The important differentials for monostotic Paget's are primary or metastatic bone tumors, chronic bone infection, fibrous dysplasia, etc. In those cases, bone biopsy can be helpful in establishing the diagnosis. Bone biopsy should be avoided in weight-bearing bone because there is a risk of fracture and other complications [45].

Radionuclide bone scanning is a more sensitive test than a plain x-ray in identifying early disease. It helps to determine the extent of the disease and may also identify the affected bones, which are not associated with symptoms. The Endocrine Society guidelines do not recommend repeating the bone scan as a follow-up testing modality to confirm remission as biochemical markers of bone turnover have good correlation with disease activity when compared to bone scan [44].

In advanced cases, computed tomography (CT) scan or magnetic resonance imaging (MRI) can be performed when malignancy is suspected. They can also aid in evaluation of the patients with negative radiographs but suspected fracture and preoperative planning for corrective surgeries [47]. In uncomplicated Paget's disease of the spine, MRI may show a mixed pattern of increased or decreased T1 signal of the vertebral bodies, which correlates with the mixed osteolytic and osteoblastic phase of the disease [48]. MRI can also be of value in evaluating soft tissue component of the tumor arising from the pagetic lesion or if the patient presents with neurological symptoms in cases of spinal stenosis or cord/nerve compression.

Biochemical Markers

Serum total alkaline phosphatase (ALP) can be tested to determine the metabolic activity of the bone. In active Paget's disease, serum ALP can be elevated when the other liver enzymes are normal. In patients with liver disease, bone-specific alkaline phosphatase (BSAP) can be obtained.

ALP can be normal in some cases [49]. In those circumstances also, BSAP should be checked. Elevated BSAP indicates high bone turnover. Bone turnover markers are also helpful in monitoring the response to the treatment and to follow the evolution of the disease in untreated patients as it has a good correlation with disease activity.

ALP is a less expensive test and is more readily available as compared to BSAP. After initiation of therapy, ALP falls more slowly, and a clear response is noted in 4–8 weeks [45].

Procollagen type 1 N-terminal propeptide (P1NP) is another marker of bone formation, which can be used when other liver function tests are abnormal as there may be up to 20% cross-reactivity of antibodies to liver ALP with bone ALP [44]. In a recently published meta-analysis, P1NP was found to be the best marker to assess the disease activity both initially and after treatment with bisphosphonates [50]. However, the limited availability of P1NP is a consideration.

Markers of bone resorption such as serum C-telopeptide (CTx) or urine N-telopeptide (NTx) can also be tested to estimate the bone metabolic activity and monitor the response to treatment. The advantage of the resorption markers over the bone formation marker is the faster demonstration of decrease in bone resorption than bone formation after treatment.

In a recent publication [51], two molecular tests has been developed which can predict the Paget's disease phenotype better than the bone turnover markers alone. Further studies are needed before the molecular tests can be used in clinical practice.

Treatment

The goals of treatment include normalization of bone turnover, improving patient's symptoms, slowing down or halting disease progression, as well as lowering the risk of complications if possible.

Pharmacological therapy should be offered to patients who fall into one of the following categories: those with active disease who are symptomatic; those whose bone scintigraphy is consistent with Paget's disease involving weight-bearing bones, spine, skull, or other areas where complications can occur (with or without having an elevated bone marker such as ALP); those who have pagetic bone involvement adjacent to major joints; those undergoing planned surgery involving bony areas affected by Paget's; as well as those with hypercalcemia associated with immobilization who have polyostotic disease [44, 52].

Although bisphosphonates, the major therapeutic agents for Paget's disease, reduce bone pain, the notion that bisphosphonate therapy will reduce hard end points remains unproven. This was addressed in the PRISM Trial. In this trial, intensive bisphosphonate therapy was compared to symptomatic therapy in 1324 patients. The patients in the symptomatic group were only treated with analgesics or anti-inflammatory drugs if they had pagetic bone pain and only received bisphosphonates if they did not respond (tiludronate and etidronate were the first-line bisphosphonate treatment in this group). The intensive group received repeated courses of bisphosphonates (risedronate was the first-line treatment in the intensive treatment group) irrespective of symptoms with the aim of reducing and normalizing ALP. The end points of the study included fracture, orthopedic surgery, quality of life, bone pain, and hearing threshold. The median follow-up was 3 years. The ALP level was significantly lower in the intensive treatment group starting at 4 months post initiation of treatment and remained significantly lower throughout the study ($p < 0.001$), but there was no statistically significant difference between the two groups in the end points listed above [53]. However this study had several limitations including the use of less potent treatment therapies in the symptomatic arm as well as the fact that when the study was conducted, zoledronic acid was not available. This is an important point, and in the upcoming sections, we will review the efficacy of the more potent bisphosphonates, including zoledronic acid, for the treatment.

Currently there are only two classes of medications that are approved by the US Food and Drug Administration (FDA) for treatment of Paget's disease of the bone: bisphosphonates and calcitonin.

Bisphosphonates: General Considerations

Paget's disease of the bone is characterized by high bone turnover, and therefore the treatment options that are commonly used target osteoclasts, with the aim of reducing bone turnover. The bisphosphonate nucleus consists of two phosphate groups joined by a central carbon atom. Bisphosphonates bind avidly to the bone and can remain there for years. During bone resorption, bisphosphonates are taken up by osteoclasts and inhibit the enzyme farnesyl pyrophosphate which in turn can have an adverse effect on osteoclasts and lead to osteoclast apoptosis. Different bisphosphonates have different potencies depending on the bisphosphonate's affinity for hydroxyapatite or skeletal uptake [44]. The bisphosphonates can be further categorized as those that contain nitrogen (which include zoledronic acid, pamidronate, risedronate, alendronate, ibandronate, and neridronate), and this group of bisphosphonates are the main agents used for treatment of Paget's disease of the bone [44, 52, 54].

It is important to ensure appropriate laboratory testing is conducted and abnormalities addressed prior to initiation of treatment with bisphosphonates to minimize adverse treatment outcomes. The laboratory evaluation should include serum calcium, creatinine, phosphorous, and 25-hydroxyvitamin D level (25-OHD). If vitamin D deficiency is present, normalization of 25-OHD is important prior to initiating bisphosphonate therapy to minimize risk of hypocalcemia. Serum parathyroid hormone level (PTH) is helpful for further evaluation in patients who have an abnormal calcium level. PTH level would be expected to be low in patients with hypercalcemia due to immobilization in patients with Paget's bone disease [55]. Patients need to take oral bisphosphonates as directed to ensure optimizing absorption and minimizing potential side effects. Some guidelines recommend evaluation by a dentist when possible. For patients who require extensive dental work, it is important that the dental work is addressed prior to initiation of bisphosphonate therapy to ensure proper healing and reducing the risk of osteonecrosis of the jaw, a rare complication of bisphosphonate therapy [56, 57].

Bisphosphonates: Etidronate

Etidronate was the first bisphosphonate to be used for treatment of Paget's disease of the bone. It is administered 400 mg/day orally for 6 months [44, 52, 58]. There are numerous studies looking at the efficacy of etidronate for treatment of Paget's disease [44, 52, 59]; however, in this chapter, we will mainly focus on the more potent bisphosphonates that are primarily used for the treatment of Paget's disease.

Bisphosphonates: Alendronate

Alendronate is one of the main oral bisphosphonates that is used for the treatment of Paget's. In a double-blind, randomized trial, a mix of patients some of whom were bisphosphonate naïve, others not, received either alendronate 40 mg a day (27 patients) or placebo (28 patients) for 6 months. Overall, there was a 78% response rate (normalization of ALP or ≥60% decrease ALP from baseline) in the alendronate group. ALP had normalized in 12% of the patients at 3 months and 48% at 6 months. Radiographic assessment showed 46% of the patients in the alendronate group had improvement of osteolysis compared to 4% in the placebo group, and the difference was significantly different at 6 months ($P = 0.0.2$). In a small subset of biopsied patients, bone histology showed that indices of bone formation and resorption in pagetic bone were significantly lower in the alendronate group without evidence of defective demineralization. There was no significant change in the pagetic bone pain between the two groups. The main side effect experienced by patients included upper gastrointestinal symptoms [60].

In a 6-month study comparing alendronate to etidronate, alendronate proved to be more effective than etidronate both on reductions in ALP and lower risk of osteomalacia [61].

Bisphosphonates: Risedronate

Risedronate is the other oral bisphosphonate that is commonly used for the treatment of Paget's disease. In an open-label, multicenter study, 162 patients with Paget's disease of the bone (some previously bisphosphonate treated, some not) were treated with risedronate 30 mg a day for 84 days followed by no treatment for 112 days. This cycle was repeated once if ALP did not normalize or if it increased from nadir value by ≥25%. At the end of the first cycle, the mean percentage of ALP decline was 65.7%, and at the end of the second cycle, it was 69.1% ($p < 0.001$ compared to baseline). During the entire study, 54% of the patients had normalization of ALP. Of the patients who had been on prior therapy, 91% responded to risedronate, and 54% had normalization of ALP. There was a significant decline in pagetic bone pain during the study ($P < 0.001$). The most commonly reported side effects were headache, diarrhea, dyspepsia, and constipation. The results of this study showed risedronate to be an effective treatment for Paget's disease of the bone [62].

When compared to etidronate, risedronate caused a greater decrease in pain, sharper fall in ALP, and lower relapse rate [63].

Bisphosphonates: Pamidronate

Pamidronate is given as an intravenous infusion (IV) and is one of the main IV bisphosphonates that is used for the treatment of Paget's disease of the bone. In a 2-year study, 71 patients with Paget's disease without prior history of bisphosphonate treatment received IV pamidronate. The patients were subdivided based on disease severity as having mild, moderate, or severe disease, and the dose of pamidronate increased with increasing disease severity. ALP level declined after pamidronate treatment, and those who had mild to moderate disease had a better response (normalization of ALP occurred in 43/49 patients at 6 months) compared to those with more severe disease (normalization of ALP occurred in 3/13 patients at 6 months). Relapse rates varied with disease severity, 6% with mild severity, 39% with moderate severity, and 62% with severe disease. Pain scores and osteolytic lesions improved as well [64].

In another study, pamidronate decreased ALP by 63% ($p < 0.0001$), and normalization of ALP occurred in 50 patients (the patients with a lower ALP level had a higher rate of achieving ALP normalization) [65].

Alendronate was more efficacious than pamidronate in both previously bisphosphonate-treated and drug-naïve people in lowering ALP [66].

Bisphosphonates: Zoledronic Acid

Zoledronic acid is administered as a once-a-year 5 mg infusion, and it has become the preferred treatment for Paget's disease of the bone [44]. In a randomized, double-blind, controlled 6-month trial, the effectiveness of a 15-min infusion of 5 mg of zoledronic acid (182 patients) was compared to 60 days of risedronate 30 mg/day (175 patients). Therapeutic response was defined as normalization of ALP or a reduction of at least 75% in total ALP excess (the difference between midpoints of the reference range). Bone biopsies were performed after double tetracycline labeling.

At the end of the study, 96% of patients had therapeutic response compared to 74.3% of the risedronate group ($p < 0.001$). The time to first therapeutic response was significantly shorter with zoledronic acid (64 days versus 89 days for risedronate). ALP normalized in 88.6% of the zoledronic acid group compared to 57.9% in the risedronate group. The response rate to zoledronic acid was consistent regardless of disease severity and prior treatment history. At 3 months, pain scores improved in both groups. The patients who met therapeutic response were eligible for trial extension. The median follow-up at the end of the core study was 190 days, and during that time, 25.6% of the patients in the risedronate group had a loss of therapeutic response compared to 0.9% in the zoledronic acid group ($P < 0.001$).

A small subset of patients had bone biopsies and there was no defective bone mineralization. The main side effect reported in the zoledronic acid group was flu-like symptoms, and eight patients developed hypocalcemia (two were symptomatic). One patient developed symptomatic hypocalcemia in the risedronate group. The rates of gastrointestinal side effects were similar in both groups [55]. This greater response to zoledronic acid compared to risedronate was confirmed in another study [67].

Registry data from 98 patients with Paget's disease who had been treated with 5 mg intravenous infusion of zoledronic acid were reviewed to assess response rates over a 3-year period. At 1 year, 93.3% of the patients remained in remission, 89.5% at 2 years, and 91.6% at 3 years [68].

In a 15-month randomized clinical study, pamidronate (30 mg IV for 2 consecutive days every 3 months) was compared to zoledronic acid (4 mg IV). The primary end point was normalization of ALP or 75% reduction of total ALP excess at 6 months. In the zoledronic acid group, 97% of the patients reached the primary end point compared to 45% of the patients in the pamidronate group. In the zoledronic group, 93% of the patients had normalization of ALP compared to 35% in the pamidronate group. At 12- and 15-month follow-up, ALP remained in the normal range in 79% and 65% of the zoledronic acid treatment group, respectively [69].

In a 3-year extension study of Paget's Disease: Randomized Trial of Intensive versus Symptomatic Management (PRISM) trial, 270 patients were enrolled in the intensive treatment group (this time zoledronic acid was the first-line bisphosphonate), and 232 patient continued in the symptomatic treatment group (bisphosphonate treatment was only given for bone pain). The primary outcome was fractures, and some of the secondary outcomes included orthopedic procedures, quality of life, and bone pain. The ALP level was significantly lower in the intensive group on entry to the study, and the margin of difference between the groups increased over the course of the study. There were no differences in quality-of-life measures, bone pain, fracture risk, or orthopedic procedures [70]. So again, while it seems reasonable that decrease in bone turnover should prevent complications, clinical trial data proving this has not yet been published.

In an open-label study, 14 patients (7 female and 7 male) with active Paget's disease of the bone who were resistant to other bisphosphonates were treated with zoledronic acid. There was an 81% decrease in post-therapy ALP level after zoledronic acid. Continued remission was seen for as long as 60 months. One patient showed lack of remission despite two doses of zoledronic acid administered 1 year apart (the patient had a 68% decrease in ALP level and 62% but failed to go into remission) [71]. Zoledronic acid appears to be effective in majority of cases of bisphosphonate resistance, but more data is necessary to see if this trend will hold true as more patients are treated with zoledronic acid [71–74].

Other Bisphosphonates

Other bisphosphonates have also been used for treatment of Paget's disease of the bone such as ibandronate, tiludronate, and clodronate. However use of these agents is very limited and the data from these studies will not be reviewed here.

Calcitonin

Calcitonin is a peptide hormone produced by the C-cells in the thyroid and can directly bind to a receptor on osteoclasts and reduce bone turnover [44]. Calcitonin is administered 100 U subcutaneously daily. Calcitonin treatment over several months can lead to 50% reduction in ALP, and lower doses of 50–100 U every other day can be used for maintenance. Several factors have led to calcitonin falling out of favor for the treatment for Paget's disease including lack of robust biochemical and clinical response, lack of sustained response to treatment once the medication is stopped, the need for daily injections, the side effects associated with the medication, as well as the better efficacy of newer therapies (as noted above). Calcitonin is mainly used in patients who are not able to tolerate bisphosphonates or if there is a contraindication to bisphosphonate treatment [44, 52].

Denosumab

Denosumab (human monoclonal antibody to RANK ligand) is being evaluated as a possible treatment option for Paget's disease of the bone. More data is necessary to assess the therapeutic efficacy of this agent for Paget's disease and can potentially be used as a second-line treatment option for those intolerant to bisphosphonate treatment [75–79].

Back to the Patient

This patient has symptomatic Paget's disease with enlarging skull, hearing loss, and back pain, though the latter could certainly be multifactorial. If calcium, vitamin D, and creatinine are normal, he should be given either oral of intravenous bisphosphonate.

References

1. De Deuxchaisnes CN, Krane SM. Paget's disease of bone: clinical and metabolic observations. Medicine. 1964;43:233–66.
2. Altman RD, Bloch DA, Hochberg MC, Murphy WA. Prevalence of pelvic Paget's disease of bone in the United States. J Bone Miner Res. 2000;15(3):461–5.
3. Gardner MJ, Guyer PB, Barker DJ. Paget's disease of bone among British migrants to Australia. Br Med J. 1978;2(6149):1436–7.
4. Gomez Acotto C, Mautalen CA. European origin of patients with Paget's disease of bone in the Buenos Aires area. Eur J Epidemiol. 2001;17(5):409–11.
5. Gennari L, Di Stefano M, Merlotti D, Giordano N, Martini G, Tamone C, et al. Prevalence of Paget's disease of bone in Italy. J Bone Miner Res. 2005;20(10):1845–50.
6. Barker DJ, Chamberlain AT, Guyer PB, Gardner MJ. Paget's disease of bone: the Lancashire focus. Br Med J. 1980;280(6222):1105–7.
7. Guyer PB, Chamberlain AT. Paget's disease of bone in two American cities. Br Med J. 1980;280(6219):985.
8. Siris ES, Ottman R, Flaster E, Kelsey JL. Familial aggregation of Paget's disease of bone. J Bone Miner Res. 1991;6(5):495–500.
9. Barker DJ, Clough PW, Guyer PB, Gardner MJ. Paget's disease of bone in 14 British towns. Br Med J. 1977;1(6070):1181–3.
10. Cooper C, Dennison E, Schafheutle K, Kellingray S, Guyer P, Barker D. Epidemiology of Paget's disease of bone. Bone. 1999;24(5 Suppl):3s–5s.
11. Collins DH. Paget's disease of bone; incidence and subclinical forms. Lancet (London, England). 1956;271(6933):51–7.
12. Ralston SH. Clinical practice. Paget's disease of bone. N Engl J Med. 2013;368(7):644–50.
13. Eekhoff ME, van der Klift M, Kroon HM, Cooper C, Hofman A, Pols HA, et al. Paget's disease of bone in The Netherlands: a population-based radiological and biochemical survey – the Rotterdam study. J Bone Miner Res. 2004;19(4):566–70.
14. Morales-Piga AA, Bachiller-Corral FJ, Abraira V, Beltran J, Rapado A. Is clinical expressiveness of Paget's disease of bone decreasing? Bone. 2002;30(2):399–403.
15. Harvey L, Gray T, Beneton MN, Douglas DL, Kanis JA, Russell RG. Ultrastructural features of the osteoclasts from Paget's disease of bone in relation to a viral aetiology. J Clin Pathol. 1982;35(7):771–9.
16. Menaa C, Barsony J, Reddy SV, Cornish J, Cundy T, Roodman GD. 1,25-Dihydroxyvitamin D3 hypersensitivity of osteoclast precursors from patients with Paget's disease. J Bone Miner Res. 2000;15(2):228–36.
17. Cundy T, Reid IR. Paget's disease of bone. Clin Biochem. 2012;45(1–2):43–8.
18. Seton M, Choi HK, Hansen MF, Sebaldt RJ, Cooper C. Analysis of environmental factors in familial versus sporadic Paget's disease of bone – the New England registry for Paget's disease of bone. J Bone Miner Res. 2003;18(8):1519–24.

19. Siris ES. Epidemiological aspects of Paget's disease: family history and relationship to other medical conditions. Semin Arthritis Rheum. 1994;23(4):222–5.
20. Merlotti D, Gennari L, Galli B, Martini G, Calabro A, De Paola V, et al. Characteristics and familial aggregation of Paget's disease of bone in Italy. J Bone Miner Res. 2005;20(8):1356–64.
21. Morales-Piga AA, Rey-Rey JS, Corres-Gonzalez J, Garcia-Sagredo JM, Lopez-Abente G. Frequency and characteristics of familial aggregation of Paget's disease of bone. J Bone Miner Res. 1995;10(4):663–70.
22. Chung PY, Beyens G, Boonen S, Papapoulos S, Geusens P, Karperien M, et al. The majority of the genetic risk for Paget's disease of bone is explained by genetic variants close to the CSF1, OPTN, TM7SF4, and TNFRSF11A genes. Hum Genet. 2010;128(6):615–26.
23. Albagha OM, Wani SE, Visconti MR, Alonso N, Goodman K, Brandi ML, et al. Genome-wide association identifies three new susceptibility loci for Paget's disease of bone. Nat Genet. 2011;43(7):685–9.
24. Beauregard M, Gagnon E, Guay-Belanger S, Morissette J, Brown JP, Michou L. Identification of rare genetic variants in novel loci associated with Paget's disease of bone. Hum Genet. 2014;133(6):755–68.
25. Singer FR. Paget's disease of bone-genetic and environmental factors. Nat Rev Endocrinol. 2015;11(11):662–71.
26. Mills BG, Singer FR, Weiner LP, Holst PA. Cell cultures from bone affected by Paget's disease. Arthritis Rheum. 1980;23(10):1115–20.
27. Rebel A, Basle M, Pouplard A, Malkani K, Filmon R, Lepatezour A. Towards a viral etiology for Paget's disease of bone. Metab Bone Dis Relat Res. 1981;3(4–5):235–8.
28. Tan A, Ralston SH. Clinical presentation of Paget's disease: evaluation of a contemporary cohort and systematic review. Calcif Tissue Int. 2014;95(5):385–92.
29. Falchetti A, Masi L, Brandi ML. Paget's disease of bone: there's more than the affected skeletal – a clinical review and suggestions for the clinical practice. Curr Opin Rheumatol. 2010;22(4):410–23.
30. Bone HG. Nonmalignant complications of Paget's disease. J Bone Miner Res. 2006;21(Suppl 2):P64–8.
31. Shah M, Shahid F, Chakravarty K. Paget's disease: a clinical review. Br J Hosp Med (London, England: 2005). 2015;76(1):25–30.
32. Franck WA, Bress NM, Singer FR, Krane SM. Rheumatic manifestations of Paget's disease of bone. Am J Med. 1974;56(5):592–603.
33. Rubin DJ, Levin RM. Neurologic complications of Paget disease of bone. Endocr Pract. 2009;15(2):158–66.
34. Monsell EM. The mechanism of hearing loss in Paget's disease of bone. Laryngoscope. 2004;114(4):598–606.
35. Fisher EW. Rhinological manifestations of Paget's disease of bone (Osteitis deformans). J Cranio-Maxillo-Facial Surg. 1990;18(4):169–72.
36. Anand IS, Florea VG. High output cardiac failure. Curr Treat Options Cardiovasc Med. 2001;3(2):151–9.
37. Wermers RA, Tiegs RD, Atkinson EJ, Achenbach SJ, Melton LJ 3rd. Morbidity and mortality associated with Paget's disease of bone: a population-based study. J Bone Miner Res. 2008;23(6):819–25.
38. Heistad DD, Abboud FM, Schmid PG, Mark AL, Wilson WR. Regulation of blood flow in Paget's disease of bone. J Clin Invest. 1975;55(1):69–74.
39. Arnalich F, Plaza I, Sobrino JA, Oliver J, Barbado J, Pena JM, et al. Cardiac size and function in Paget's disease of bone. Int J Cardiol. 1984;5(4):491–505.
40. Laroche M, Delmotte A. Increased arterial calcification in Paget's disease of bone. Calcif Tissue Int. 2005;77(3):129–33.
41. Strickberger SA, Schulman SP, Hutchins GM. Association of Paget's disease of bone with calcific aortic valve disease. Am J Med. 1987;82(5):953–6.
42. Mangham DC, Davie MW, Grimer RJ. Sarcoma arising in Paget's disease of bone: declining incidence and increasing age at presentation. Bone. 2009;44(3):431–6.

43. Tan A, Ralston SH. Paget's disease of bone. QJM : Mon J Assoc Phys. 2014;107(11):865–9.
44. Singer FR, Bone HG 3rd, Hosking DJ, Lyles KW, Murad MH, Reid IR, et al. Paget's disease of bone: an endocrine society clinical practice guideline. J Clin Endocrinol Metab. 2014;99(12):4408–22.
45. Lyles KW, Siris ES, Singer FR, Meunier PJ. A clinical approach to diagnosis and management of Paget's disease of bone. J Bone Miner Res. 2001;16(8):1379–87.
46. Bachiller-Corral J, Diaz-Miguel C, Morales-Piga A. Monostotic Paget's disease of the femur: a diagnostic challenge and an overlooked risk. Bone. 2013;57(2):517–21.
47. Al-Rashid M, Ramkumar DB, Raskin K, Schwab J, Hornicek FJ, Lozano-Calderon SA. Paget disease of bone. Orthop Clin N Am. 2015;46(4):577–85.
48. Morales HMR. Imaging findings of Paget's disease of the spine. Clin Neuroradiol. 2015;25(3):225–32.
49. Balani A, Marda SS. Images in clinical medicine. Paget's disease of bone. N Engl J Med. 2016;374(13):1264.
50. Al Nofal AA, Altayar O, BenKhadra K, Qasim Agha OQ, Asi N, Nabhan M, et al. Bone turnover markers in Paget's disease of the bone: a systematic review and meta-analysis. Osteoporos Int. 2015;26(7):1875–91.
51. Guay-Belanger S, Simonyan D, Bureau A, Gagnon E, Albert C, Morissette J, et al. Development of a molecular test of Paget's disease of bone. Bone. 2016;84:213–21.
52. Siris ES, Lyles KW, Singer FR, Meunier PJ. Medical management of Paget's disease of bone: indications for treatment and review of current therapies. J Bone Miner Res. 2006;21(Suppl 2):P94–8.
53. Langston AL, Campbell MK, Fraser WD, MacLennan GS, Selby PL, Ralston SH. Randomized trial of intensive bisphosphonate treatment versus symptomatic management in Paget's disease of bone. J Bone Miner Res. 2010;25(1):20–31.
54. Ralston SH, Langston AL, Reid IR. Pathogenesis and management of Paget's disease of bone. Lancet (London, England). 2008;372(9633):155–63.
55. Reid IR, Miller P, Lyles K, Fraser W, Brown JP, Saidi Y, et al. Comparison of a single infusion of zoledronic acid with risedronate for Paget's disease. N Engl J Med. 2005;353(9):898–908.
56. Khan A, Morrison A, Cheung A, Hashem W, Compston J. Osteonecrosis of the jaw (ONJ): diagnosis and management in 2015. Osteoporos Int. 2016;27(3):853–9.
57. Adler RA, El-Hajj Fuleihan G, Bauer DC, Camacho PM, Clarke BL, Clines GA, et al. Managing osteoporosis in patients on long-term bisphosphonate treatment: report of a task force of the American Society for Bone and Mineral Research. J Bone Miner Res. 2016;31(10):1910.
58. Delmas PD, Meunier PJ. The management of Paget's disease of bone. N Engl J Med. 1997;336(8):558–66.
59. Roux C, Gennari C, Farrerons J, Devogelaer JP, Mulder H, Kruse HP, et al. Comparative prospective, double-blind, multicenter study of the efficacy of tiludronate and etidronate in the treatment of Paget's disease of bone. Arthritis Rheum. 1995;38(6):851–8.
60. Reid IR, Nicholson GC, Weinstein RS, Hosking DJ, Cundy T, Kotowicz MA, et al. Biochemical and radiologic improvement in Paget's disease of bone treated with alendronate: a randomized, placebo-controlled trial. Am J Med. 1996;101(4):341–8.
61. Siris E, Weinstein RS, Altman R, Conte JM, Favus M, Lombardi A, et al. Comparative study of alendronate versus etidronate for the treatment of Paget's disease of bone. J Clin Endocrinol Metab. 1996;81(3):961–7.
62. Siris ES, Chines AA, Altman RD, Brown JP, Johnston CC Jr, Lang R, et al. Risedronate in the treatment of Paget's disease of bone: an open label, multicenter study. J Bone Miner Res. 1998;13(6):1032–8.
63. Miller PD, Brown JP, Siris ES, Hoseyni MS, Axelrod DW, Bekker PJ. A randomized, double-blind comparison of risedronate and etidronate in the treatment of Paget's disease of bone. Paget's Risedronate/Etidronate Study Group. Am J Med. 1999;106(5):513–20.
64. Gutteridge DH, Retallack RW, Ward LC, Stuckey BG, Stewart GO, Prince RL, et al. Clinical, biochemical, hematologic, and radiographic responses in Paget's disease following intravenous pamidronate disodium: a 2-year study. Bone. 1996;19(4):387–94.

65. Tucci JR, Bontha S. Intravenously administered pamidronate in the treatment of Paget's disease of bone. Endocr Pract. 2001;7(6):423–9.
66. Walsh JP, Ward LC, Stewart GO, Will RK, Criddle RA, Prince RL, et al. A randomized clinical trial comparing oral alendronate and intravenous pamidronate for the treatment of Paget's disease of bone. Bone. 2004;34(4):747–54.
67. Hosking D, Lyles K, Brown JP, Fraser WD, Miller P, Curiel MD, et al. Long-term control of bone turnover in Paget's disease with zoledronic acid and risedronate. J Bone Miner Res. 2007;22(1):142–8.
68. Devogelaer JP, Geusens P, Daci E, Gielen E, Denhaerynck K, Macdonald K, et al. Remission over 3 years in patients with Paget disease of bone treated with a single intravenous infusion of 5 mg zoledronic acid. Calcif Tissue Int. 2014;94(3):311–8.
69. Merlotti D, Gennari L, Martini G, Valleggi F, De Paola V, Avanzati A, et al. Comparison of different intravenous bisphosphonate regimens for Paget's disease of bone. J Bone Miner Res. 2007;22(10):1510–7.
70. Tan A, Goodman K, Walker A, Hudson J, MacLennan GS, Selby PL, et al. Long-term randomized trial of intensive versus symptomatic management in Paget's disease of bone: the PRISM-EZ study. J Bone Miner Res. 2017;32(6):1165–73.
71. Tucci JR. Zoledronic acid therapy of patients with Paget disease of bone resistant to or with unsustained remission following prior bisphosphonate therapy. Endocr Pract. 2015;21(10):1111–6.
72. Watts RA, Skingle SJ, Bhambhani MM, Pountain G, Crisp AJ. Treatment of Paget's disease of bone with single dose intravenous pamidronate. Ann Rheum Dis. 1993;52(8):616–8.
73. Gutteridge DH, Ward LC, Stewart GO, Retallack RW, Will RK, Prince RL, et al. Paget's disease: acquired resistance to one aminobisphosphonate with retained response to another. J Bone Miner Res. 1999;14(Suppl 2):79–84.
74. Reid IR, Brown JP, Levitt N, Roman Ivorra JA, Bachiller-Corral J, Ross IL, et al. Re-treatment of relapsed Paget's disease of bone with zoledronic acid: results from an open-label study. Bonekey Rep. 2013;2:442.
75. Michou L, Brown JP. Emerging strategies and therapies for treatment of Paget's disease of bone. Drug Des Dev Ther. 2011;5:225–39.
76. Polyzos SA, Singhellakis PN, Naot D, Adamidou F, Malandrinou FC, Anastasilakis AD, et al. Denosumab treatment for juvenile Paget's disease: results from two adult patients with osteoprotegerin deficiency ("Balkan" mutation in the TNFRSF11B gene). J Clin Endocrinol Metab. 2014;99(3):703–7.
77. Reid IR, Sharma S, Kalluru R, Eagleton C. Treatment of Paget's disease of bone with Denosumab: case report and literature review. Calcif Tissue Int. 2016;99(3):322–5.
78. Grasemann C, Schundeln MM, Hovel M, Schweiger B, Bergmann C, Herrmann R, et al. Effects of RANK-ligand antibody (denosumab) treatment on bone turnover markers in a girl with juvenile Paget's disease. J Clin Endocrinol Metab. 2013;98(8):3121–6.
79. Schwarz P, Rasmussen AQ, Kvist TM, Andersen UB, Jorgensen NR. Paget's disease of the bone after treatment with Denosumab: a case report. Bone. 2012;50(5):1023–5.

Chapter 9
Hypophosphatasia

Rod Marianne Arceo-Mendoza, Anne Margarette Bacal, and Pauline M. Camacho

Case

A 55-year-old postmenopausal Caucasian woman presented for bone health evaluation with a history of recurrent metatarsal stress fractures. She recalls seeing a podiatrist at age 51 for a spontaneous left fourth metatarsal fracture that healed slowly over a 6-month period. Spontaneous right fifth and left fifth metatarsal fractures occurred 1 year later, for which she subsequently underwent open reduction and internal fixation, for worsening pain. She also reports long-standing bone pain in her hips and thighs. She follows with her PCP for intermittent headaches.

On further history, she reports losing several "baby" teeth prematurely as a child. She also required extensive dental work for numerous dental caries. She also recalls being told she had gait abnormality as a child and started walking late, compared to her peers of the same age.

She denies any known family history of bone disorder but recalls that her mother sustained a foot fracture at age 50, which also healed slowly.

Laboratory findings revealed low serum alkaline phosphatase (ALP) activity of 12 IU/liter (normal, 30–105 IU/liter). Pyridoxal-5-phosphate was measured by high-performance liquid chromatography and was 49.9 μg/l. A value above 18.5 μg/l is considered to be elevated. Bone-specific alkaline phosphatase (BSAP) was also measured by immunochemiluminometric assay and was low at 5 ug/L (normal postmenopausal female range, 0–22 μg/L). Biochemical findings were consistent with hypophosphatasia.

R. M. Arceo-Mendoza (✉) · A. M. Bacal · P. M. Camacho
Division of Endocrinology and Metabolism, Loyola University Medical Center, Loyola University Osteoporosis and Metabolic Bone Disease Center, Maywood, IL, USA
e-mail: rmmendoza@lumc.edu; Annemargarette.Bacal@lumc.edu; PCAMACH@lumc.edu

P. M. Camacho (ed.), *Metabolic Bone Diseases*,
https://doi.org/10.1007/978-3-030-03694-2_9

Mutation analysis revealed a heterozygous defect in exon 10 of *TNSALP* (*ALPL*). Her bone densitometry demonstrated low bone mass. Teriparatide was then started and injected daily for 2 years. Patient's serum ALP increased while receiving teriparatide. Sequential imaging demonstrated fracture healing. BMD remained stable on follow-up. Her pain improved and no further fractures were sustained.

Introduction

Hypophosphatasia (HPP) is an inherited metabolic bone disease from deficient activity of tissue-nonspecific isoenzyme of alkaline phosphatase (TNSALP). This condition was first described in 1948 by Dr. John C Rathbun, with a pediatric patient presenting with rickets and seizures, and was found to have low alkaline phosphatase activity in serum, bone, and other tissues at autopsy [1]. During the past several years, clinical understanding about HPP has steadily increased. Diagnostic and management options had evolved, and HPP has now become more treatable [2].

Hypophosphatasia affects 1 in 100,000 live births [1]. It affects approximately 500–600 known individuals in the United States [3]. In European populations, the prevalence of severe HPP has been estimated at 1 in 300,000 [1]. Hypophosphatasia varies in severity and presents throughout all life stages, prenatal to adulthood. However, a common feature of hypophosphatasia across all age groups is reduced serum alkaline phosphatase leading to defective bone mineralization.

Pathogenesis

In humans, three genes encode for tissue-specific alkaline phosphatase expressed in intestinal, placental, and germ cell tissues: ALPLI, ALPP, and ALPPL2, respectively. A fourth gene, the ALPL gene, encodes for tissue-nonspecific alkaline phosphatase (TNSALP) expressed in the skeleton, liver, kidney, and developing teeth. Loss of function mutation in ALPL gene leads to hypophosphatasia, which is either autosomal dominant or autosomal recessive. Mutation in the ALPL gene alters the configuration of the TNSALP crucial for stability and enzymatic function [4]. TNSALP hydrolyzes inorganic pyrophosphate (PPi) which is a strong inhibitor of mineralization. This, in turn, produces inorganic phosphate and together with calcium form hydroxyapatite crystals that comprise the bone matrix.

Clinical Features

Hypophosphatasia clinically presents in different forms of severity ranging from nonspecific symptoms in adults to very severe perinatal form including death in utero. Hypophosphatasia is primarily classified based on the age of diagnosis into six different subtypes: perinatal lethal, prenatal benign, infantile, childhood, adult, and odontohypophosphatasia. Perinatal forms and most infantile forms are autosomal recessive, while perinatal benign, childhood, adult, and odontohypophosphatasia can be either autosomal recessive or autosomal dominant; the more severe the disease is, the more often it is subject to recessive inheritance [2].

Perinatal Lethal

This is the most severe form of hypophosphatasia manifesting in utero with severe skeletal hypomineralization and is almost always lethal soon after birth. Skull bones can appear mineralized only centrally, osteochondral spurs are present in forearms and legs, and limbs appear short and deformed. Infants die at birth or in the first few days of life due to severe respiratory distress from chest deformities and lung hypoplasia [5].

Prenatal Benign

Radiographic features overlap with perinatal lethal. In particular, ultrasound findings such as poor skeletal mineralization, limb bowing, and short femurs cannot reliably differentiate the benign from the lethal form. However, spontaneous improvement is noted from the third trimester of pregnancy and maybe even normal at birth.

Infantile

Infants born with this form of hypophosphatasia appear healthy at birth, and clinical manifestations appear at 6 months of life such as poor feeding, inadequate weight gain, hypotonia, wide fontanels, and rachitic deformities [6]. Mortality is approximately 50% of cases, and vitamin B6-dependent seizures are linked to poor prognosis [2].

Childhood

In most cases, childhood hypophosphatasia becomes evident after 1 year of age and presentation can vary. Childhood hypophosphatasia may present earlier, and clinical features may overlap with infantile hypophosphatasia. Signs and symptoms include rickets, skeletal deformities, gait abnormalities, fractures, delayed walking, weakness, and bone and joint pain. Loss of teeth before 5 years of age is often the first apparent symptom and may lead to early diagnosis.

Adult

This form of hypophosphatasia appears after middle age and often presents with pain due to stress fractures or pseudofractures. Hip or thigh pain can indicate femoral pseudofractures that usually occur proximally and laterally in the subtrochanteric region. Patients can also present with nonspecific symptoms. In an analysis of 38 patients with adult hypophosphatasia, musculoskeletal pain and recurring headaches showed the highest prevalence of clinical symptoms with 60% and 55%, respectively [7]. Low bone mass and fractures due to adult hypophosphatasia may lead to a wrong diagnosis of primary osteopenia or osteoporosis and can lead to inappropriate treatment with bisphosphonates [5].

Odontohypophosphatasia

This is the least severe form of hypophosphatasia presenting with dental alterations in tooth shape, structure, and color. It involves premature loss of primary teeth, primary teeth impaction, delayed eruption of teeth, and severe dental caries. A case series demonstrated that individual patients with isolated dental manifestation of hypophosphatasia in childhood may later develop into childhood and adult form of the disease with frequent fractures and chronic pain [8].

Diagnosis

Hypophosphatasia is diagnosed through combined history, physical examination, and laboratory and radiographic findings. Low alkaline phosphatase should prompt suspicion for hypophosphatasia. Genetic analysis is available to confirm the diagnosis in doubtful cases by detecting a mutation in the ALPL gene. Abnormal growth plates, fractures, and wide open cranial sutures can be seen in infantile and childhood hypophosphatasia, whereas metatarsal stress fractures, pseudofractures of the femur, osteopenia, and chondrocalcinosis can be seen in adult hypophosphatasia.

In general, those patients with severe forms of the disease present with lower serum ALP level.

Other conditions may also present with low serum alkaline phosphatase. These include hypothyroidism, pregnancy, anemia, and drug administration.

Management

Hypophosphatasia involves medical treatment, surgical repair, and enzyme replacement therapy.

Enzyme replacement therapy with asfotase alfa was approved in 2015 for treatment of pediatric-onset hypophosphatasia. Asfotase alfa is a bone-targeted TNSALP replacement with clinical efficacy in perinatal, infantile, and childhood-onset hypophosphatasia; however its benefits have yet to be shown for adult form of hypophosphatasia [9]. The most common adverse effect of asfotase alfa is injection site reaction which can manifest as erythema, pain, discoloration, swelling, pruritus, and bruising [7].

Use of teriparatide (recombinant human parathyroid hormone PTH 1–34) for adult hypophosphatasia was first reported in 2007 which showed fracture repair with a reduction in pain and increased serum alkaline phosphatase activity [10]. Teriparatide is an anabolic agent used to reduce fracture risk in women with osteoporosis. It also increases bone mineral density and bone formation. It is administered daily as a subcutaneous injection. A number of published case reports [10, 11] demonstrate improvement and resolution of metatarsal stress fractures in adults with HPP. However, the benefit of its use remains to be fully elucidated.

References

1. Whyte MP. Hypophosphatasia – aetiology, nosology, pathogenesis, diagnosis and treatment. Nat Rev Endocrinol. 2016;12(4):233–46.
2. Mornet E. Hypophosphatasia. Metabolism. 2018;82:142–55.
3. Shapiro JR, Lewiecki EM. Hypophosphatasia in adults: clinical assessment and treatment considerations. J Bone Miner Res. 2017;32(10):1977–80.
4. Millan JL, Whyte MP. Alkaline phosphatase and hypophosphatasia. Calcif Tissue Int. 2016;98(4):398–416.
5. Bianchi ML. Hypophosphatasia: an overview of the disease and its treatment. Osteoporos Int. 2015;26(12):2743–57.
6. Whyte MP, Zhang F, Wenkert D, et al. Hypophosphatasia: validation and expansion of the clinical nosology for children from 25 years experience with 173 pediatric patients. Bone. 2015;75:229–39.
7. Kishnani PS, Rush ET, Arundel P, et al. Monitoring guidance for patients with hypophosphatasia treated with asfotase alfa. Mol Genet Metab. 2017;122(1–2):4–17.
8. Mori M, Dearmey SL, Weber TJ, Kishnani PS. Case series: odontohypophosphatasia or missed diagnosis of childhood/adult-onset hypophosphatasia? – Call for a long-term follow-up of premature loss of primary teeth. Bone Rep. 2016;5:228–32.
9. Schmidt T, Mussawy H, Rolvien T, et al. Clinical, radiographic and biochemical characteristics of adult hypophosphatasia. Osteoporos Int. 2017;28(9):2653–62.
10. Whyte MP, Mumm S, Deal C. Adult hypophosphatasia treated with teriparatide. J Clin Endocrinol Metab. 2007;92(4):1203–8.
11. Camacho PM, Mazhari AM, Wilczynski C, Kadanoff R, Mumm S, Whyte MP. Adult hypophosphatasia treated with teriparatide: report of 2 patients and review of the literature. Endocr Pract. 2016;22(8):941–50.

Chapter 10
Osteogenesis Imperfecta

Ruchita Patel and Pauline M. Camacho

Case

A 45-year-old Caucasian male with dwarfism referred for management of osteogenesis imperfecta type III. He has had has many fractures from minimal stress in adolescence and 13 surgeries since age 3, including a loose rod in his left lower extremity. Last fracture was at age 21 years. He is mainly wheelchair bound but able to stand with upper extremity strength. There's no family history of osteoporosis. He has loss height over the years and admits to a poor intake of dietary calcium. He does not take any vitamin D or calcium supplementation.

On exam, he is 3 ft tall and weighs 71 lbs. He has short stature, bluish sclera (Fig. 10.1), brown translucent teeth with spacing in between (Fig. 10.2), and normal hearing. He has kyphoscoliosis and pectus excavatum. He has joint and long bone deformities (Figs. 10.3 and 10.4) with palpable edge of rod of left lower extremity that was tender. He had noticeable thinning of the skin in his extremities (Fig. 10.5).

His metabolic bone workup revealed: bone-specific alkaline phosphatase of 41.7 ug/L and continues to stay in the 30s throughout years of follow-up, vitamin D 25 OH 22 ng/mL, TSH 1.49 uu/mL (0.40–4.60), 24 urine calcium 205 mg/24 h, total calcium 8.8 (8.9–10.3 mg/dL), ionized calcium 1.14 (1.15–1.30 mmol/L), and total alkaline phosphatase 142 (30–110 IU/L). Around age 50 years, he had his first CTX level drawn and it was 495 (87–345 pg/mL).

R. Patel
Department of Endocrinology, Diabetes and Metabolism, Advocate Christ Medical Center, Oak Lawn, IL, USA

P. M. Camacho (✉)
Division of Endocrinology and Metabolism, Loyola University Medical Center, Loyola University Osteoporosis and Metabolic Bone Disease Center, Maywood, IL, USA
e-mail: pcamach@lumc.edu

P. M. Camacho (ed.), *Metabolic Bone Diseases*,
https://doi.org/10.1007/978-3-030-03694-2_10

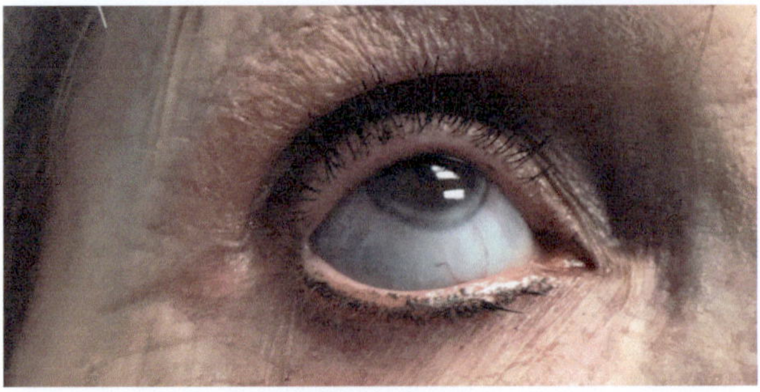

Fig. 10.1 Bluish, gray sclera

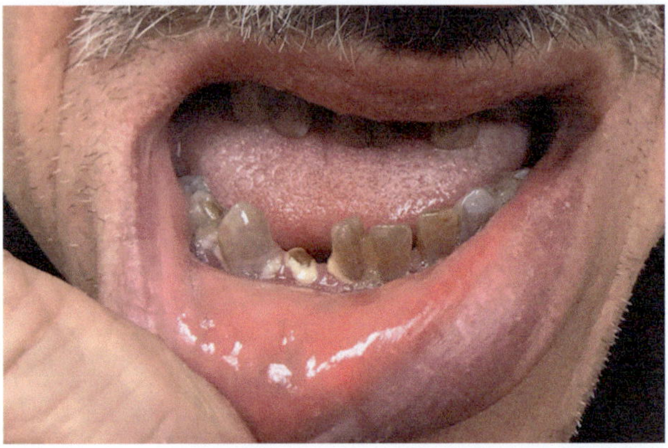

Fig. 10.2 Teeth of patient, findings seen in dentinogenesis imperfecta

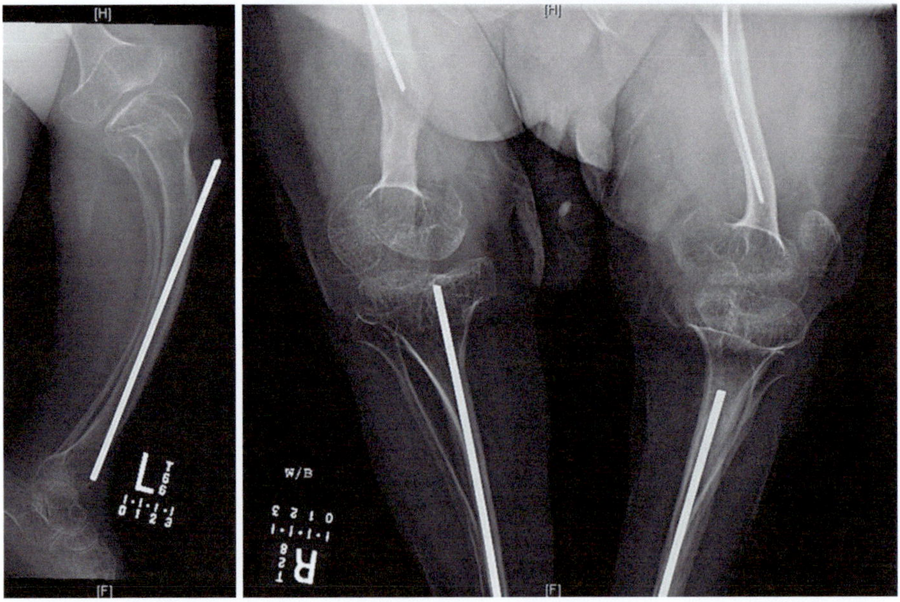

Figs. 10.3 and 10.4 Patient's long bone deformities

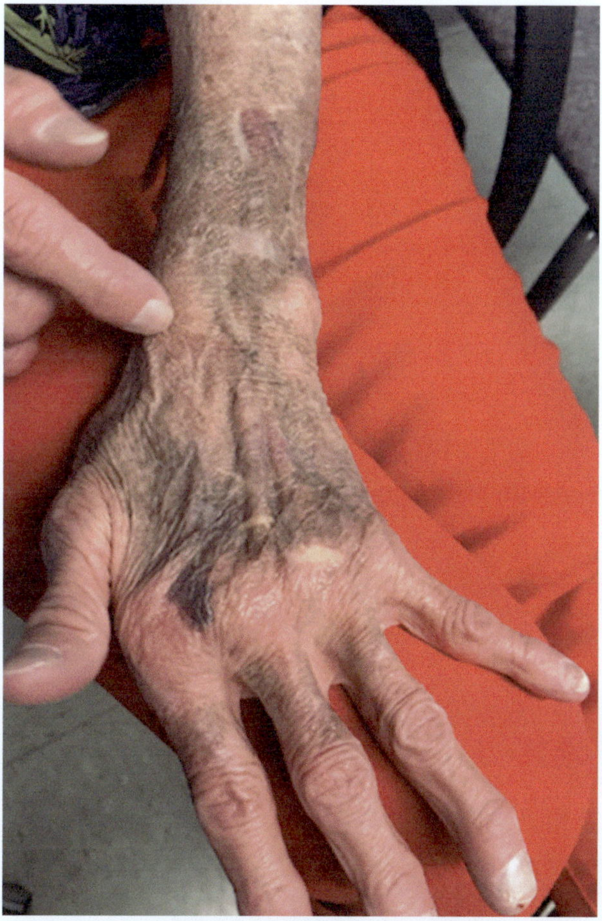

Fig. 10.5 Findings seen with thinning of the skin, easy bruisability

He had a DXA scan (Figs. 10.6 and 10.7) completed that showed a T score of −5.7 at lumbar spine and T score −6.0 at femoral neck. For vitamin D insufficiency, he was started on ergocalciferol 50,000 units monthly and advised to increase his dietary intake of calcium to about 1200 mg/day. Given his history of fractures and DXA findings, he was offered PO bisphosphonate for treatment but the patient declined. During follow-up, he did not have any recurrent fractures and so has not been placed on any antiresorptive therapy or anabolic therapy. Given his extensive deformities, no further DXA monitoring is needed but we are ensuring that his dietary intake of calcium and vitamin D levels are sufficient.

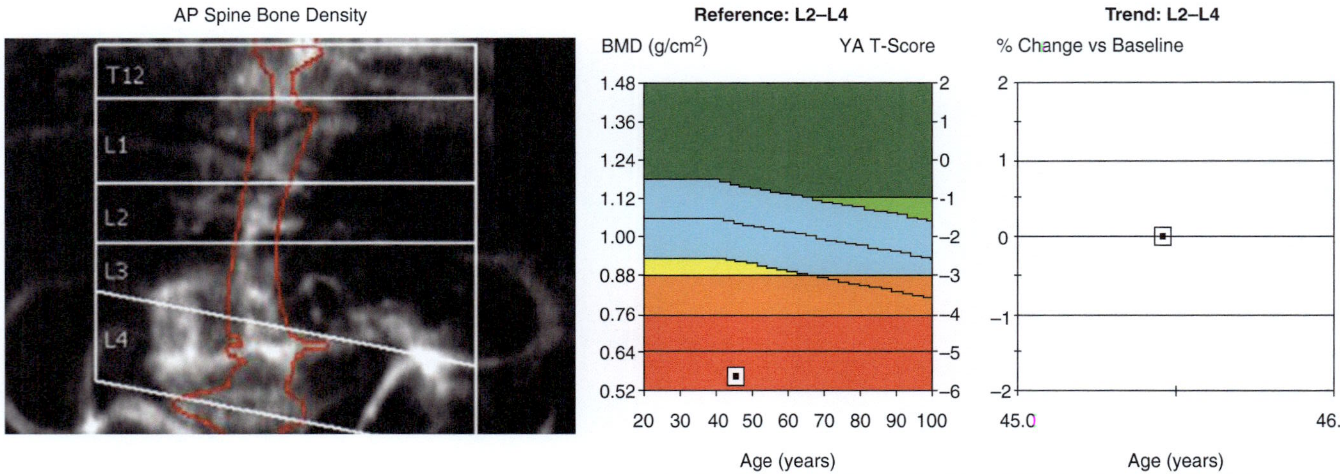

Region	BMD[1] (g/cm²)	Young-Adult[2] T-Score	Age-Matched[3] Z-Score
L1	0.403	–6.3	–4.7
L2	0.486	–6.3	–4.6
L3	0.517	–6.0	–4.4
L4	0.616	–5.2	–3.6
L1–L2	0.434	–6.4	–4.7
L1–L3	0.464	–6.2	–4.6
L1–L4	0.520	–5.8	–4.2
L2–L3	0.505	–6.1	–4.5
L2–L4	0.560	–5.7	–4.0
L3–L4	0.578	–5.5	–3.9

Fig. 10.6 Lumbar spine DXA for patient on GE Lunar machine

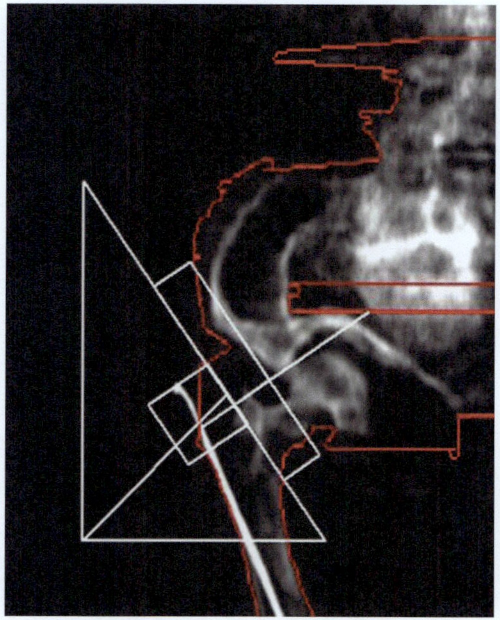

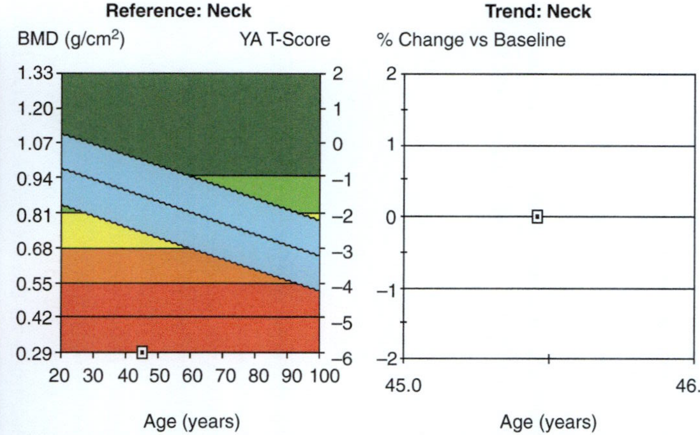

Region	BMD[1] (g/cm²)	Young-Adult[2] T-Score	Age-Matched[3] Z-Score
Neck	0.295	−6.0	−4.4
Wards	0.088	−6.7	−4.9
Troch	0.000	-	-
Shaft	0.370	-	-
Total	0.315	−5.5	−4.2

HAL chart results unavailable

Trend:Neck				
Measured Date	Age (years)	BMD[1] (g/cm²)	Change vs Previous (%)	Change vs Previous (%/yr)
11/22/2006	45.4	0.295	-	-

COMMENTS:

Fig. 10.7 Hip DXA for patient on GE Lunar machine

Introduction

Osteogenesis imperfecta (OI) is a rare group of metabolic bone disorders that are characterized by defects in connective tissue presenting with bone fragility in early childhood and affect about 1/13,500–15,000 births [1, 2]. Mutations in the genes that encode type I collagen lead to the development of OI, mainly *COL1A1* and *COL1A2*. Mutations in these genes affect the ability of the chains to fold into a trimer. In recent times, OI also encompasses additional genes discovered to be involved in the posttranslational modification of type I collagen, bone cell signaling, and regulation of bone matrix homeostasis [3].

Classification (Table 10.1)

Type I collagen is the most prevalent collagen in the bone matrix, with two a1 chains (encoded by COL1A1 gene) and one a2 chain (encoded by COL1A2 gene). Its precursor, type I procollagen, undergoes posttranslational modifications, which leads to fibril formation. The defects in the genes and proteins in this process lead to the various types of OI [2]. Sillence first proposed the classification of OI in 1979, based on clinical and radiographic characteristics[4]. There were four categories: type I, nondeforming with blue sclera OI; type II, perinatally lethal OI; type III, progressively deforming OI; and type IV, moderate and severe OI [5]. About 85–90% of OI cases are caused by autosomal dominant mutations in the *COL1A1* or *COL1A2* genes [2, 5]. Types V through XI have been included but are based on different criteria from types I to IV. Type V OI is inherited via an autosomal dominant manner and defined by bone histology, along with clinical and radiographic signs [4, 6]. It is associated with a defect in the *IFITM5* gene. Typically a triad with radiodense metaphyseal band, hypertrophic callus at fractures or surgical sites, and calcification of forearm interosseous membrane is seen; along with variable sclerae [4, 6]. Type VI is inherited autosomal recessively and bone histology shows a mineralization defect in *SERPINF1*. Bone histology has distinctive lamellae findings with "fish-scale" appearance. Clinically, these individuals have moderate to severe skeletal disease, along with slightly elevated alkaline phosphatase levels [4, 7]. Type VII OI is also inherited in an autosomal recessive manner, with defects in *CRTAP* gene (cartilage-associated protein). Clinically, patients will have rhizomelia and moderate bone disease. It can be lethal in those with null mutations in the *CRTAP* gene [4, 8]. Type VIII OI has some overlap with type VII. It is inherited autosomal recessively, and there are enzymatic defects in prolyl 3-hydroxylase 1 (P3H1), which is encoded by the gene *LEPRE1*. Clinically, those individual with null mutations in LEPRE1 have white sclera, growth deficiency, and undermineralization. Thus, they may look similar to those with OI types II and III [4, 8]. Type IX OI is caused by defects in peptidyl-prolyl cis-trans isomerase (PPIB). Mutations in this gene

Table 10.1 Classification of osteogenesis imperfecta – combining Sillence classification and newer autosomal recessive types

Type	Inheritance pattern	Clinical presentation	Genes/ proteins involved
I	AD	Mildest; blue sclera; may have hearing loss; possible dentinogenesis imperfecta; joint hyperlaxity; fractures in childhood, aortic regurgitation	*COL1A1*
II	AD	Lethal in the perinatal period; premature births, small for gestational age; long bones are osteoporotic; blue/gray sclera; die of pulmonary causes	*COL1A1/ COL1A2*
III	AD	Triangular facies; severe bone dysplasia; dozens to hundreds of fractures; growth deficiency; final stature is close to prepubertal stage; most develop scoliosis; develop respiratory problems; "popcorn" appearance of metaphyses and epiphyses	*COL1A1/ COL1A2*
IV	AD	Variable sclera; many fractures per year in childhood but decrease after puberty; bowing of long bones; short stature; go on to develop osteoporosis; scoliosis	*COL1A1/ COL1A2*
V	AD	Radiodense metaphyseal band; hypertrophic callus at fractures; calcification of forearm interosseous membrane; variable sclera	*IFITM5 (Bril)*
VI	AR	Moderate to severe skeletal disease; slightly elevated alkaline phosphatase;	*SERPINF1 (PEDF)*
VII	AR	Rhizomelia, moderate skeletal disease; lethal form includes white sclera, rhizomelia, small to normal cranium	*CRTAP*
VIII	AR	White sclera; growth deficiency; rhizomelia; "popcorn" metaphyses	*LEPRE1 (P3HI)*
IX	AR	Moderate skeletal disease; white sclera; growth deficiency	*PPIB (CyPB)*
X	AR	Severe/lethal; dentinogenesis imperfecta; skin bullae; pyloric stenosis; hearing loss; blue sclera; renal stones	*SERPINH1 (HSP47)*
XI	AR	Normal to gray sclera; fractures of long bones; platyspondyly; scoliosis; encompasses Bruck syndrome[a] and Kuskokwim syndrome[b]; variable congenital contractures	*FKBP10*

AD autosomal dominant, *AR* autosomal recessive
[a]Bruck syndrome: osteogenesis imperfecta with congenital joint contractures
[b]Kuskokwim syndrome: congenital contracture syndrome

causing premature stop codons are similar to lethal forms of types VII and VIII [4, 9, 10]. Type X OI is a very rare autosomal recessive disorder caused by defects in the endoplasmic reticulum localized collagen chaperone *HSP47*. It is usually lethal with dentinogenesis imperfecta, skin bullae, and pyloric stenosis [4, 11]. Finally, type XI OI is another autosomal recessive form related to defects in FKBP10. This has been known to lead to progressive deformities associated with long bone fractures, scoliosis, and platyspondyly [4, 12]. In addition, has been associated with congenital contractures [13, 14].

Clinical Presentation

Individuals with OI have brittle bones with skeletal deformities (bowing deformities) and growth retardation. The severe forms of OI can present with stillbirth or multiple fractures early on in life, whereas the milder forms have lower rates of fractures in adult individuals. However, in the milder forms, fractures can occur postpartum or postmenopausal [2].

Skeletal Manifestations

Skeletal manifestations include macrocephaly, flat midface and triangular facies, dentinogenesis imperfecta, pectus excavatum or carinatum, barrel chest, and scoliosis or kyphosis [15]. Radiographs include osteopenia, long bone bowing, undertubulation and metaphyseal flaring, thin ribs, narrow thoracic apex, and vertebral compressions [15]. In terms of fractures, vertebral fractures are very common. Rib fractures are common in the severe forms, which lead to the chest wall deformities. Long bone fractures have variable presentations and usually occur in the tibia and fibula of children with the milder forms. Dentinogenesis imperfecta involves a defect in the formation of dentin that is frequently seen in OI, with a prevalence of 28% [3, 16]. In this disorder, teeth are discolored, translucent and wear prematurely. In addition, the roots are short and dentine is hypertrophic with destruction of the pulp. Primary teeth are affected more than permanent teeth and can lead to malocclusion and delayed tooth eruption [3, 16]. In terms of bone mineral density (BMD), patients with OI have lower areal BMD secondary to smaller bone size and lower volumetric BMD. Histomorphometric studies in children with OI have shown decreased cancellous bone volume due to a reduced trabecular number and thickness [17].

Extraskeletal Manifestations

Individuals with OI develop several other comorbidities and phenotypic features. Hearing loss is prevalent in about 50% of adult patients with OI, with a combination of conductive and sensorineural hearing loss. Blue/gray sclera is seen in type I OI, the mildest form of OI. The color can be stable for remainder of life or decrease in darkness over time. In addition, there is hyperlaxity of joints in up to 66–70% of patients [18]. More than half of patients will report a history of joint dislocation. However, with aging, joint hypermobility tends to decrease due to stiffening and mechanical effects of skeletal deformities. Hypercalciuria was seen in 36% of children with OI in a small study. During follow-up of 12 of those patients in the initial study, 8 still had hypercalciuria 4 years later, and urinary calcium levels correlated with severity of skeletal disease [19, 20]. Cardiovascular complications are common in patients with OI as well. Patients with OI have impairment in right ventricular and left ventricular systolic and diastolic dysfunction [21]. Given the type 1 collagen production defect in patients with OI; heart valves are also affected and patients subsequently develop valvulopathies, along with increased aortic diameter. These abnormalities may manifest with aortic root dilatation, aortic regurgitation, or mitral regurgitation [22, 23]. Finally, individuals with OI can have neurological symptoms. These include headaches with movement, trigeminal neuralgia, difficulty with balance, leg and arm weakness, and hydrocephalus [2, 3].

Treatment

Treatment in OI is focused on a multifaceted approach with not only reducing bone pain, but to reduce incidence of fracture, improve mobility, manage activities of daily living (ADL's), and manage extraskeletal manifestations. In addition to medical or surgical therapy, a physical rehabilitation team is vital for best results in these individuals.

Calcium and Vitamin D

There is a lot of literature to support the adequate intake of vitamin D and calcium in order to achieve optimal bone health in metabolic bone diseases. Unfortunately, there is a paucity of randomized trials to support the use in patients with OI. However, cross-sectional studies indicate that vitamin D 25 OH correlate positively with lumbar spine areal BMD [24, 25]. A randomized trial did not show benefit of high-dose supplementation of vitamin D3 (2000 IU vs. 400 IU) in BMD measurement at 1 year, only in achieving higher vitamin D 25 OH levels [26]. Therefore, it is recommended that intake of calcium and vitamin D3 is up to 1300 mg/day and about 600–800 IU/day depending on age and weight of the individual [27].

Bisphosphonates

As opposed to the central dogma of standard osteoporosis treatment in postmenopausal women and men over the age of 50 years, where mainstay therapies can decrease the risk of future fractures, treatment for individuals with OI bone-specific medications is more restricted. Indications for treatment include presence of vertebral fractures independent of lumbar spine BMD z-score or at least two or three low trauma fractures by the age of 10 or 18 years with lumbar spine z-scores of less than or equal to –2.0 [28]. Adults with OI are recommended to start pharmacotherapy if they have a fragility fracture and/or T scores less than or equal to −2.5.

Bisphosphonates are the most commonly used therapy for the treatment of postmenopausal osteoporosis, osteoporosis in men, and even glucocorticoid-induced osteoporosis. They bind on bone surface and induce cell death to osteoclasts, decreasing bone remodeling, thereby increasing bone mineralization and subsequently BMD. Bisphosphonates cannot change the type I collagen defects seen in this inherited disorder but do reduce the high turnover and increase bone volume, even if it's of impaired quality [15]. There have been multiple randomized controlled trials showing the reduced fracture incidence at vertebral and non-vertebral sites when using alendronate, risedronate, or zoledronic acid. However given the heterogeneity of the trials, there was not consistent reduction in fracture rates. Also, the studies did not conclusively show an improvement in bone-related pain and functional mobility [29].

Denosumab

The use of denosumab, a monoclonal antibody inhibiting the actions of RANK-L, was first in type VI. In a series of four children, who were unable to have suppressed urinary resorption markers while on previous bisphosphonate therapy, denosumab led to normalization of resorption markers when given every 3 months with a dose of 1 mg/kg of body weight [30]. Most of the studies regarding denosumab for treatment have been done on patients with previous history bisphosphonate use prior to administration of denosumab. Therefore, no data about rebound fractures in this population have been published. There does not appear to be a correlation with quality of life and pain relief with the use of denosumab during a 48 week study [31]. However, during a 2-year period, four patients with type VI OI had not only increase in areal BMD with reduced fracture rates, but a slight increase in mobility and reduced bone pain following doses of denosumab, but symptoms would recur when next injection was due every 12 weeks [32]. In a study that included female adult patients with OI, at 24 months, there was a 14.7% and 15.1% increase in lumbar spine BMD and hip BMD, respectively, without any fractures [33].

Teriparatide

Teriparatide has been approved for the treatment of postmenopausal osteoporosis and for osteoporosis in men. In recent years, it has been used as treatment of osteoporosis in adults with OI. Initially teriparatide was used in the mildest form of OI, type I, and found to have a statistically significant improvement in BMD of lumbar spine over 18 months (n = 13) after patients suffered vertebral fractures while on bisphosphonates for at least 2 years. Additionally, serum bone markers for formation and resorption also increased [34]. This was replicated in the largest placebo-controlled trial to date with 98 patients with an increase in proximal femur and lumbar spine areal BMD over 18 months. Vertebral volumetric BMD also increased, again confirming that anabolic therapy does increase bone mass in these individuals despite defects in type I collagen production. Unfortunately, the trial was not powered enough to assess fracture risk [35, 36]. Sclerostin is an inhibitor of the Wnt signaling pathway and therefore leads to decreased bone formation. Mouse studies have shown promising results of anti-sclerostin antibodies, and so the first randomized phase 2a trial of the anti-sclerostin antibody, BPS804 ($n = 14$), showed a statistically significant increase in bone formation markers and areal BMD and lowered CTX-1 from baseline. The medication was well tolerated [37] but future studies are pending regarding further use in humans.

Conclusion

Osteogenesis imperfecta is a rare genetically inherited disorder involved in mostly defects in type I collagen production. The different types have distinct phenotypes, with milder forms to severe forms, depending on which genes are involved. It is the most common cause of osteoporosis in children. Management of an individual involves support from multiple medical specialties along with physiotherapy. Pharmacological therapy exists for treatment of osteoporosis or those at high risk of fractures, but fracture prevention data on long bone fractures is not robust with some therapies. More research needs to be done in this specific population of people, as there are many unanswered questions.

References

1. Stoll C, Dott B, Roth M-P, Alembik Y. Birth prevalence rates of skeletal dysplasias. Clin Genet. 2008;35(2):88–92. https://doi.org/10.1111/j.1399-0004.1989.tb02912.x.
2. Tournis S, Dede AD. Osteogenesis imperfecta – a clinical update. Metabolism. 2017; https://doi.org/10.1016/j.metabol.2017.06.001.
3. Harrington J, Sochett E, Howard A. Update on the evaluation and treatment of osteogenesis imperfecta. Pediatr Clin N Am. 2014;61(6):1243–57. https://doi.org/10.1016/j.pcl.2014.08.010.
4. Marini JC. Osteogenesis imperfecta. In: Primer on the metabolic bone diseases and disorders of mineral metabolism. Ames: Wiley; 2013. p. 822–9. https://doi.org/10.1002/9781118453926.ch99.
5. Palomo T, Vilaça T, Lazaretti-Castro M. Osteogenesis imperfecta. Curr Opin Endocrinol Diabetes Obes. 2017;24(6):381–8. https://doi.org/10.1097/MED.0000000000000367.
6. Rauch F, Moffatt P, Cheung M, et al. Osteogenesis imperfecta type V: marked phenotypic variability despite the presence of the *IFITM5* c.−14C>T mutation in all patients. J Med Genet. 2013;50(1):21–4. https://doi.org/10.1136/jmedgenet-2012-101307.
7. Glorieux FH, Ward LM, Rauch F, Lalic L, Roughley PJ, Travers R. Osteogenesis imperfecta type VI: a form of brittle bone disease with a mineralization defect. J Bone Miner Res. 2002;17(1):30–8. https://doi.org/10.1359/jbmr.2002.17.1.30.

8. Ward LM, Rauch F, Travers R, et al. Osteogenesis imperfecta type VII: an autosomal recessive form of brittle bone disease. Bone. 2002;31(1):12–8. http://www.ncbi.nlm.nih.gov/pubmed/12110406. Accessed 1 July 2018
9. Pyott SM, Schwarze U, Christiansen HE, et al. Mutations in PPIB (cyclophilin B) delay type I procollagen chain association and result in perinatal lethal to moderate osteogenesis imperfecta phenotypes. Hum Mol Genet. 2011;20(8):1595–609. https://doi.org/10.1093/hmg/ddr037.
10. van Dijk FS, Nesbitt IM, Zwikstra EH, et al. PPIB mutations cause severe osteogenesis imperfecta. Am J Hum Genet. 2009;85(4):521–7. https://doi.org/10.1016/j.ajhg.2009.09.001.
11. Christiansen HE, Schwarze U, Pyott SM, et al. Homozygosity for a missense mutation in SERPINH1, which encodes the collagen chaperone protein HSP47, results in severe recessive osteogenesis imperfecta. Am J Hum Genet. 2010;86(3):389–98. https://doi.org/10.1016/j.ajhg.2010.01.034.
12. Alanay Y, Avaygan H, Camacho N, et al. Mutations in the gene encoding the RER protein FKBP65 cause autosomal-recessive osteogenesis imperfecta. Am J Hum Genet. 2010;86(4):551–9. https://doi.org/10.1016/j.ajhg.2010.02.022.
13. McPherson E, Clemens M. Bruck syndrome (osteogenesis imperfecta with congenital joint contractures): review and report on the first North American case. Am J Med Genet. 1997;70(1):28–31. http://www.ncbi.nlm.nih.gov/pubmed/9129737. Accessed 5 July 2018
14. Barnes AM, Duncan G, Weis M, et al. Kuskokwim syndrome, a recessive congenital contracture disorder, extends the phenotype of *FKBP10* mutations. Hum Mutat. 2013;34(9):1279–88. https://doi.org/10.1002/humu.22362.
15. Forlino A, Marini JC. Osteogenesis imperfecta. Lancet. 2016;387(10028):1657–71. https://doi.org/10.1016/S0140-6736(15)00728-X.
16. O'Connell AC, Marini JC. Evaluation of oral problems in an osteogenesis imperfecta population. Oral Surg Oral Med Oral Pathol Oral Radiol Endod. 1999;87(2):189–96. http://www.ncbi.nlm.nih.gov/pubmed/10052375. Accessed 1 July 2018
17. Rauch F, Travers R, Parfitt AM, Glorieux FH. Static and dynamic bone histomorphometry in children with osteogenesis imperfecta. Bone. 2000;26(6):581–9. https://doi.org/10.1016/S8756-3282(00)00269-6.
18. Arponen H, Mäkitie O, Waltimo-Sirén J. Association between joint hypermobility, scoliosis, and cranial base anomalies in paediatric Osteogenesis imperfecta patients: a retrospective cross-sectional study. BMC Musculoskelet Disord. 2014;15(1):428. https://doi.org/10.1186/1471-2474-15-428.
19. Chines A, Petersen DJ, Schranck FW, Whyte MP. Hypercalciuria in children severely affected with osteogenesis imperfecta. J Pediatr. 1991;119(1 Pt 1):51–7. http://www.ncbi.nlm.nih.gov/pubmed/2066859. Accessed 2 July 2018
20. Chines A, Boniface A, McAlister W, Whyte M. Hypercalciuria in osteogenesis imperfecta: a follow-up study to assess renal effects. Bone. 1995;16(3):333–9. http://www.ncbi.nlm.nih.gov/pubmed/7786636. Accessed 2 July 2018
21. Radunovic Z, Steine K. Prevalence of cardiovascular disease and cardiac symptoms: left and right ventricular function in adults with osteogenesis imperfecta. Can J Cardiol. 2015;31(11):1386–92. https://doi.org/10.1016/j.cjca.2015.04.016.
22. Lamanna A, Fayers T, Clarke S, Parsonage W. Valvular and aortic diseases in osteogenesis imperfecta. Heart Lung Circ. 2013;22(10):801–10. https://doi.org/10.1016/j.hlc.2013.05.640.
23. Ashournia H, Johansen FT, Folkestad L, Diederichsen ACP, Brixen K. Heart disease in patients with osteogenesis imperfecta — a systematic review. Int J Cardiol. 2015;196:149–57. https://doi.org/10.1016/j.ijcard.2015.06.001.
24. Edouard T, Glorieux FH, Rauch F. Predictors and correlates of vitamin D status in children and adolescents with osteogenesis imperfecta. J Clin Endocrinol Metab. 2011;96(10):3193–8. https://doi.org/10.1210/jc.2011-1480.

25. Edouard T, Glorieux FH, Rauch F. Relationship between vitamin D status and bone mineralization, mass, and metabolism in children with osteogenesis imperfecta: histomorphometric study. J Bone Miner Res. 2011;26(9):2245–51. https://doi.org/10.1002/jbmr.413.
26. Plante L, Veilleux L-N, Glorieux FH, Weiler H, Rauch F. Effect of high-dose vitamin D supplementation on bone density in youth with osteogenesis imperfecta: a randomized controlled trial. Bone. 2016;86:36–42. https://doi.org/10.1016/j.bone.2016.02.013.
27. Nutrition – Osteogenesis Imperfecta Foundation | OIF.org. http://www.oif.org/site/PageServer?pagename=Nutrition. Accessed 2 July 2018.
28. Ward LM, Konji VN, Ma J. The management of osteoporosis in children. Osteoporos Int. 2016;27(7):2147–79. https://doi.org/10.1007/s00198-016-3515-9.
29. Dwan K, Phillipi CA, Steiner RD, Basel D. Bisphosphonate therapy for osteogenesis imperfecta. In: Basel D, editor. Cochrane database of systematic reviews. Chichester: Wiley; 2014. p. CD005088. https://doi.org/10.1002/14651858.CD005088.pub3.
30. Semler O, Netzer C, Hoyer-Kuhn H, Becker J, Eysel P, Schoenau E. First use of the RANKL antibody denosumab in osteogenesis imperfecta type VI. J Musculoskelet Neuronal Interact. 2012;12(3):183–8. http://www.ncbi.nlm.nih.gov/pubmed/22947550. Accessed 2 July 2018
31. Hoyer-Kuhn H, Stark C, Franklin J, Schoenau E, Semler O. Correlation of bone mineral density on quality of life in patients with osteogenesis imperfecta during treatment with denosumab. Pediatr Endocrinol Rev. 2017;15(Suppl 1):123–9. https://doi.org/10.17458/per.vol15.2017.hsf.correlationbonemineraldensity.
32. Hoyer-Kuhn H, Netzer C, Koerber F, Schoenau E, Semler O. Two years' experience with denosumab for children with osteogenesis imperfecta type VI. Orphanet J Rare Dis. 2014;9:145. https://doi.org/10.1186/s13023-014-0145-1.
33. Uehara M, Nakamura Y, Takahashi J, et al. Efficacy of denosumab for osteoporosis in three female patients with osteogenesis imperfecta. Tohoku J Exp Med. 2017;242(2):115–20. https://doi.org/10.1620/tjem.242.115.
34. Gatti D, Rossini M, Viapiana O, et al. Teriparatide treatment in adult patients with osteogenesis imperfecta type I. Calcif Tissue Int. 2013;93(5):448–52. https://doi.org/10.1007/s00223-013-9770-2.
35. Leali PT, Balsano M, Maestretti G, et al. Efficacy of teriparatide vs neridronate in adults with osteogenesis imperfecta type I: a prospective randomized international clinical study. Clin Cases Miner Bone Metab. 2017;14(2):153–6. https://doi.org/10.11138/ccmbm/2017.14.1.153.
36. Orwoll ES, Shapiro J, Veith S, et al. Evaluation of teriparatide treatment in adults with osteogenesis imperfecta. J Clin Invest. 2014;124(2):491–8. https://doi.org/10.1172/JCI71101.
37. Glorieux FH, Devogelaer J-P, Durigova M, et al. BPS804 anti-sclerostin antibody in adults with moderate osteogenesis imperfecta: results of a randomized phase 2a trial. J Bone Miner Res. 2017;32(7):1496–504. https://doi.org/10.1002/jbmr.3143.

Chapter 11
Tumor-Induced Osteomalacia

Mark Anthony Sandoval

Abbreviations

CT	Computed tomography
DOTANOC	1,4,7,10-Tetraazacyclododecane -D-Phe[1]-1-Nal[3]-octreotide
DOTATATE	1,4,7,10-Tetraazacyclododecane-1,4,7,10-tetraacetic acid octreotate
DOTATOC	1,4,7,10-Tetraazacyclododecane-N,N,N,N-tetraacetic-acid-D-Phe[1] -Tyr[3] –octreotide
FDG	Fluorodeoxyglucose
FGF	Fibroblast growth factor
HYNIC-TOC	Hydrazinonicotinyl-Tyr3-Octreotide
MEPE	Matrix extracellular phosphoglycoprotein
MIBI	Methoxyisobutylisonitrile
MRI	Magnetic resonance imaging
NPT	Sodium-phosphate cotransporter
OOM	Oncogenic osteomalacia
PET	Positron emission tomography
PMT	Phosphaturic mesenchymal tumor
PMTMCT	Phosphaturic mesenchymal tumor, mixed connective tissue variant
sFRP-4	Secreted frizzled-related protein 4
SPECT	Single photon emission computed tomography
TIO	Tumor-induced osteomalacia
TmP/GFR	Tubular maximum reabsorption of phosphate corrected for glomerular filtration rate
TRP	Tubular phosphate reabsorption

M. A. Sandoval (✉)
Department of Physiology and Section of Endocrinology, Diabetes and Metabolism,
Department of Medicine, College of Medicine and Philippine General Hospital,
University of the Philippines Manila, Manila, Philippines
e-mail: mssandoval1@up.edu.ph

P. M. Camacho (ed.), *Metabolic Bone Diseases*,
https://doi.org/10.1007/978-3-030-03694-2_11

Introduction

Tumor-induced osteomalacia (TIO) is an interesting paraneoplastic syndrome wherein bone formation is affected by the secretion by a tumor of a phosphaturic substance. The condition is also known as oncogenic osteomalacia (OOM). Being a paraneoplastic syndrome, the causative tumor does not cause symptoms via mechanical means but via overproduction of a biologically active substance which affects another organ. The causative tumor is of varied histologies but is usually a benign mesenchymal neoplasm. The biologically active substance is a phosphaturic hormone now identified to be fibroblast growth factor 23 (FGF23). The affected organ is the bone. The clinical presentation is due the resultant bone disease since the causative tumor is usually asymptomatic.

The diagnosis is entertained when there are typical symptoms, hypophosphatemia discovered during adulthood, absence of a family history of hypophosphatemia, renal phosphate wasting, low 1,25 dihydroxy vitamin D, high FGF23, and typical radiographic changes in the bone. A search for the causative tumor should then be done. Cure is possible when the causative tumor is completely excised.

Case

A 31-year-old Filipino male consulted for progressive hunchback deformity, marked loss of height, and bone pains.

Five years prior to consult, he started to have low back pain for which he consulted a local physician. He was given pain relievers but pain persisted. Spine x-rays were done then which apparently showed normal results. Two years prior to consult, he started to have bone pains not anymore limited to the back. He is able to walk around the house but would have difficulty walking long distances. He has been to many doctors in their hometown but none were able to provide with relief from pain. On consult, his bone pains have become so severe that sitting up from a lying position or even turning in bed would bring him so much pain. He also started to develop kyphosis and that he has become shorter by 14 cm (Fig. 11.1).

He has no previous fracture. He has no other known illnesses. He is not taking glucocorticoids, levothyroxine, or anticonvulsants. There is no similar illness in the family. He is a social alcoholic drinker. He is a previous smoker who has stopped several years ago. His work is usually outdoors. He is not a vegetarian. He is married and has three biological children, the youngest being 3 years old.

He has no constitutional symptoms such as fever, weight loss, anorexia, or malaise. He also does not have dyspnea despite the kyphosis. He mentioned having decreased morning penile erections but continues to shave his facial hair every 2–3 days.

On physical exam, he is awake, coherent, and conversant. He is seen initially wheelchair-borne. When asked to stand, gross sagittal balance was compensated by

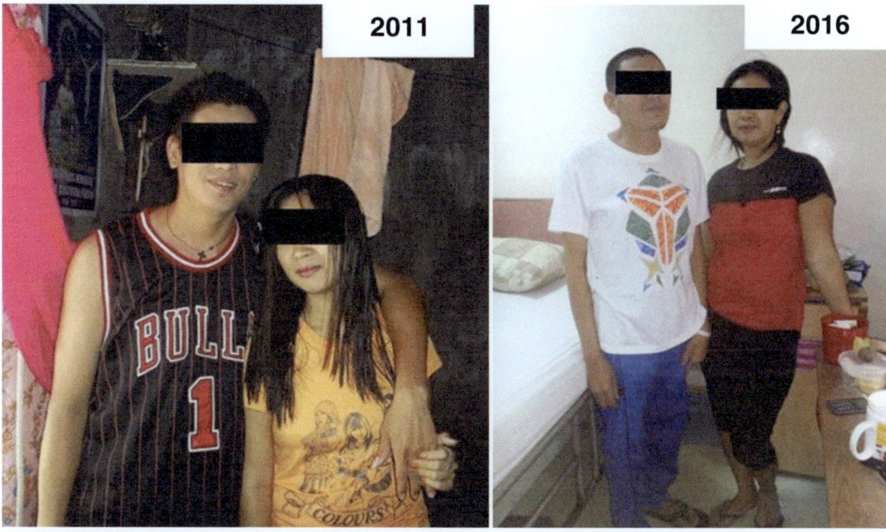

Fig. 11.1 The patient was 175 cm tall, far taller than her wife prior to this illness (2011) (left). By 2016, he is 161 cm and is now only slightly taller than his wife (right). (Courtesy of Dr. Mark Anthony Sandoval)

hip extension and partial knee flexion. He had to hyperextend his cervical spine to have parallel vision. He can ambulate with assistance around the room. Vital signs are as follows: heart rate 92/min, respiratory rate 22/min, BP 130/90 mmHg, and temperature 36.8C. He weighs 55.5 kg. His present height is 161 cm. His known tallest height achieved is 175 cm. He had no neck mass nor goiter. Confrontation testing revealed a normal visual field.

There is a 3 × 3 cm red fleshy soft tissue mass on the floor of the mouth just posterior to the right lateral mandibular incisor and creating a diastema between the right central and lateral mandibular incisors (Fig. 11.2). The mass is not bleeding and had no necrotic areas. When asked, the patient mentioned that this mass has been there for the past 4 years and is not bothering him. He did not initially mention this during the history taking as he thought this had no correlation with his complaints.

There is thoracic kyphosis and pectus carinatum (Fig. 11.3). There is no gynecomastia and no galactorrhea. Pulmonary, cardiac, and abdominal exams are normal. There are no gross deformities of the extremities. There are no subcutaneous masses palpated. There are normal-sized external genitalia with bilaterally descended testes, each approximately 25 g. There is adequate facial, axillary, and pubic hair.

Spine x-ray (Fig. 11.4) showed marked thoracic kyphosis with a Cobb angle of 60° measured from T2 vertebra to T11 vertebra. There were consequent costal and sternal deformities. There is moderate flattening of the superior thoracic vertebrae (vertebra plana). MRI of the spine also demonstrated the exaggerated kyphosis at the thoracic region and also revealed end plate deformities of almost all vertebrae (Fig. 11.5).

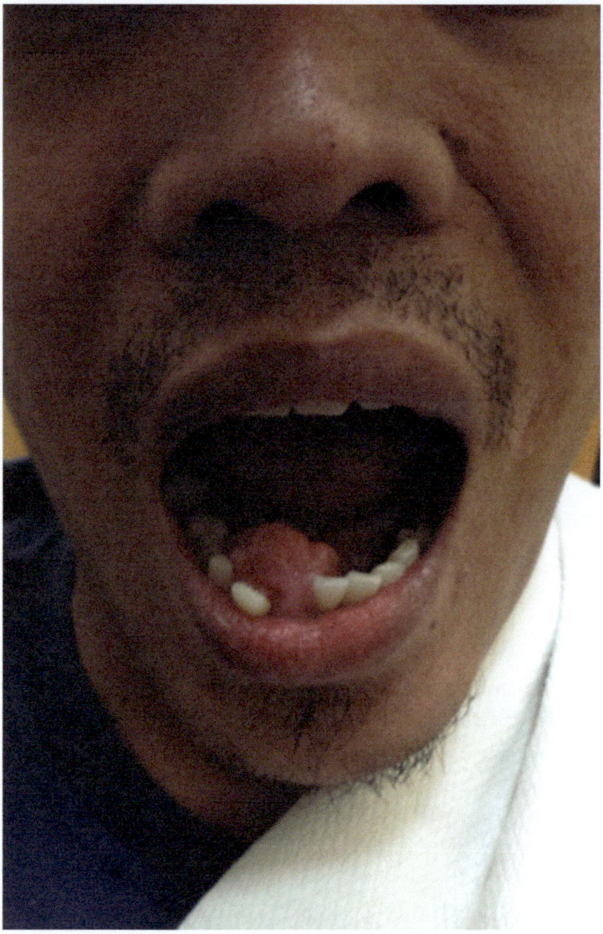

Fig. 11.2 An oral mandibular mass just posterior to the right central and lateral anterior incisors. (From Sandoval et al. [43])

Work-up for metabolic bone disease revealed serum calcium to be in the range of 2.38–2.65 mmol/L (normal 2.10–2.55), while serum phosphorus was low at a range of 0.28–0.64 mmol/L (normal: 0.81–1.49). Serum creatinine was normal at 58.34 umol/L. Intact parathyroid hormone was high at 173.5 pg/mL (normal: 10–65). Alkaline phosphatase was elevated at 243 IU/L (normal: 38–126). Serum testosterone, luteinizing hormone, and prolactin were normal.

Initial consideration was primary hyperparathyroidism based on one elevated serum calcium level, consistently low serum phosphorus, and elevated intact PTH. Attempts to localize the excess PTH were done, but neck ultrasound and parathyroid scintigraphy both failed to show enlarged or hyperfunctioning parathyroid glands.

Serum 25-hydroxy vitamin D was low at 13.86 nmol/L (normal: >80).

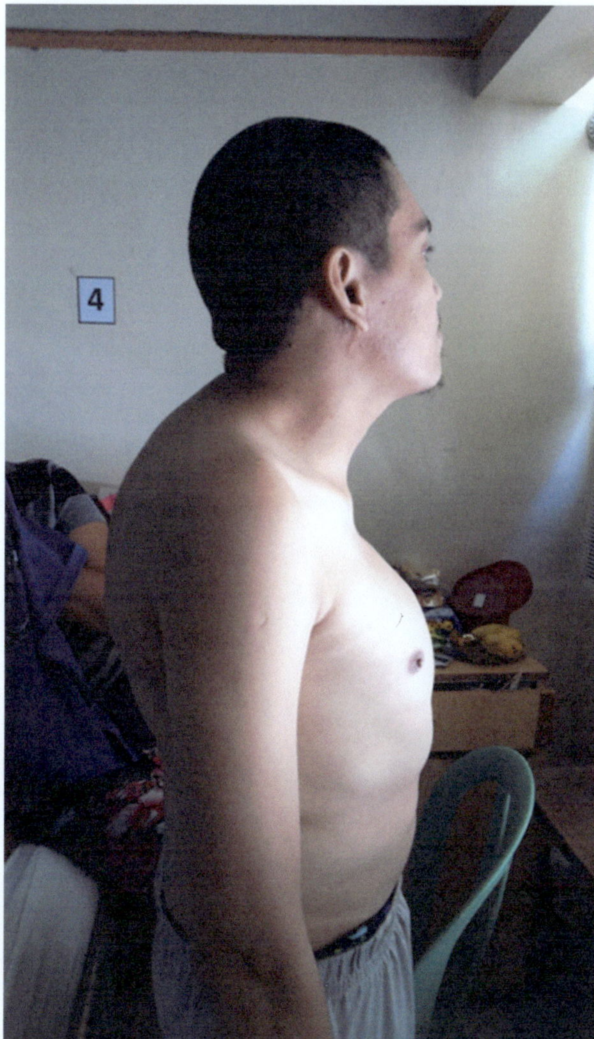

Fig. 11.3 Severe kyphosis with resultant pectus carinatum. (From Sandoval et al. [43])

Skeletal survey x-ray showed generalized osteopenia. There were transverse lucencies traversing part of the cortex oriented at right angles to the long axis of the fourth metacarpals, fourth metatarsals, and ulnae (Fig. 11.6). These are called Looser zones or pseudofractures. There was also endosteal scalloping of the right humerus (Fig. 11.7). These x-ray findings are typical of osteomalacia.

Dual emission x-ray absorption bone densitometry showed markedly low z-scores for the lumbar spine (−4.8), right femoral neck (−5.0), left femoral neck (−4.6), and distal 33% of the left forearm (−4.4%).

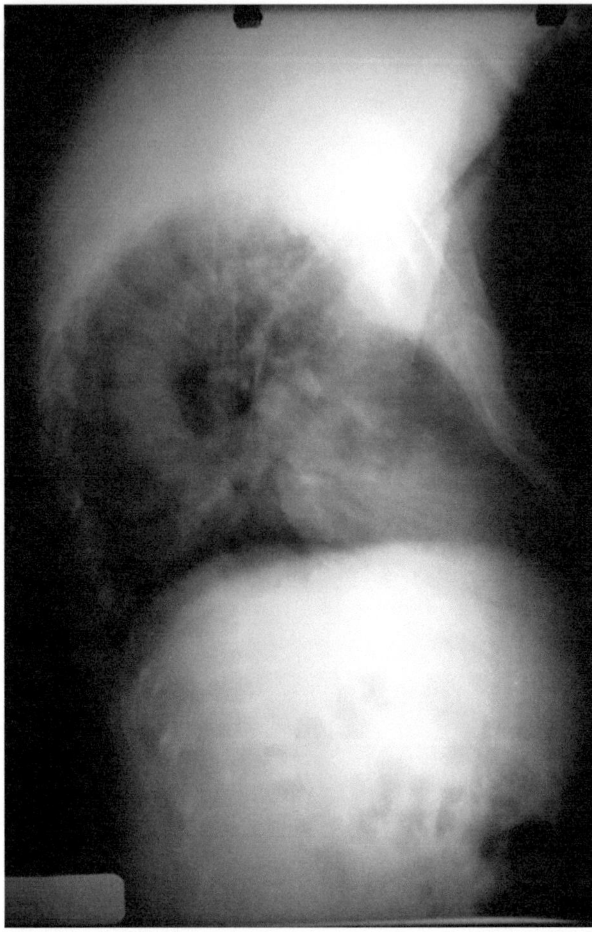

Fig. 11.4 Lateral thoracic spine x-ray showing severe kyphosis. (From Sandoval et al. [43])

Measures of renal phosphate wasting were determined. Tubular phosphate reabsorption (TRP) was 0.8745, while tubular maximum reabsorption of phosphate corrected for glomerular filtration rate (TmP/GFR) was low at 0.54 mmol/L (normal for his sex and age: 1.00–1.35). These results suggest that serum phosphorus is low because of renal phosphate wasting.

Vitamin D deficiency was considered along with the inherited or genetic causes of osteomalacia such as X-linked hypophosphatemic rickets (XLHR), autosomal dominant hypophosphatemic rickets (ADHR), and autosomal recessive hypophosphatemic rickets (ARHR), but the rapid onset of symptoms and the lack of family history of a similar illness made these unlikely.

Incision biopsy of the oral mass was performed with the expectation that it would be an expansile lytic lesion of bone (also known as a brown tumor) which is seen in primary hyperparathyroidism. Microscopic findings, however, showed a hypercel-

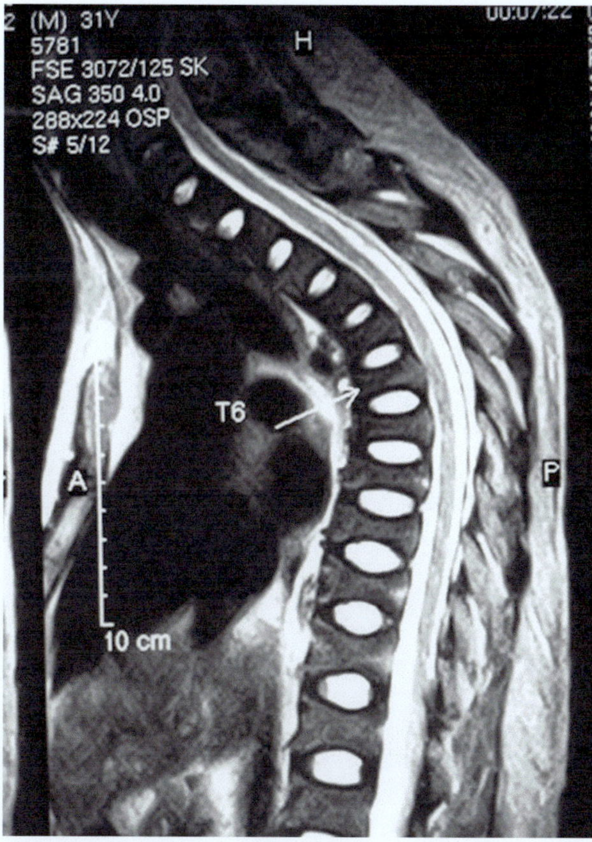

Fig. 11.5 MRI of the thoracic spine (sagittal view) showing severe kyphosis. (From Sandoval et al. [43])

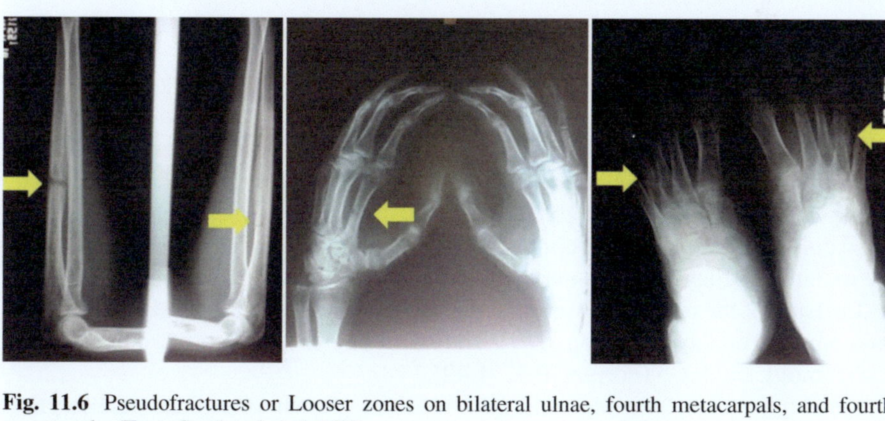

Fig. 11.6 Pseudofractures or Looser zones on bilateral ulnae, fourth metacarpals, and fourth metatarsals. (From Sandoval et al. [43])

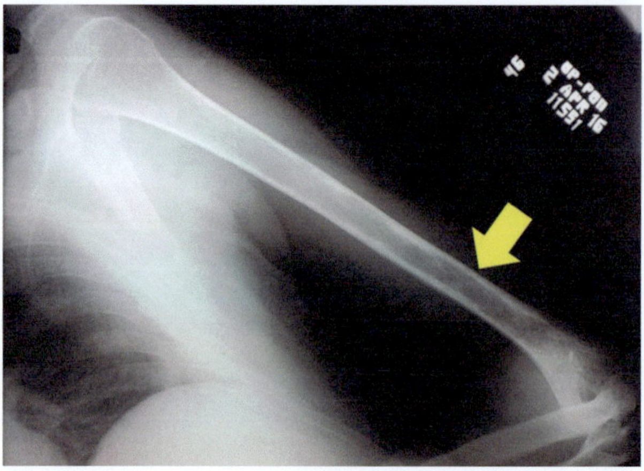

Fig. 11.7 Endosteal scalloping of the right humerus. (From Sandoval et al. [43])

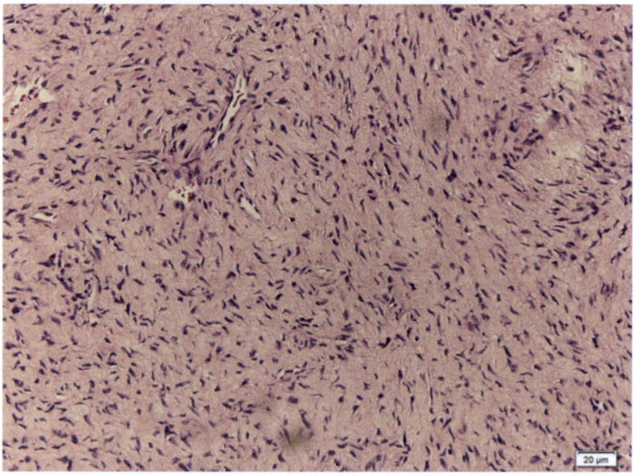

Fig. 11.8 Incision biopsy of the oral mass showing a hypercellular lesion of spindly fibroblasts in a whorl-like or storiform pattern, diagnosed to be a peripheral fibroma. H&E stain, × 200 magnification. (Courtesy of Dr. Mark Anthony Sandoval)

lular lesion composed of spindly fibroblasts arranged in whorl-like or storiform pattern. This was assessed to be a peripheral fibroma (Fig. 11.8).

To prove that the oral mass is the culprit, phosphorus supplementation and administration of cholecalciferol and calcitriol were intentionally withheld. His dietary intake was also not modified. We wanted to observe if renal phosphate wasting would decrease and if serum phosphorus level would increase with removal of the oral mass being the sole intervention.

Excision of the oral mass was done. Serum phosphorus immediately increased to 0.66 mmol/L on day 1 post-op, 0.91 mmol/L on day 2, 1.09 mmol/L on day 3, and 1.06 mmol/L on day 5 (normal: 0.81–1.49).

Renal phosphate wasting was also resolved. Renal phosphate reabsorption increased to normal with TPR increasing to 0.933 and TmP/GFR to 1.1699 mmol/L.

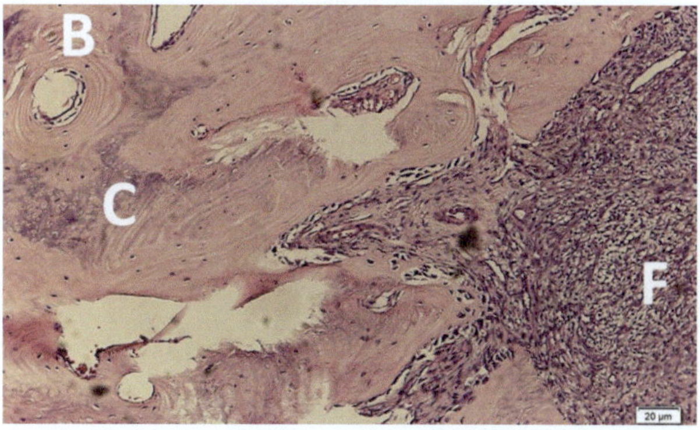

Fig. 11.9 Excision biopsy of the oral mass showing a hypercellular lesion composed of spindly fibroblasts (F) with areas of the cartilage (C) and bone (B). Final histopathologic diagnosis is peripheral ossifying fibroma. H&E, ×100 magnification. (From Sandoval et al. [43])

Resolution of these metabolic parameters after removal of the oral fibroma with no other intervention proves that the oral fibroma is indeed the cause of the hypophosphatemia and hyperphosphaturia. Demonstration of an elevated FGF23 preoperatively and resultant decrease postoperatively will confirm that the tumor does produce FGF23 and that this is the culprit hormone. However, measurement of FGF23 could not be performed as the assay is not available in our country.

Microscopic examination of the excised oral mass showed the same hypercellular lesion composed of spindly fibroblasts in a storiform pattern. There were areas in the tumor that showed the bone and cartilage as well. Final histologic diagnosis is a peripheral ossifying fibroma (Fig. 11.9).

The patient was sent home on calcium ascorbate 150 mg + calcium monohydrogen phosphate 500 mg tablet twice daily and cholecalciferol 7000 IU per day orally.

One month after discharge, bone pains have been resolved making the patient ambulatory again. He can already move around without any assistance and is already able to ride a motorcycle, simple things that he was not able to do before because of the severe bone pains. The kyphosis remains, however. Repeat serum phosphorus taken 2 months postsurgery is normal at 1.49 mmol/L, and 25-hydroxy vitamin D has slightly increased from 13.86 to 20.20 nmol/L.

(Case reprinted from Sandoval et al. [43].)

Epidemiology

The disease affects men and women equally. Being an acquired condition, the affected individuals are usually adults, with the onset usually in the fourth and fifth decades of life. Diagnosis and localization of the offending tumor could be challenging with the average time to diagnosis from the onset of symptoms ranging from 4 to 7 years (see Table 11.1) [26, 28, 55].

Table 11.1 Epidemiologic characteristics of patients with tumor-induced osteomalacia as described in three studies

Characteristics	Jiang et al. [28] Setting: China *n* = 39	Yu et al. [55] Setting: China *n* = 17	Jagtap et al. [26] Setting: India (*n* = 9)
Male: female distribution	19:20	8:9	3:6
Average age at diagnosis, years	42 (range: 20–69)	46.6 (range: 23–67)	37.5 (range: 8–65)
Average time from onset of symptoms to diagnosis, years	6.7 (range: 1.5–28)	4.0 (range 1–20)	7.67 (range: 1–25)

Pathophysiology

The causative tumor secretes a phosphaturic substance or a phosphatonin. This phosphate-excreting hormone has not been identified until 2001 when a team from Japan identified a phosphaturic substance, fibroblast growth factor 23 (FGF23) from a hemangiopericytoma [46].

FGF23 causes low serum phosphate levels in two ways. First, it inhibits the sodium-phosphate cotransporter 2a and 2c (NPT2a and NPT2c) in the proximal tubules of the kidney, causing inhibition of phosphate reabsorption. This then leads to renal phosphate wasting and eventual lowering of serum concentrations of phosphate. Secondly, FGF23 inhibits the enzyme 1 alpha hydroxylase present in the kidneys. This enzyme converts 25-hydroxy vitamin D to the active form 1,25 dihydroxy vitamin D. The inhibition of this enzyme causes low levels of 1,25 (OH)2 vitamin D. Additionally, FGF23 stimulates the enzyme 24-alpha hydroxylase which converts 1,25 dihydroxy vitamin D to 1,24,25 trihydroxy vitamin D which is not active. Thus, the effect on these two enzymes leads to a lower 1,25 dihydroxy vitamin D level which then leads to decreased absorption of phosphorus from the gastrointestinal tract [11, 17].

FGF23 exerts its effects when it attaches to the FGFR1c-aKlotho complex. FGFR1c is a receptor common to several FGFs, but aKlotho is needed as a co-receptor for FGF23 to exert its effects [31].

FGF23 is the most often measured phosphatonin among patients with TIO. FGF7 is also a phosphatonin and has also been found to be elevated in the serum of one particular patient with TIO [5].

There are other molecules which have been experimentally shown to inhibit renal phosphate reabsorption. Hence, they can also be considered as phosphatonins. Secreted frizzled-related protein 4 (sFRP-4) and matrix extracellular phosphoglycoprotein (MEPE) are frequently expressed in causative tumors of patients with TIO. Both have been demonstrated to inhibit sodium-dependent phosphate transport in opossum kidney cells and promoted excretion of phosphate by the kidneys when given to rats [7, 41]. However, elevated levels of these substances have not yet been demonstrated in serum of patients affected with TIO.

When serum phosphate is low, bone formation is impaired since phosphorus, together with calcium, is a component of hydroxyapatite. Impairment of bone for-

Table 11.2 Common symptoms reported by patients with TIO as described in three different studies

	Jiang et al. [28]	Yu et al. [55]	Hu et al. [25]
	$n = 39$	$n = 17$	$n = 14$
Symptom	Frequency	Frequency	Frequency
Muscle weakness/fatigue	100%	100%	64%
Bone pain	100%	100%	86%
Trouble walking/debilitated condition	100%	100%	86%
Pathological fractures/stress fractures	84.6	100%	
Reduced height	64.1%		

mation then leads to the clinical manifestations such as bone pain, bone deformities, and fractures.

Clinical Presentation

Patients with TIO usually manifest with symptoms due to the bone disease and not due to the causative tumor. The causative tumor is usually small, may not be palpable, and does not present with pain or mass effect symptoms.

The most common symptoms are muscle weakness or fatigue, bone pain, and trouble walking (see Table 11.2). Patients may also present with reduced height due to spinal deformities. Fractures, whether clinically apparent or only discovered through radiographs, are also common. Table 11.2 shows the most common symptoms reported by patients with TIO [25, 28, 55].

Laboratory Features

Biochemical

The one laboratory result that will give a clue that the bone disease is of metabolic origin is persistent hypophosphatemia. This finding should trigger the clinician to conduct subsequent tests [21].

Hypophosphatemia is due to renal phosphate wasting. Thus, measures of renal tubular reabsorption of phosphate will be low. Renal tubular reabsorption of phosphate can be expressed either as tubular phosphate reabsorption (TRP) or as tubular maximum reabsorption of phosphate corrected for glomerular filtration rate (TmP/GFR). Both measures require determination of phosphorus and creatinine in both serum and urine. The formulae, derived from Payne [38], are as follows:

$$\text{TRP} = 1 - \frac{\text{Serum creatinine} \times \text{Urine phosphate}}{\text{Urine creatinine} \times \text{Serum phosphate}}$$

The normal range of values for TRP is 85–95%.

The computation of TmP/GFR is dependent on the computed TRP.

If TRP is less than or equal to 0.86,

$$\text{TmP} / \text{GFR} = \text{TRP} \times \text{serum phosphate}$$

If TRP is greater than 0.86,

$$\text{TmP} / \text{GFR} = \text{serum phosphate} \times \frac{0.3 \times \text{TRP}}{1 - (0.8 \times \text{TRP})}$$

When doing these computations, careful attention must be placed to ensure that the levels of phosphate and creatinine in serum and urine are expressed in the same units.

Serum 25-hydroxy vitamin D is normal while serum 1,25 dihydroxy vitamin D is low. This is due to impaired conversion of 25-hydroxy vitamin D to its active form. Serum calcium and creatinine are expected to be normal.

Parathyroid hormone is normal but may be elevated as a compensatory response to the low active vitamin D levels, a condition known as secondary hyperparathyroidism.

Alkaline phosphatase is likewise elevated due to the increased osteoblastic activity that is associated with the condition.

Being the hormone that causes the phosphaturia, FGF23 is expected to be elevated. There was a case, however, that reported that FGF23 measured from a peripheral vein was found to be normal on two determinations. However, FGF23 was found to be high in the vein where the tumor was draining. Specifically, FGF23 was high in the right femoral vein with the causative tumor eventually being localized at the plantar aspect of the right foot. This case teaches that if other indicators point to TIO, the diagnosis must not be abandoned if peripherally circulating levels are found to be normal [3].

Aside from FGF23, another phosphatonin, FGF7, may be elevated. There has been a case wherein both FGF7 and FGF23 are elevated. In this case, selective venous catheterization showed that FGF7 was the more abundant phosphatonin being 9.5 times elevated, while FGF23 was only 1.12 times increased in the femoral vein of the side where the tumor is suspected [5].

Radiologic

Skeletal radiographs will reveal the changes in the bone brought about by the chronically low circulating levels of phosphorus. The most common skeletal changes on radiography are vertebral compression fractures which explain the loss of height experienced by many patients (see Table 11.3).

Table 11.3 Radiographic findings in patients with TIO and their frequency of occurrence

	Jiang et al. [28]	Yu et al. [55]
	$n = 39$	$n = 17$
Radiographic finding	Frequency	Frequency
Vertebral compression fractures	74.4%	58.8%
Pelvis deformities	38.5%	47.1%
Femur fracture		41.2%
Pseudofractures or Looser zones	30.8%	35.3%
Blurred pubic symphysis	10.3%	

Pseudofractures, also known as Looser zones, are linear lucencies of the cortex that are oriented perpendicular to the long axis of the affected bones. These and the other radiographic features in Table 11.3 can also be seen in patients who have osteomalacia from other etiologies. Hence, these are not specific for TIO alone.

Bone Mineral Density

Bone mineral density measured by dual-energy x-ray absorptiometry (DXA) is decreased as a result of deficient mineralization.

Bone Scan

Bone scan using Tc99m methylene diphosphonate may show the characteristic finding in patients with osteomalacia – increased uptake in the costochondral junctions corresponding to the scintigraphic equivalent of the physical examination finding of a rachitic rosary (Fig. 11.10).

Bone scan also shows uptake in multiple sites due to increased osteoblastic activity. It is important to note that these may be confused with bone metastases which appear the same way [47]. It is catastrophic to make a diagnosis of metastatic bone disease in someone who does not harbor cancer but who just complains of bone pains, which is the typical presentation of someone with TIO. Thus, the findings on bone scan must be interpreted depending on the clinical context.

Localization of Tumors

Localization of the causative tumor would be straightforward if the tumor is palpable and in an accessible area. However, only less than half of tumors can be localized by physical examination alone [28]. Table 11.4 shows the location of the tumors

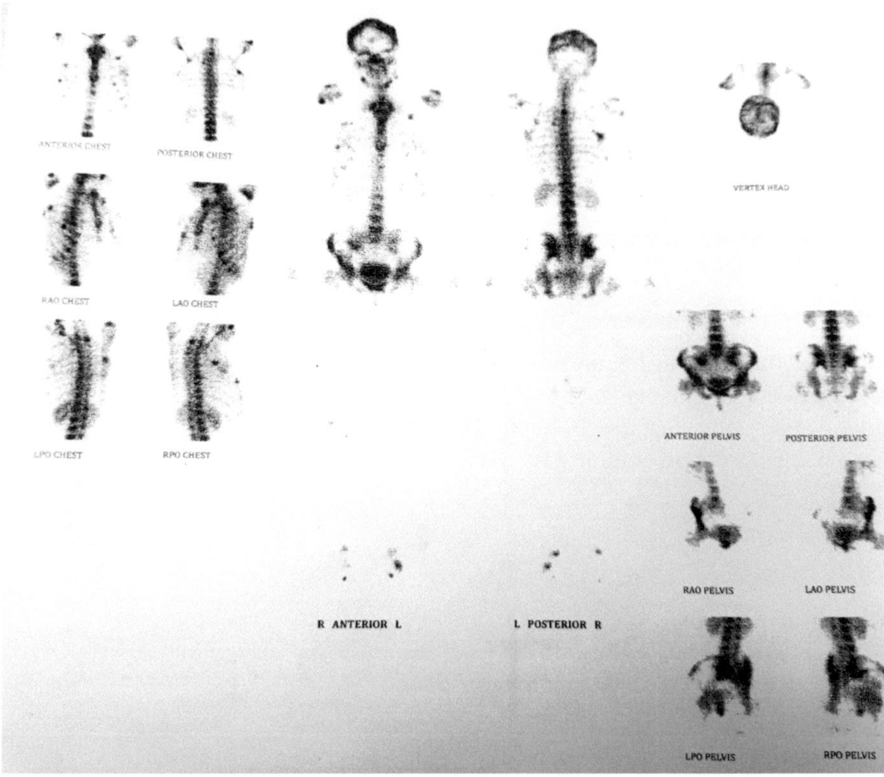

Fig. 11.10 ^{99}m-Technetium-hydroxymethylene diphosphonate bone scintigraphy in tumor-induced osteomalacia showing multiple areas of increased uptake. This appearance can be misinterpreted as multiple bone metastases. Photo credits to Dr. Maria Carrissa Abigail Roxas of the Section of Endocrinology, Diabetes and Metabolism, Department of Medicine, Philippine General Hospital, University of the Philippines Manila, Manila, Philippines

Table 11.4 Location of tumors causing TIO by region of the body

	Jiang et al. [28]	Yu et al. [55]
	$n = 39$	$n = 17$
Location	Frequency	Frequency
Lower extremities	56%	59%
Head	31%	24%
Thorax	5%	
Upper extremities	5%	
Hip	3%	12%
Abdomen		6%

according to region of the body. It must be noted that some tumors may be multifocal or present in more than one site (2% of patients) [23, 28, 42].

It is the tumors' usually occult location and possible multifocality that necessitate the conduct of imaging tests for most patients with suspected TIO.

The tumors may be found in the soft tissue and in the bone. In the soft tissue, they can be found in the heel pad, thigh, and popliteal fossa, among others. When in the bone, they have been found in the acetabulum, greater trochanter, distal femur, fibular head, and vertebral body [4, 18]. When present in the bone, majority of tumors (82%) were in the epiphyses [50]. They can also be found in the craniofacial sinuses [25].

Functional and anatomical imaging tests need to be done to know the location of the tumor. It has been recommended to perform functional imaging tests first followed by anatomical imaging tests, the latter being able to confirm the presence of a mass if functional imaging shows increased focal radiotracer uptake [50] (Fig. 11.11).

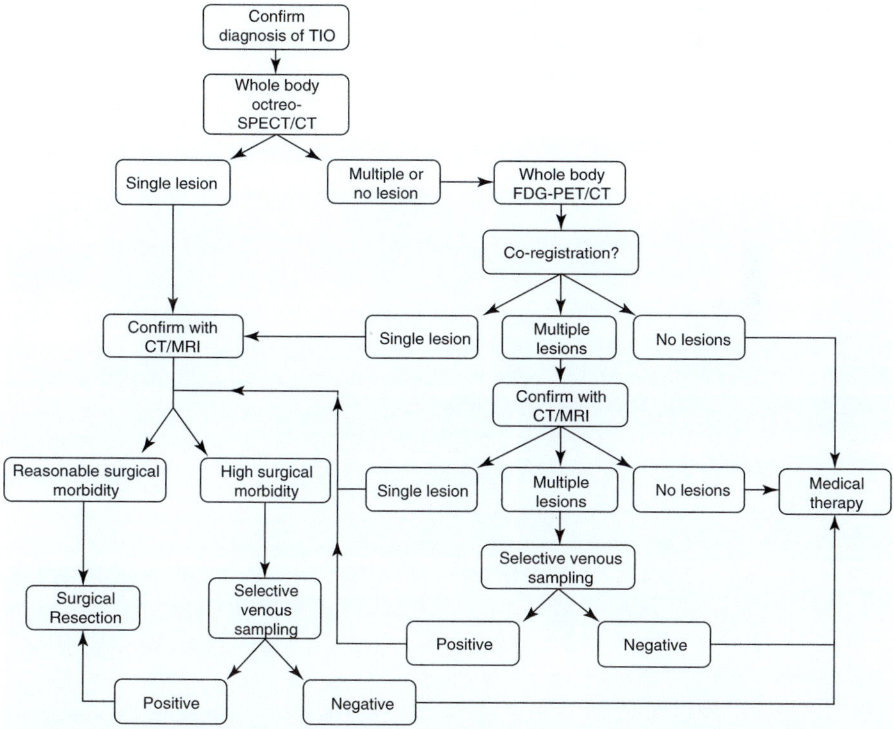

Fig. 11.11 Algorithm for systematic approach to localizing tumors in tumor-induced osteomalacia. After confirming a clinical and biochemical picture of tumor-induced osteomalacia, we recommend obtaining functional imaging as a first step in tumor localization. Octreo-SPECT (SPECT-CT if available) is the recommended initial screening imaging test, as it was shown to have greater specificity and sensitivity than FDG-PET/CT. If a single lesion suspicious for TIO is found and it is confirmed on anatomical imaging and carries a reasonable surgical morbidity, surgical resection is recommended. If multiple lesions or no lesions are found on octreo-SPECT, FDG-PET/CT should follow. This may help to identify a lesion that was not initially seen on octreo-SPECT (as in Fig. 11.3) or help to confirm a lesion seen on octreo-SPECT. If appropriate, proceed to anatomical imaging with CT and/or MRI. If the area with the suspected lesion entails high surgical morbidity, or if multiple lesions are identified, selective venous sampling is recommended to confirm or rule out the tumor. If no lesion is found or a suspected lesion(s) is not confirmed on venous sampling, medical therapy is recommended. (From Chong et al. [9])

Functional Imaging Tests (Figs. 11.12, 11.13, and 11.14)

Functional imaging tests demonstrate uptake by the tumor of a radioisotope-labeled substance. These include scintigraphy, single photon emission computed tomography (SPECT), and positron emission tomography (PET). These functional imaging tests can make use of any of the following radiotracers [2, 20, 22, 27, 28, 29, 50]:

- ^{111}In-pentetreotide
- ^{99m}Tc octreotide
- ^{68}Ga DOTATATE (^{68}Gallium 1,4,7,10-tetraazacyclododecane-1,4,7,10-tetraacetic acid octreotate)
- ^{68}Ga DOTANOC (^{68}Ga 1,4,7,10-tetraazacyclododecane -D-Phe^{1}-1-Nal^{3}-octreotide)
- ^{68}Ga DOTATOC (^{68}Ga 1,4,7,10-Tetraazacyclododecane-N,N,N,N-tetraacetic-acid-D-Phe^{1} -Tyr^{3} –octreotide)

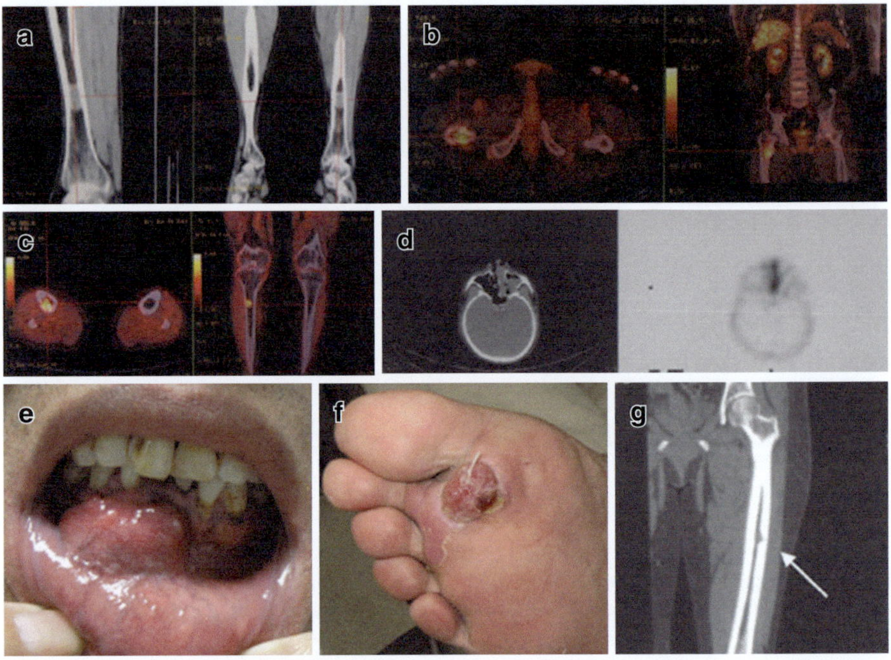

Fig. 11.12 Localization of tumor-induced osteomalacia tumors. (**a**) Patient 9: 18F-fluorodeoxyglucose (^{18}F-FDG) positron emission tomography/computed tomography (PET/CT) (a neoplasm with negative ^{18}F-FDG uptake). (**b**) Patient 2: ^{18}F-FDG-PET/CT (a neoplasm with high ^{18}F-FDG uptake). (**c**) Patient 12: ^{18}F-FDG-PET/CT (a neoplasm with high ^{18}F-FDG uptake). (**d**) Patient 16: ^{99m}Tc-octreotide scintigraphy (a neoplasm in the left nasal cavity). (**e**) Patient 11: physical examination (a neoplasm in the mandible). (**f**) Patient 6: physical examination (a neoplasm in the foot). (**g**) Patient 13: magnetic resonance imaging (a neoplasm in the left femur). (From Yu et al. [55])

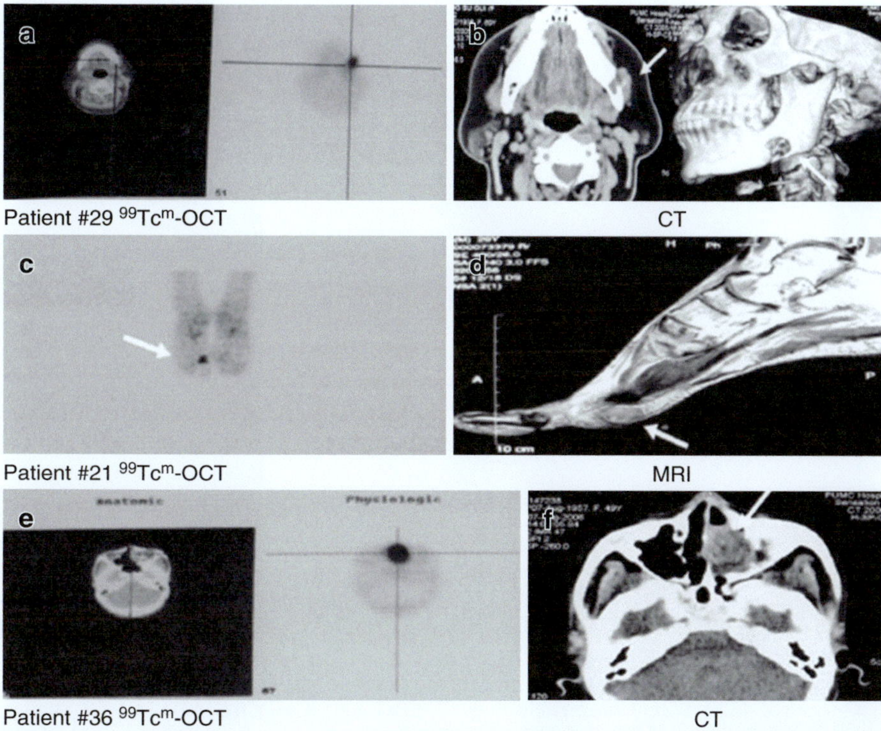

Fig. 11.13 Localization of causative tumors using functional and anatomic imaging modalities. (**a**) shows increased radiotracer uptake on the left jaw using technetium-99 m octreotide scan, while (**b**) shows the same mass as seen on CT scan. (**c**) shows increased radiotracer uptake near the right big toe which was confirmed to be a mass on MRI as seen in (**d**). (**e**) shows increased radiotracer uptake on the left ethmoid area, again confirmed to be a mass in (**f**) by CT scan. (From Jiang et al. [28])

- ^{99m}Tc-HYNIC-TOC (^{99mTc}-Hydrazinonicotinyl-Tyr3-Octreotide)
- 18F-Fluorodeoxyglucose
- ^{99m}Tc MIBI (^{99m}Tc Methoxyisobutylisonitrile)
- ^{201}Th

The first six radiotracers in the list above are octreotide-based. Their utility lies in the fact that causative tumors express the somatostatin receptor. DOTATATE is said to have a high affinity for SSTR2 which is the type predominantly expressed in causative tumors. In fact, it has been suggested that ^{68}Ga DOTATATE may be a better radioisotope than ^{18}F fluorodeoxyglucose when performing PET/computed tomography (CT) since there were tumors that did not take up ^{18}F FDG but took up ^{68} Ga DOTATATE [2, 14, 24].

A practical advice to follow is to make sure that the entire body be included in the functional imaging procedure, from head to toe and to include the elbows, hands, knees, and feet since the causative tumor may be in these areas (Agarwal et al. 2015; [10, 32]).

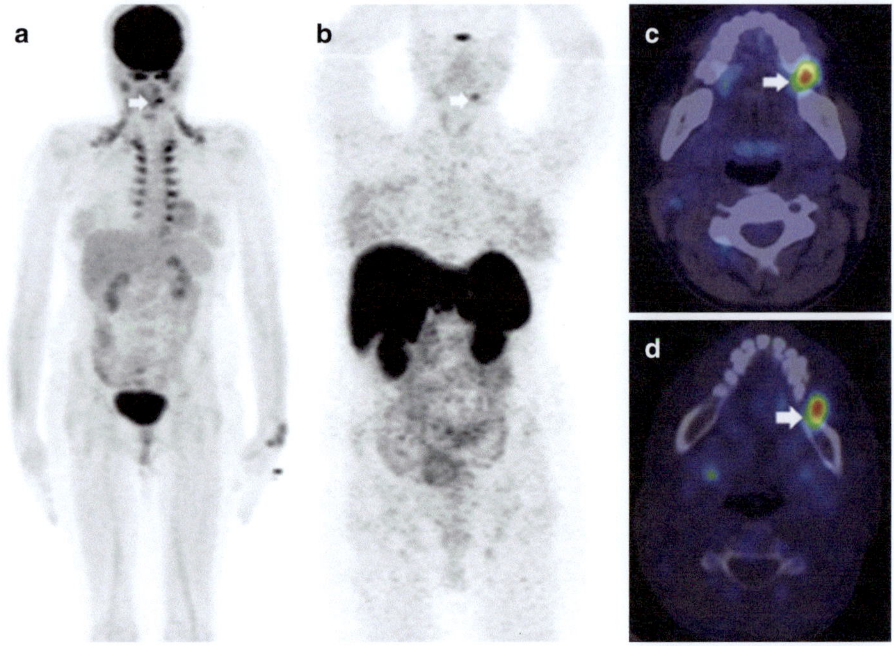

Fig. 11.14 A 30-year-old woman with generalized body pain and weakness for 3 years and FGF-23 C-terminal 452.6 RU/mL underwent both ^{18}F-FDG and ^{68}Ga DOTATATE PET/CT studies. ^{18}F-FDG-PET/CA (**a**) and ^{68}Ga DOTATATE PET/CT (**b**) MIP images show focus of abnormal tracer uptake on the left side of the chin (arrow). ^{18}F-FDG-PET/CT (**c**) and ^{68}Ga DOTATATE PET/CT (**d**) transaxial-fused images localize the abnormal uptake to an ill-defined lesion in the left second molar region in the mandible (arrow). Subsequently guided MRI was performed, which showed lytic lesion in the mandible corresponding to the PET abnormality. Histopathology from the mandibular lesion was consistent with ameloblastic fibroma, a neoplasm of odontogenic epithelium and mesenchymal tissues. (From Agrawal et al. [2])

Functional imaging using ^{99m}Tc octreotide scan may give false-positive results in cases where there is inflammation or fractures. Inflammation may give a false-positive result since the somatostatin receptor can also be found in lymphocytes. Thus, it is prudent to do anatomical imaging as well to confirm the presence of a mass since patients with TIO are already prone to fractures by virtue of decreased mineralization.

Anatomical Imaging Tests

Anatomical imaging tests include ultrasound, computed tomography (CT) scan, and magnetic resonance imaging (MRI). Concordance of the findings of anatomical and imaging tests is 95–100% [28].

Selective Venous Catheterization

In cases where the findings on functional and anatomical imaging remain inconclusive, selective venous catheterization with measurement of FGF23 can help localize the tumors [16]. This procedure relies on the fact that each of our body's veins has a defined area of the body from which it receives deoxygenated blood. Measurement of a high level of the hormone in a specific vein gives away the site of the source of the excess hormone. Veins which show FGF23 values that are at least 1.6× higher than that of the general circulation represent the venous drainage of the causative tumor [4] (Figs. 11.15 and 11.16).

It has been proposed that selective venous sampling be done in patients with only one tumor on anatomical imaging but for which surgery carries a significant morbidity, or for patients with multiple tumors on imaging in order to demonstrate which of these are hormonally overfunctioning [9].

Etiology

The causative tumors range in size from as small as 1 cm to as large as 14 cm, with a median greatest diameter of 3 cm [25]. The causative tumors are of varied histologies but they are usually mesenchyme-derived. Immunoreactivity to vimentin proves their mesenchymal origin (Weidner et al. 1987).

A pathologic study of 17 tumors that were associated with osteomalacia showed that these tumors can be grouped into four categories according on their histologic features: phosphaturic mesenchymal tumor, osteoblastoma-like, nonossifying fibroma-like, and ossifying fibroma-like. The first category, PMT, was composed of primitive-appearing spindle-shaped cells. The tumor stroma contained microcystic structures, clusters of osteoclast-like giant cells, blood vessels, and areas of the poorly developed cartilage and bone. The tumors in the last three categories can be classified based on their histologic resemblance with the other known mesenchymal tumors (Weidner et al. 1987; [53]).

Up to two-thirds of tumors causing TIO are classified pathologically as phosphaturic mesenchymal tumors [25] (Fig. 11.17). Table 11.5 shows the various histologic types of tumors that have been shown to cause TIO.

There are also individual case reports that showed the following as causing TIO as well: [4, 12, 26, 27, 30, 34–36, 44, 51]

- Anaplastic thyroid cancer [1]
- Angiofibroma
- Angiolipoma
- B-cell non-Hodgkin's lymphoma
- Chondroblastoma
- Chondrosarcoma

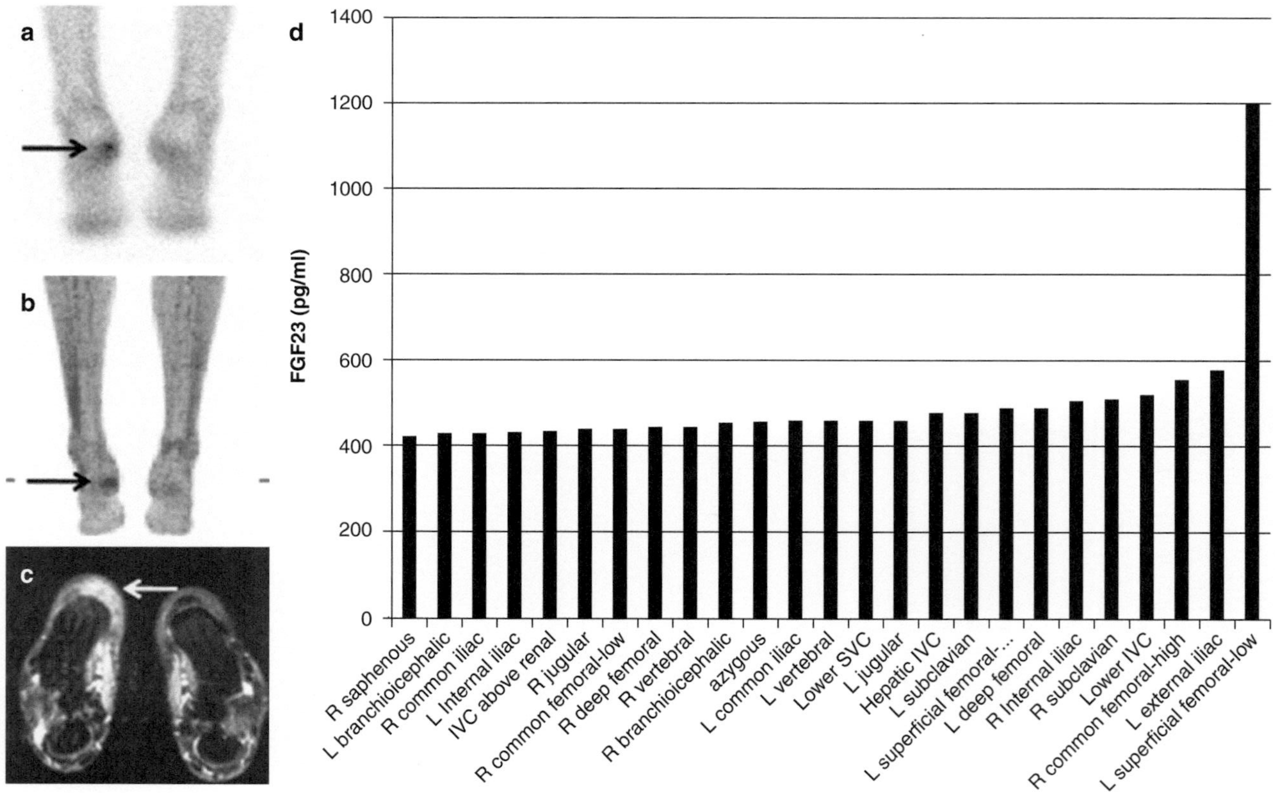

Fig. 11.15 Example of a positive result on selective venous sampling. A suspicious lesion was identified by indium-111 pentetreotide scintigraphy (**a**) and FDG-PET scan (**b**) that correlated with an ill-defined lesion in the flat pad of the heel on MRI (**c**). Surgical removal of the fat pad would entail an extensive procedure that involved the translocation of a vascularized muscle flap from the arm. The results of the selective venous sampling measurements of FGF-23, which confirmed that the lesion was the FGF-23-secreting lesion, are shown (**d**). The tumor is indicated by arrows. (From Andreopoulou et al. [4])

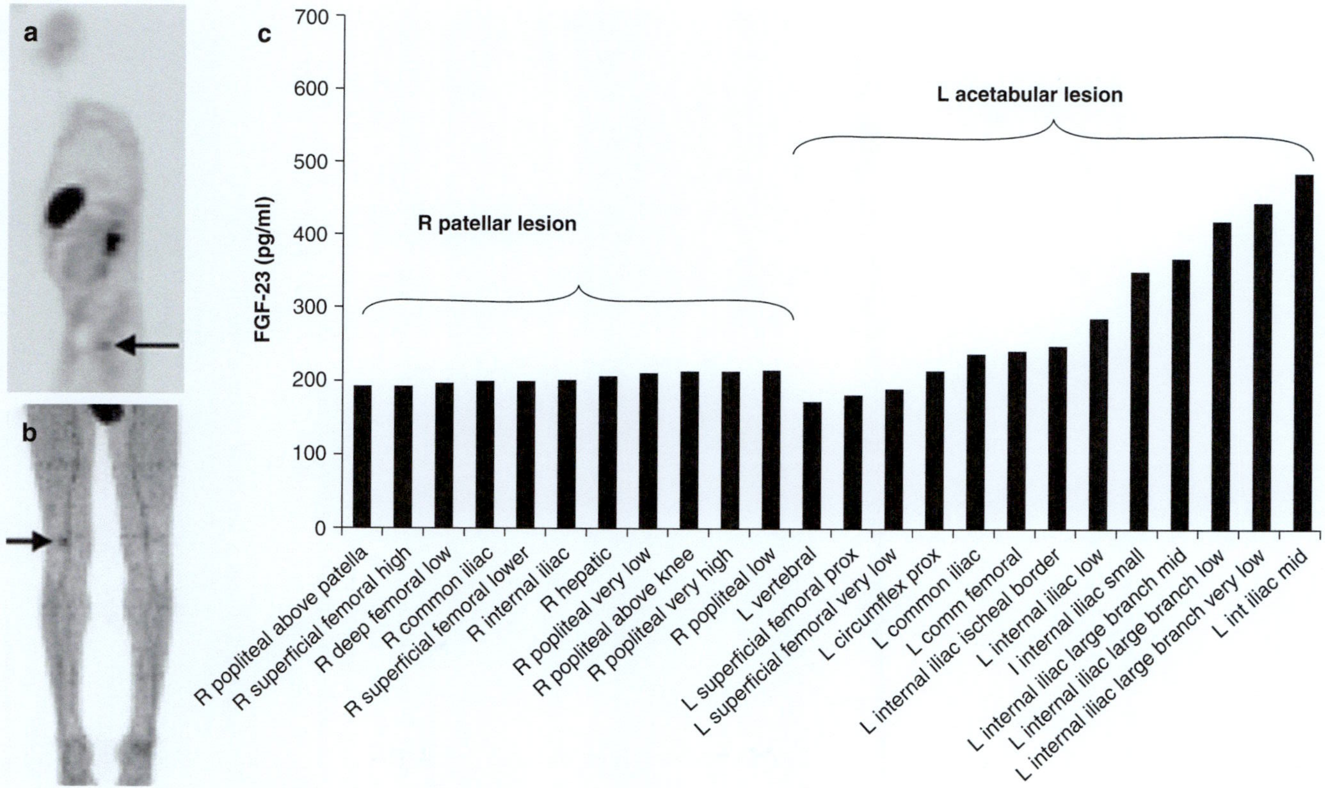

Fig. 11.16 Example of a venous sampling that distinguished between multiple positive images. FDG-PET imaging identified suspicious lesions in both the acetabulum (**a**) and the patella (**b**) that were suspicious for the FGF-23-secreting tumor. The results of the selective venous sampling measurements of FGF-23 (**c**) confirmed that the lesion in the acetabulum was the FGF-23-secreting tumor. The suspicious lesions are indicated by the arrows. This was confirmed by surgical removal and resolution of hypophosphatemia. (From Andreopoulou et al. [4])

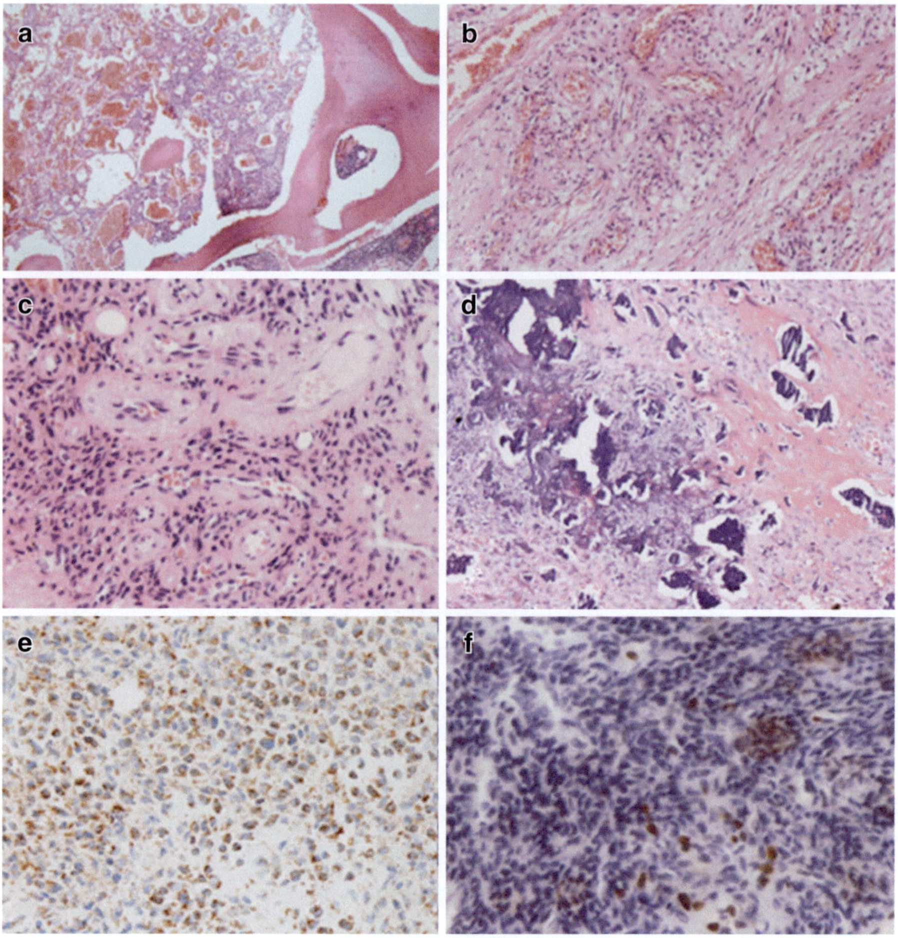

Fig. 11.17 (**a–f**) Tumor-induced osteomalacia histopathology. (**a**) The tumor cells infiltrated between bone trabeculae (×100). (**b**) Tumor cells were very bland, spindle to stellate in shape (×100). (**c**) A very well-developed capillary network was typically present (×100). (**d**) The matrix of the tumor was calcified in an unusual "grungy" fashion (×100). (**e**) Tumor cells were positive for FGF-23 (×200). (**f**) Some tumor cells were positive for Ki67 (×400). (From Wang et al. [50])

Table 11.5 Histologic types of tumors that cause TIO and their frequency [25]

Histology	Frequency
Phosphaturic mesenchymal tumor (PMT)	69%
Phosphaturic mesenchymal tumor, mixed connective tissue variant (PMTMCT)	15%
Odontogenic fibroma	8%
Hemangiopericytoma	3%
Giant cell tumor of a tendon	3%
Malignant tumors (2 PMTs and 1 PMTMCT)	8%

- Dermatofibroma
- Epidermal nevus
- Fibroma
- Fibrosarcoma
- Fibrous histiocytoma, both benign and malignant forms
- Giant cell tumor
- Glomangiopericytoma
- High-grade serous ovarian carcinoma
- Neurilemmoma
- Neurofibroma
- Osteoblastoma
- Osteosarcoma
- Prostate carcinoma
- Schwannoma
- Sclerosing hemangiomas
- Small cell carcinoma of the lung
- Unicameral bone cyst

Most tumors mentioned above are benign in behavior and histology. However, there are observations of tumors which are histologically benign but behave aggressively characterized by multiple recurrences. A tumor described by Yavropoulou et al. [54] expressed receptors for other growth factors, namely, platelet-derived growth factor (PDGF) and vascular endothelial growth factor (VEGF), which may have made it behave aggressively.

It must be emphasized that the presence of a phosphaturic mesenchymal tumor may not necessarily result to hypophosphatemia and osteomalacia [52]. In fact, there are cases wherein a PMT even expressed FGF23 mRNA, yet the patient did not have osteomalacia [13].

Treatment

Surgery

Complete removal of the causative tumor by surgery cures the disease.

When present in long bones, curettage and segmental resection are two surgical options (Fig. 11.18). Curettage is the surgical choice when removal of the tumor will result to significant postoperative morbidity for the patient such as when it could lead to impairment of joint function. Otherwise, segmental resection is the preferred approach. Both curettage and segmental resection lead to similar rates of complete resection (67% and 80%, respectively). However, recurrence rate was higher in those who underwent curettage (50%) compared to those who underwent segmental resection (0%) [50].

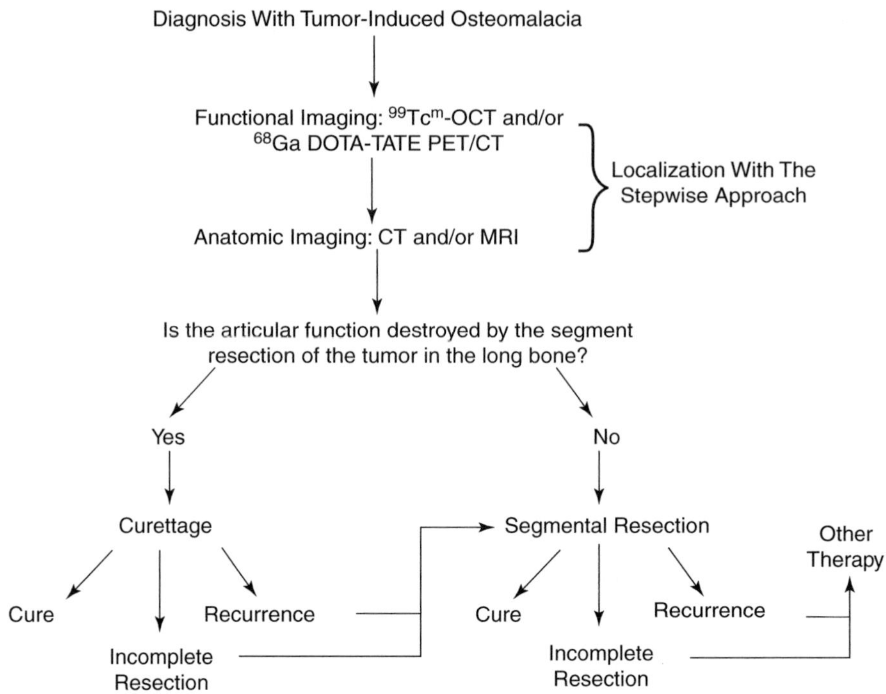

Fig. 11.18 Flowchart showing surgical treatments of tumor-induced osteomalacia lesions in long bones. (From Wang et al. [50])

In patients in whom FGF23 can be measured before and after resection of the causative tumor, FGF23 normalizes in as short as 2–24 h, since the half-life of FGF23 is only 45 min [33]. Normalization of serum phosphorus then follows, occurring within 2–5 days after surgery. Ninety percent of patients will have normal serum phosphorus levels after 5 days from surgery [28] (Figs. 11.19 and 11.20). In cases where complete resection is not achieved, serum phosphorus remains low suggesting continued oversecretion of FGF23.

Pharmacologic

In patients who cannot undergo surgery or where complete resection of the causative tumor is not possible, there are several pharmacologic agents which can be used.

Administration of phosphorus can increase serum phosphorus levels, but high doses are not tolerated due to the occurrence of diarrhea. Calcitriol, being the active form of vitamin D that is decreased in TIO patients, is also helpful in normalizing serum phosphorus levels by increasing intestinal phosphate absorption. Intravenous

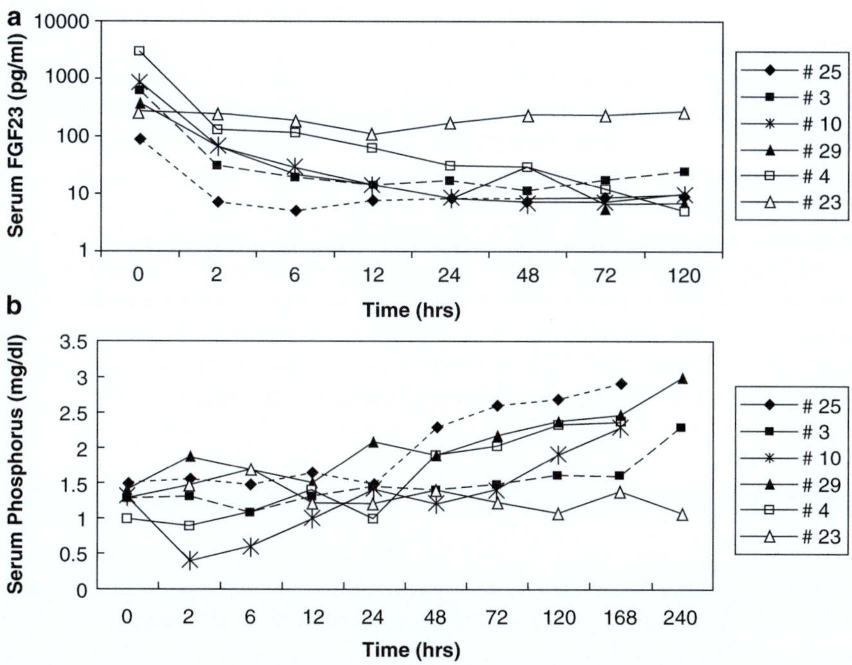

Fig. 11.19 Changes in serum FGF-23 and phosphorus concentrations before and after surgery in six TIO Chinese patients. Note: the normal range for serum FGF-23 10–50 pg/mL,(101,103) for serum phosphorus 2.2–4.2 mg/dL. (From Jiang et al. [28])

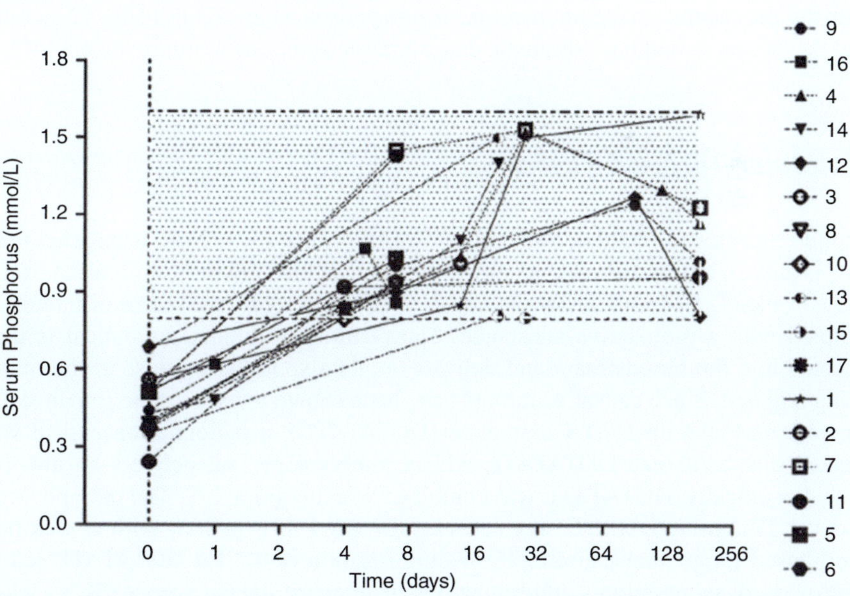

Fig. 11.20 Changes in serum phosphorus concentrations before and after surgery in 17 Chinese tumor-induced osteomalacia patients. The *shaded area* represents the normal range for serum phosphorus concentration. (From Yu et al. [55])

dipyridamole, a known vasodilator, can also be an option since it reduces fractional excretion of phosphorus and increases TmP/GFR. However, it did not result to an increase in serum phosphate levels [37]. Octreotide inhibits FGF23 secretion since tumors causing TIO express the somatostatin receptor, which is also the reason why they light up on octreotide scintigraphy. Octreotide has been shown to decrease renal phosphate excretion, increase the threshold for renal tubular reabsorption of phosphate, and increase serum phosphate levels [45]. Cinacalcet has also been tried successfully in patients with TIO. It inhibits parathyroid hormone (PTH) secretion and leads to a reduction in renal phosphate excretion. Thus, this led to a reduction in the dose of phosphorus supplementation needed to maintain normal or near-normal serum phosphorus levels. It is important to emphasize, however, that cinacalcet does not suppress FGF23 production by the causative tumor. The resulting decrease in PTH level only eased the phosphaturia in TIO patients [19].

Tumor-Directed Therapy

CT-guided percutaneous ethanol and cryoablation is also an option for patients in whom the location of the tumor will make surgery very debilitating. In this procedure, a cannula is guided into the lesion using an imaging modality, in this case a CT scan, and it is through this cannula that ethanol is administered and a cryoablation probe is introduced. Cryoablation therapy is carried out using the freeze-thaw-freeze procedure for 10 min–5 min–10 min. This method has been shown to promptly decrease FGF23 levels and normalize serum phosphate levels. Successful treatment with this procedure can maintain normal serum phosphate levels until after 12 months, and the patient would have dramatic densitometric and clinical improvement [48].

Molecular-Targeted Therapy

Peptide receptor radionuclide therapy (PRRT), a form of molecular-targeted therapy, is also an option for patients in whom the causative tumor is difficult to excise fully. In PRRT, a peptide known to attach or be taken up by the tumor of interest is coupled with a radioactive substance. The resulting radiopharmaceutical is then injected into the bloodstream and delivers an ablative radiation dose to the tumor being targeted. Since causative tumors have been shown to express the somatostatin receptor and take up DOTA octreotate (DOTATATE), a radiopharmaceutical was created that combines DOTATATE with a radioisotope that delivers an ablative dose. Specifically, DOTATATE was combined with lutetium-177. The radiopharmaceutical 177Lu-DOTATATE was successfully tried in a patient with a recurrent skull-based tumor that caused TIO. Administration of 177Lu-DOTATATE led to improvement in symptoms and reductions in standard uptake values (SUV) when surveillance PET scans using ^{18}F-FDG and ^{68}Ga DOTATATE were serially done [6].

Anti-FGF23 Antibody

A promising treatment option is the administration of anti-FGF23 antibody. A phase 2 clinical study is already underway investigating the effects of KRN23, a humanized anti-FGF23 antibody, on patients with TIO. Preliminary data show that this anti-FGF23 antibody increased serum phosphorus, TmP/GFR, and 1,25 dihydroxy vitamin D after 24 weeks of monthly subcutaneous administration [8, 15].

A phase I randomized placebo-controlled clinical trial has already been done among patients with X-linked hypophosphatemic rickets (XLHR) who also have elevated FGF23 levels similar to patients with TIO. In this particular study, KRN23, a humanized anti-FGF23 antibody, has been demonstrated to increase maximum renal tubular threshold for phosphate reabsorption, serum phosphate, and 1,25 dihydroxy vitamin D levels in human subjects. Intravenous and subcutaneous routes are both effective. Intravenous administration has a faster onset of action but has a shorter duration of effect, while subcutaneous administration resulted in a slower onset of action but a more sustained duration of effect. It may just be a matter of time that anti-FGF23 antibody therapy be used and found effective in patients with TIO as well (Carpenter et al. 2014; [15]).

Prognosis

As mentioned earlier, the reduction in FGF23 and normalization of serum phosphate levels occur in just a matter of days after successful removal of the causative tumor. These can be maintained if the disease does not recur.

With longer follow-up after successful resection, bone pain can be expected to disappear in 1–2 months, while patients can already be expected to walk by 0.5–3.5 months [25].

If radiographic changes are monitored, Looser zones or pseudofractures are expected to resolve in as short as 6 months. From being radiolucent linear lesions, these become mineralized as shown by a radiopaque appearance (Fig. 11.21) [39, 56].

Dual emission x-ray absorptiometry can also be repeated with normalization of bone density being expected in as short as 16 weeks (Fig. 11.22) [39, 40].

Summary

- Tumor-induced osteomalacia is an acquired disease of the bone that occurs due to oversecretion of the phosphaturic hormone FGF23 by a functioning tumor.
- Clinical features are similar to other causes of osteomalacia such as bone pains, bone deformities, and bone weakness.

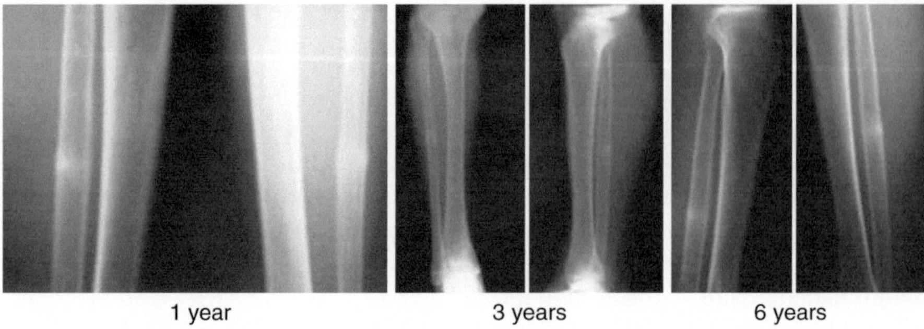

Fig. 11.21 Radiography of the right leg 1, 3, and 6 years after tumor resection. A sclerotic focal area deforming the cortical profile of the middle third of the right fibula can be seen on both anterior-posterior and lateral projections. (From Piemonte et al. [39])

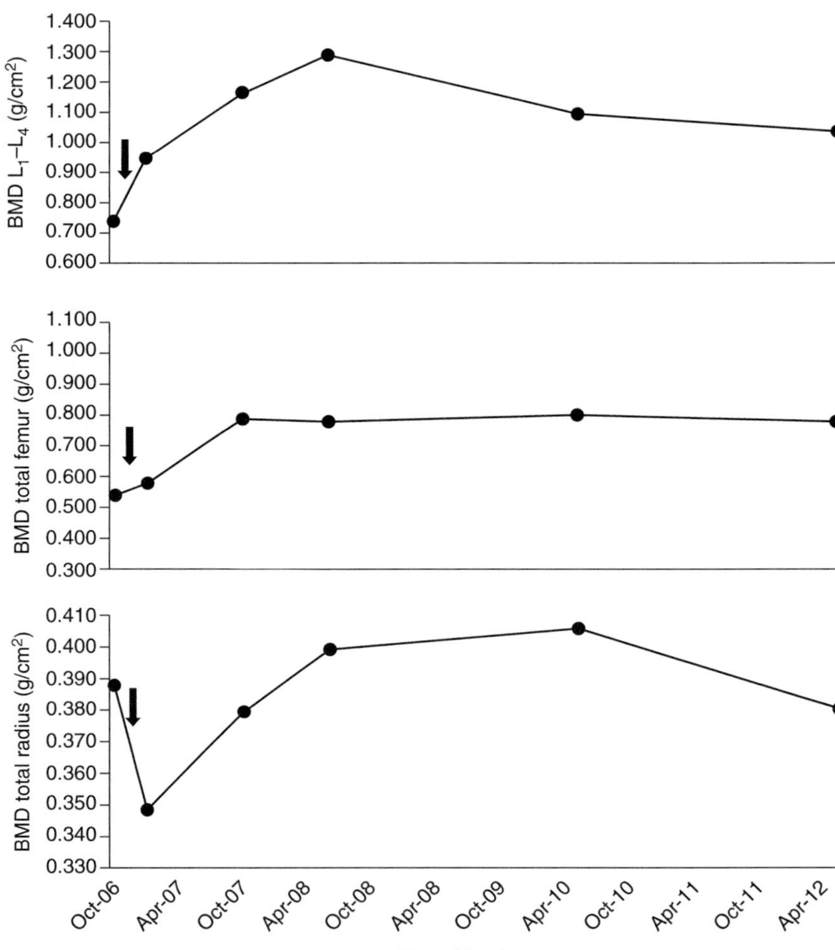

Fig. 11.22 Changes of lumbar, femoral, and radial BMD after tumor resection. The arrow indicates the date of surgery. (From Piemonte et al. [39])

- Laboratory hallmarks are hypophosphatemia, phosphaturia, and low 1,25 dihydroxy vitamin D.
- The causative tumor must be located by a combination of physical examination and functional and anatomical imaging tests.
- Cure is possible and prognosis is favorable when the causative tumor is excised.
- When surgery is not possible or carries significant postoperative morbidity, a variety of pharmacologic agents and tumor-directed therapies can be employed.

References

1. Abate EG, Bernet V, Cortese C, Garner HW. Tumor induced osteomalacia secondary to anaplastic thyroid carcinoma: a case report and review of the literature. Bone Rep. 2016;5:81–5. https://doi.org/10.1016/j.bonr.2015.11.004.
2. Agrawal K, Bhadala S, Mittal BR, Shukla J, Sood A, Bhattacharya A, et al. Comparison of 18F-FDG and 68Ga DOTATATE PET/CT in localization of tumor causing oncogenic osteomalacia. Clin Nucl Med. 2015;40(1):e6–e10.
3. Amblee A, Uy J, Senseng C, Hart P. Tumor-induced osteomalacia with normal systemic fibroblast growth factor-23 level. Clin Kidney J. 2014;7:186–9. https://doi.org/10.1093/ckj/sfu004.
4. Andreopoulou P, Dumitrescu CE, Kelly MH, Brillante BA, Cutler Peck CM, Wodajo FM, et al. Selective venous catheterization for the localization of phosphaturic mesenchymal tumors. J Bone Miner Res. 2011;26(6):1295–302. https://doi.org/10.1002/jbmr.316.
5. Bansal S, Khazim K, Suri R, Martin D, Werner S, Fanti P. Tumor induced osteomalacia: associated with elevated circulating levels of fibroblast growth factor-7 in addition to fibroblast growth factor-23. Clin Nephrol. 2015; https://doi.org/10.5414/CN108596.
6. Basu S, Fargose P. 177Lu-DOTATATE PRRT as promising new treatment approach in recurrent skull base phosphaturic mesenchymal tumor causing paraneoplastic oncogenic osteomalacia: a potential therapeutic application of PRRT beyond NET. J Nucl Med Technol. First published online September 15. 2016; https://doi.org/10.2967/jnmt.116.177873.
7. Berndt TJ, Schiavi S, Kumar R. "Phosphatonins" and the regulation of phosphorus homeostasis. Am J Physiol Ren Physiol. 2005;289:F1170–82. https://doi.org/10.1152/ajprenal.00072.2005.
8. Carpenter TO, Miller PD, Weber TJ, Peacock M, Ruppe MD, Insogna K, Osei S, Luca D, Skrinar A, San Martin J, Jan de Beur S. Effects of KRN23, an ant-FGF23 antibody on patients with tumor-induced osteomalacia and epidermal nevus syndrome: results from an ongoing phase 2 study. 2016. http://www.ultragenyx.com/file.cfm/22/docs/Carpenter_2016_ASBMR_Oral_TIO_Final.pdf. Accessed 8 Jan 2017.
9. Chong WH, Andreoupoulou P, Chen CC, Reynolds J, Guthrie L, Kelly M, et al. Tumor localization and biochemical response to cure in tumor-induced osteomalacia. J Bone Miner Res. 2013;28(6):1386–98. https://doi.org/10.1002/jbmr.1881.
10. Chong WH, Yavuz S, Patel SM, Chen CC, Collins MT. The importance of whole body imaging in tumor-induced osteomalacia. J Clin Endocrinol Metab. 2011;96(12):3599–600. https://doi.org/10.1210/jc.2011-1757.
11. Drezner MK, Feinglos MN. Osteomalacia due to a 1a,25-dihydroxycholecalciferol deficiency: association with a giant cell tumor of bone. J Clin Invest. 1977;60:1046–53.
12. Elderman JH, Wabbijn M, de Jongh F. Hypophosphataemia due to FGF-23 producing B cell non-Hodgkin's lymphoma. BMJ Case Rep. 2016; https://doi.org/10.1136/bcr-2015-213954.
13. Ellis MB, Gridley D, Lal S, Nair GR, Feiz-Irfan I. Phosphaturic mesenchymal tumor of the brain without tumor-induced osteomalacia in an 8-year-old girl: case report. J Neurosurg Pediatr. 2016; https://doi.org/10.3171/2015.9.PEDS14617.
14. El-Maouche D, Sadowski SM, Papadakis GZ, Guthrie L, Cottle-Delisie C, Merkel R, et al. 68Ga-DOTATATE for tumor localization in tumor induced osteomalacia. J Clin Endocrinol Metab. 2016;101(10):3575–81. https://doi.org/10.1210/jc.2016-2052.

15. Fukumoto S. Anti-fibroblast growth factor 23 antibody therapy. Curr Opin Nephrol Hypertens. 2014a;23(4):346–51. https://doi.org/10.1097/01.mnh.0000447012.98357.da.
16. Fukumoto S. Diagnostic modalities for FGF23-producing tumors in patients with tumor-induced osteomalacia. Endocrinol Metab. 2014b;29:136–43. https://doi.org/10.3803/EnM.2014.29.2.136.
17. Fukumoto S. FGF23: phosphate metabolism and beyond. IBMS BoneKey. 2010;7(8):268–78. https://doi.org/10.1138/20100458.
18. Gandhi GY, Shah AA, Wu KJ, Gupta V, Shoraka AR. Tumor-induced osteomalacia caused by primary fibroblast growth factor 23 secreting neoplasm in axial skeleton: a case report. Case Rep Endocrinol. 2012; https://doi.org/10.1155/2012/185454.
19. Geller JL, Khosravi A, Kelly MH, Riminucci M, Adams JS, Collins MT. Cinacalcet in the management of tumor-induced osteomalacia. J Bone Miner Res. 2007;22(6):931–7. https://doi.org/10.1359/JBMR.070304.
20. Haeusler G, Freilinger M, Dominkus M, Egerbacher M, Amann G, Kolb A, et al. Tumor-induced hypophosphatemic rickets in an adolescent boy—clinical presentation, diagnosis, and histological findings in growth plate and muscle tissue. J Clin Endocrinol Metab. 2010;95(10):4511–7. https://doi.org/10.1210/jc.2010-0543.
21. Halperin F, Anderson RJ, Mulder JE. Tumor-induced osteomalacia: the importance of measuring serum phosphorus levels. Nat Clin Pract Endocrinol Metab. 2007;3(10):721–5. https://doi.org/10.1038/ncpendmet0639.
22. Hesse E, Moessinger E, Rosenthal H, Laenger F, Brabant G, Thorsten P, et al. Oncogenic osteomalacia: exact tumor localization by co-registration of positron emission and computed tomography. J Bone Miner Res. 2006;22(1):158–62. https://doi.org/10.1359/JBMR.060909.
23. Higley M, Beckett B, Schmahmann S, Dacey E, Foss E. Locally aggressive and multifocal phosphaturic mesenchymal tumors: two unusual cases of tumor-induced osteomalacia. Skelet Radiol. 2015; https://doi.org/10.1007/s00256-015-2246-x.
24. Ho CL. Ga68-DOTA peptide PET/CT to detect occult mesenchymal tumor-inducing osteomalacia: a case series of three patients. Nucl Med Mol Imaging. 2015;49:231–6. https://doi.org/10.1007/s13139-015-0328-2.
25. Hu F, Jiang C, Zhang Q, Shi H, Wei L, Wang Y, et al. Quantitative ELISA-like immunohistochemistry of fibroblast growth factor 23 in diagnosis of tumor-induced osteomalacia and clinical characteristics of the disease. Dis Markers. 2016:3176978. https://doi.org/10.1155/2016/3176978.
26. Jagtap VS, Sarathi V, Lila AR, Malhotra G, Sankhe SS, Bandgar T, et al. Tumor-induced osteomalacia: a single center experience. Endocr Pract. 2011;17(2):177–84.
27. Jain AS, Shelley S, Muthukrishnan I, Kalal S, Amalachandran J, Chandran S. Diagnostic importance of contrast enhanced F-fluorodeoxyglucose positron emission computed tomography in patients with tumor induced osteomalacia: our experience. Indian J Nucl Med. 2016;31(1):14–9. https://doi.org/10.4103/0972-3919.172344.
28. Jiang Y, Xia W, Xing X, Silva BC, Li M, Wang O, et al. Tumor-induced osteomalacia: an important cause of adult-onset hypophosphatemic osteomalacia in China: report of 39 cases and review of the literature. J Bone Miner Res. 2012;27(9):1967–75.
29. Jing H, Li F, Zhong D, Zhuang H. 99mTc-HYNIC-TOC (99mTc-Hydrazinonicotinyl-Tyr3-Octreotide) scintigraphy identifying two separate causative tumors in a patient with tumor-induced osteomalacia (TIO). Clin Nucl Med. 2013;38(8):664–7. https://doi.org/10.1097/RLU.0b013e3182996293.
30. John M, Shah NS. Hypophosphatemic rickets with epidermal nevus syndrome. Indian Pediatr. 2005;42:611–2.
31. Juppner H, Wolf M, Salusky IB. FGF23: more than a regulator of renal phosphate handling? J Bone Miner Res. 2010;25(10):2019–7. https://doi.org/10.1002/jbmr.170.
32. Kaneuchi Y, Hakozaki M, Yamada H, Hasegawa O, Tajino T, Konno S. Missed causative tumors in diagnosing tumor induced osteomalacia with 18F-FDG PET/CT: a potential pitfall of standard-field imaging. Hell J Nucl Med. 2016;19(1):46–8.

33. Khosravi A, Cutler CM, Kelly MH, Chang R, Royal RE, Sherry RM, Wodajo FM, Fedarko NS, Collins MT. Determination of the elimination half-life of fibroblast growth factor-23. J Clin Endocrinol Metab. 2007;92:2374–7. https://doi.org/10.1210/jc.2006-2865.
34. Kishida ES, Silva MAM, Pereira DC, Sanches JA, Sotto MN. Epidermal nevus syndrome associated with adnexal tumors, Spitz nevus, and hypophosphatemic vitamin D-resistant rickets. Pediatr Dermatol. 2005;22(1):48–54.
35. Lin H, Shih S, Tseng Y, Chen C, Chiu W, Hsu C, et al. Ovarian cancer-related hypophosphatemic osteomalacia—a case report. J Clin Endocrinol Metab. 2014;99(12):4403–7. https://doi.org/10.1210/jc.2014-2120.
36. Lyles KW, Berry WR, Haussler M, Harrelson JM, Drezner MK. Hypoposphatemic osteomalacia: association with prostatic carcinoma. Ann Intern Med. 1980;93(2):275–8.
37. Michaut P, Prie D, Amiel C, Friedlander G. Dipyridamole for renal phosphate leak? N Engl J Med. 1994;331(1):58–9.
38. Payne RB. Renal tubular reabsorption of phosphate (TmP/GFR): indications and interpretation. Ann Clin Biochem. 1998;35:201–6. [PubMed: 9547891].
39. Piemonte S, Romagnoli E, Cipriani C, De Lucia F, Pilotto R, Diacinti D, et al. Six-year follow-up of a characteristic osteolytic lesion in a patient with tumor-induced osteomalacia. Eur J Endocrinol. 2014;170(1):K1–4. https://doi.org/10.1530/EJE-13-0581.
40. Ratanasuwan T, Chetsurakarn S, Ongphiphadhanakul B, Damrongkitchaiporn S. A case report of tumor-induced osteomalacia: eight year followed-up. J Med Assoc Thail. 2008;91(12):1900–3.
41. Rowe PSN, Kumagai Y, Gutierrez G, Garrett IR, Blacher R, Rosen D, et al. MEPE has the properties of an osteoblastic phosphatonin and minhibin. Bone. 2004;34(2):303–19. https://doi.org/10.1016/j.bone.2003.10.005.
42. Sahoo J, Balachandran K, Kamalanathan S, Das KA, Patro DK, Halanaik D, et al. Tumor(s) induced osteomalacia—a curious case of double trouble. J Clin Endocrinol Metab. 2014;99(2):395–8. https://doi.org/10.1210/jc.2013-3791.
43. Sandoval MAS, Palermo MA, Carrillo R, Bundoc R, Carnate JM, Galsim R. Successful treatment of tumour-induced osteomalacia after resection of an oral peripheral ossifying fibroma. BMJ Case Rep. 2017; https://doi.org/10.1136/bcr-2016-218637.
44. Sauder A, Wiernek S, Dai X, Pereira R, Yudd M, Patel C, et al. FGF23-associated tumor-induced osteomalacia in a patient with small cell carcinoma: a case report and regulatory mechanism study. Int J Surg Pathol. 2015; https://doi.org/10.1177/1066896915617828.
45. Seufert J, Ebert K, Muller J, Eulert J, Hendrich C, Werner E, et al. Octreotide therapy for tumor-induced osteomalacia. N Engl J Med. 2001;345(26):1883–8.
46. Shimada T, Mizutani S, Muto T, Yoneya T, Hino R, Takeda S, et al. Cloning and characterization of FGF23 as a causative factor of tumor-induced osteomalacia. Proc Natl Acad Sci. 2001;98(11):6500–5. https://doi.org/10.1073/ypnas.101545198.
47. Sood A, Agarwal K, Shukla J, Goel R, Dhir V, Bhattacharya A, et al. Bone scintigraphic patterns in patients of tumor induced osteomalacia. Indian J Nucl Med. 2013;28(3):173–5. https://doi.org/10.4103/0972-3919.119541.
48. Tutton S, Olson E, King D, Shaker JL. Successful treatment of tumor-induced osteomalacia with CT-guided percutaneous ethanol and cryoablation. J Clin Endocrinol Metab. 2012;97(10):3421–5. https://doi.org/10.1210/jc.2012-1719.
49. Van der Rest C, Cavalier E, Kaux J-F, Krzesinski J-M, Hustinx R, Reginster J-Y, et al. Tumor-induced osteomalacia: the tumor may stay hidden! Clin Biochem. 2011;44:1264–6. https://doi.org/10.1016/j.clinbiochem.2011.07.013.
50. Wang H, Zhong D, Liu Y, Jiang Y, Qiu G, Weng X, et al. 2012Surgical treatments of tumor-induced osteomalacia lesions in long bones: seventeen cases with more than one year of follow-up. J Bone Joint Surg Am. 2015;97:1084–94. https://doi.org/10.2106/JBJS.N.01299.
51. Wang X, Mu Y. Emphasis should be placed on the diagnosis and therapy of tumor induced osteomalacia. Chin Med J. 2011;124(2):163–5. https://doi.org/10.3760/cma.j.issn.0366-6999.2011.02.001.

52. Wasserman JK, Purgina B, Lai CK, Gravel D, Mahaffey A, Bell D, et al. Phosphaturic mesenchymal tumor involving the head and neck: a report of five cases with FGFR1 fluorescence in situ hybridization analysis. Head Neck Pathol. 2016; https://doi.org/10.1007/s12105-015-0678-1.
53. Weidner N, Santa Cruz D. Phosphaturic mesenchymal tumors: a polymorphous group causing osteomalacia or rickets. Cancer. 1987;59(8):1442–54.
54. Yavropoulou MP, Gerothanasi N, Frydas A, Triantafyllou E, Poulios C, Hytiroglou P, et al. Tumor-induced osteomalacia due to a recurrent mesenchymal tumor overexpressing several growth factor receptors. Endocrinol Diab Metab Case Rep. 2015; https://doi.org/10.1530/EDM-15-0025.
55. Yu W, He J, Fu W, Wang C, Zhang Z. Reports of 17 Chinese patients with tumor-induced osteomalacia. J Bone Miner Metab. 2009; https://doi.org/10.1007/s00774-016-0756-9.
56. Zhang X, Yu Z, Tonghua L, Yao B, Zhaohuan L. Mesenchymoma associated with vitamin D-resistant hypophosphatemic osteomalacia: case report and review of literature. Chin Med J. 1980;93(6):391–9.

Chapter 12
Sclerotic Bone Disorders

Sina Jasim, Robert Wermers, and Daniel L. Hurley

Abbreviations

BMD	Bone mineral density
CKD-MBD	Chronic kidney disease-mineral and bone disorder
DXA	Dual-energy X-ray absorptiometry
HOA	Hypertrophic osteoarthropathy

Case Presentation

A 52-year-old Caucasian woman was seen in Metabolic Bone Disease Clinic for evaluation of an intermittently elevated total alkaline phosphatase and abnormal radiographs. Four years earlier, at age 48, she was diagnosed with bilateral well-differentiated (ER+, PR+, HER2 negative) multifocal infiltrating lobular breast carcinoma. Bilateral mastectomy was remarkable for clear margins and no evidence of lymphovascular invasion, but 21/21 right axillary lymph nodes were found to have metastasis with capsular invasion (left-sided lymph nodes were negative). She received both chemotherapy (four cycles of doxorubicin plus cyclophosphamide over 8 weeks, followed by four cycles of paclitaxel over 8 weeks) and subsequent right breast and chest wall radiation therapy (6000 cGy). She experienced

S. Jasim
Department of Internal Medicine and Division of Endocrinology, Metabolism and Lipid Research, Washington University School of Medicine, St. Louis, MO, USA
e-mail: s.jasim@wustl.edu

R. Wermers · D. L. Hurley (✉)
Department of Medicine and Division of Endocrinology, Diabetes, Metabolism and Nutrition, Mayo Clinic College of Medicine, Mayo Clinic, Rochester, MN, USA
e-mail: Wermers.Robert@mayo.edu; hurley.daniel@mayo.edu

P. M. Camacho (ed.), *Metabolic Bone Diseases*,
https://doi.org/10.1007/978-3-030-03694-2_12

chemotherapy-related amenorrhea. Tamoxifen was begun after completion of chemo-radiation treatment, with a plan to switch to an aromatase inhibitor at a later date. Two years after beginning Tamoxifen, she was tolerating it well without clinical evidence of recurrent disease.

Her metabolic bone history was detailed at her bone clinic evaluation. Because of groin pain with ambulation near the diagnosis of her breast cancer, a computerized tomography (CT) scan of the abdomen/pelvis was performed and noted "focal sclerosis in the T12 vertebral body and a very tiny focus of sclerosis adjacent to the superior endplate of the L4 vertebral body." CT scan of the chest was unremarkable except for the mastectomies and "indeterminate" sclerosis at T12." A technetium whole body bone scan showed nonspecific "diffuse, homogenous uptake" in the skull and long bones and degenerative changes at multiple joints without evidence of metastatic disease. Since then, she has had an intermittently elevated serum total alkaline phosphatase (150 units/L, normal reference 35–105).

Her past history is significant for tobacco smoking and a right ankle avulsion fracture after an ankle inversion injury. She denied alcohol use. There is no family history of metabolic bone disease, to include hyperparathyroidism and Paget's disease.

At the time of her metabolic bone clinic consultation, her total alkaline phosphatase was elevated at 142 U/L with normal levels for a complete blood count, electrolytes and creatinine (0.8 mg/dL, normal reference 0.6–1.1), liver tests (AST, ALT, total bilirubin), minerals (calcium, phosphorus), parathyroid hormone (47 pg/mL, normal reference 15–65), thyroid hormones (TSH and free thyroxine), albumin, and serum protein electrophoresis profile (negative for monoclonal protein). A recent 25-hydroxyvitamin D level was also in normal reference range. Her original radiographs of the chest (Fig. 12.1), whole body bone scan (Fig. 12.2), and CT scans (Fig. 12.3) were reviewed.

Introduction

Abnormal bone remodeling distorts normal bone homeostasis of coupled osteoblastic and osteoclastic activity and can result in high bone density or osteosclerosis. Bone sclerosis (trabecular bone thickening) reflects an increase in skeletal mass secondary to genetic or acquired causes (Table 12.1). We will review some of these causes, mostly the acquired ones, in this chapter.

Skeletal Dysplasia

Fibrous dysplasia is discussed in Chap. 13.

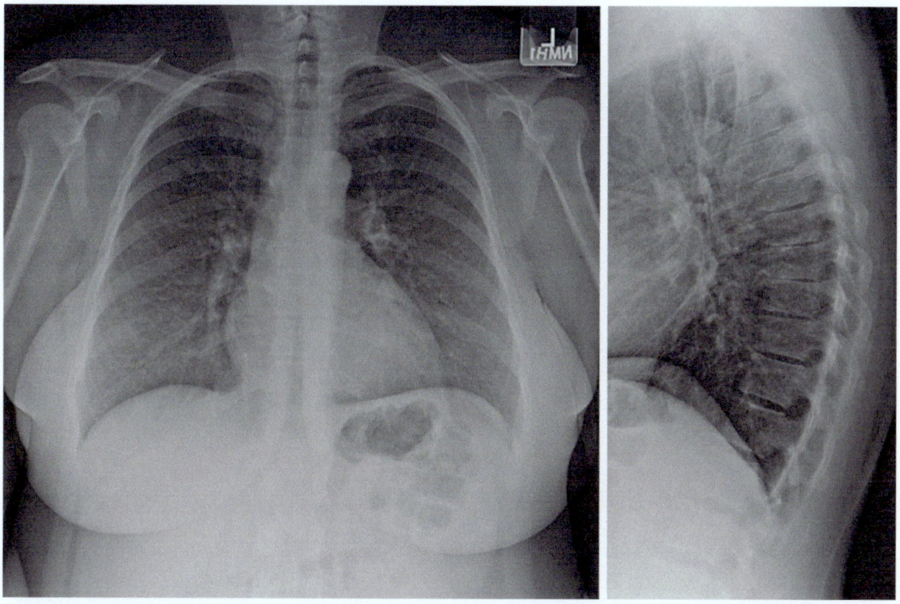

Fig. 12.1 Initial chest radiograph; anteroposterior (left) and lateral (right) views. Interpretation: Negative chest

Skeletal Dysostoses

Osteochondrodysplasia is discussed in Chap. 14.

Osteopetrosis

Osteopetrosis is a group of bone disorders due to failure of osteoclast-mediated resorption. On radiological imaging, osteopetrosis is a generalized, symmetrical increase in bone mass with possible pathological fracture of long bones. Disease severity can range from benign (autosomal dominant) in adults to malignant (autosomal recessive) in children. It can also develop secondary to infection or medications [1].

- Infantile osteopetrosis: The most severe form is autosomal recessive caused by carbonic anhydrase type II gene mutation (infantile malignant osteopetrosis). This form is usually associated with renal tubular acidosis.
  Skull bones abnormalities can lead to poor development of nasal sinuses, cranial nerve paralysis, hearing and visual loss, raised intracranial pressure, and hydrocephalus.

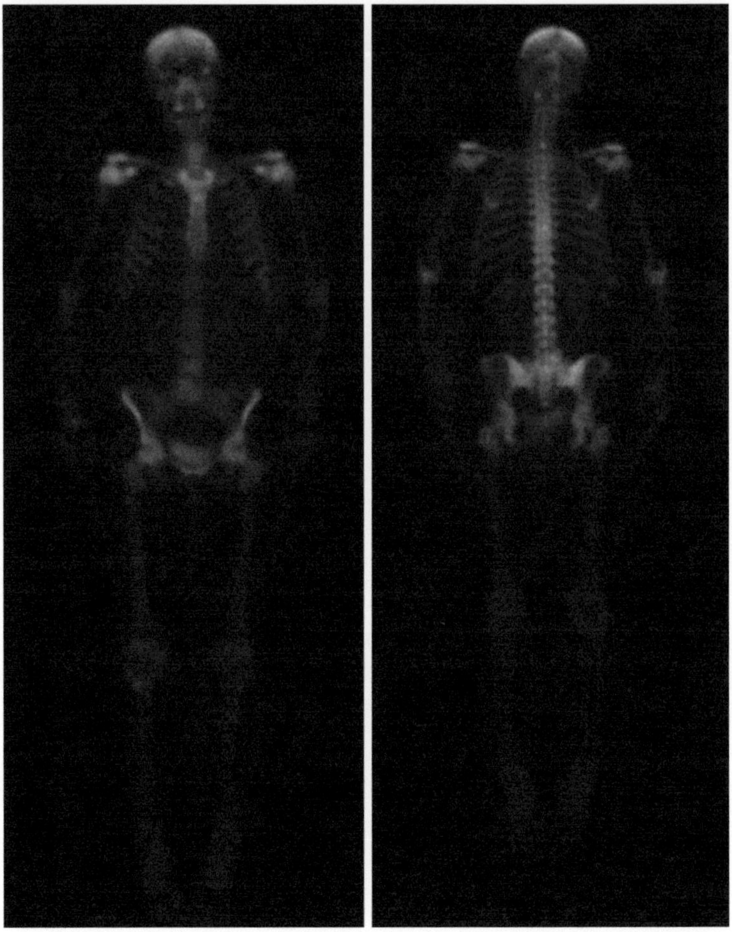

Fig. 12.2 Initial nuclear medicine (technetium 99m MDP) whole body bone scan; anterior (left) and posterior (right) views. Interpretation: Diffuse, homogenous uptake of radiotracer at the superior portion of the calvarium and (prominent) in the long bones. Degenerative changes of multiple joints in the axial and appendicular skeleton. Findings are consistent with a metabolic bone disease, without evidence of metastatic bone disease

Poor dentition and failure to thrive can ensue. An excess in osteoclast number and activity is present. Fibrosis can replace the bone marrow and lead to infection, bleeding tendency, hypersplenism, and hemolytic anemia with enlargement of the liver and spleen.

Unfortunately, no treatment is available and the disease is associated with increased morbidity and early mortality.

- Adult osteopetrosis: Usually present with brittle bones, cranial nerve palsy, carpal tunnel syndrome, and osteoarthritis. Two main forms include:

  Type 1: High bone mass due to LRP5 gene activation.

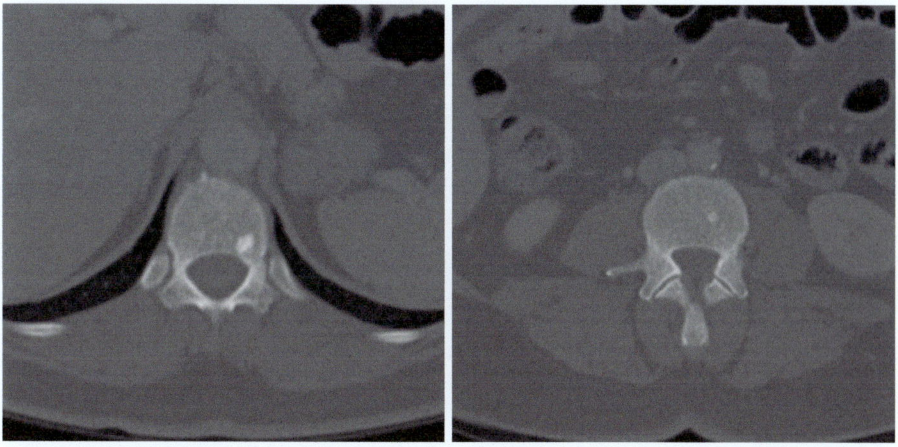

Fig. 12.3 Initial CT scans of the chest, abdomen, and pelvis; T12 (left) and L4 (right) vertebral bones. Interpretation: Bilateral mastectomies. Mild diffuse fatty liver and small hepatic dome cyst. Indeterminate focal sclerosis in the T12 vertebral body and a second tiny focus of sclerosis adjacent to the superior end plate of the L4 vertebral body. Approximately 1 cm lytic lesion in the left iliac bone adjacent to the sacroiliac joint. Findings of mild diffuse patchy sclerosis in the lumbar spine and pelvic bones are nonspecific

Table 12.1 Differential diagnosis of osteosclerosis

Skeletal dysplasias	Discussed in Chap. 13
Skeletal dysostoses	Discussed in Chap. 14
Acquired causes of osteosclerosis	Hepatitis C-associated osteosclerosis
	Heavy metal poisoning
	Excessive vitamin D or A
	Milk-alkali syndrome
	Renal osteodystrophy
	Fluorosis
	Hypertrophic osteoarthropathy
	Ionizing radiation
	Leukemia, lymphoma, myeloma, mastocytosis
	Osteomyelitis
	Paget's disease of bone
	Sarcoidosis
	Sickle cell disease
	Skeletal metastasis
Metabolic causes of osteosclerosis	Carbonic anhydrase II deficiency
	Hyper-, hypo-, and pseudohypoparathyroidism
	Hypophosphatemic osteomalacia
	X-linked hypophosphatemia

Adopted and Modified from Chap. 93. Sclerosing Bone Disorders 769 Michael P. Whyte [16]. Primer on the Metabolic Bone Diseases and Disorders of Mineral Metabolism, Eighth Edition. Edited by Clifford J. Rosen. © 2013 American Society for Bone and Mineral Research. Published 2013 by John Wiley & Sons, Inc

Type 2: Autosomal dominant osteopetrosis (Albers-Schönberg disease) caused by heterozygous mutations in the chloride channel 7 (CLCN7) gene. This disease mainly affects the spine, pelvis, and the skull base.
- Other forms of osteopetrosis are less common.

Hypocalcemia, secondary hyperparathyroidism, and high calcitriol levels are commonly seen in the infantile form. Histopathological studies have revealed increased osteoid and immature "woven" bone commonly seen in adult osteopetrosis.

Treatment options include calcium supplementation if hypocalcemia is present. High-dose glucocorticoid treatment has been administered for pancytopenia and hepatomegaly. Bone marrow transplantation (BMT) is a treatment option, especially for infantile osteopetrosis [2].

Carbonic Anhydrase II (CA II) Deficiency

This is a combination of the autosomal recessive syndrome of osteopetrosis, renal tubular acidosis, and cerebral calcification caused by a mutation of CA II encoding gene [3]. CA II is abundant in tissues such as the brain, kidney, and bones. The disease can present with recurrent fractures, failure to thrive, and developmental delay, optic nerve compression with blindness, and dental abnormalities in early childhood. Radiological images resemble those with osteopetrosis with cerebral calcification seen in childhood. BMT is the treatment of choice for osteopetrosis. Bicarbonate can be used for metabolic acidosis due to renal tubular acidosis.

Pachydermoperiostosis (Hypertrophic Osteoarthropathy; HOA)

This syndrome is characterized by abnormal proliferation of the skin and osseous tissue at the distal extremities. Clinical picture includes digital clubbing, hyperhidrosis, thickening of the skin (cutis verticis gyrata), and periostosis of bones which is usually accompanied by painful arthropathy.

Some theories of pathogenesis include localized activation of the platelet-endothelial cells and release of fibroblast growth factors; tumor production and release of factors lead to vascular proliferation, edema, and new bone formation such as vascular endothelial growth factor (VEGF) [4] and increased circulating prostaglandin PGE2.

- Primary (idiopathic) HOA: (Pachydermoperiostosis, Touraine-Solente-Gole syndrome) is a hereditary disorder caused by a mutation in the HPGD gene that encodes 15-hydroxyprostaglandin dehydrogenase, which is the primary enzyme response for prostaglandin degradation [5].

- Secondary HOA: Usually associated with lung cancer (more in adenocarcinoma), pulmonary infections, cystic fibrosis, and right-to-left cardiac shunts.

Severe periostitis cause thickening of the bones distally. Bones affected typically are the radius, ulna, tibia, and fibula, less often seen in the metacarpals and metatarsals, clavicle, pelvis, and skull base. The spine is rarely involved. Bone scanning reveals symmetrical, diffuse uptake along the cortical margins of long bones.

Treatment with nonsteroidal anti-inflammatory medications is appropriate in addition to treating the primary cause. Bisphosphonates were effective in few refractory cases [6].

Hepatitis C

The mechanism of hepatitis C-associated increased bone mass is not well understood, but it seems to be associated with disease activity and circulating levels of IGF. Trabecular, as well as periosteal and endosteal, bone thickening is seen throughout the skeleton, except the cranium. Antiresorptive therapy might be of use.

Renal Osteodystrophy

Chronic kidney disease (CKD) is commonly associated with mineral and bone metabolism abnormalities, manifested by abnormalities in calcium, phosphorus, parathyroid hormone (PTH), fibroblast growth factor 23 (FGF23), and vitamin D metabolism, bone turnover, mineralization, or extraskeletal calcification. The best way for the diagnosis and classification of bone disease in CKD is bone biopsy [7] which is invasive; therefore, we rely more on bone turnover biomarkers to have an idea about the ratio of bone formation and bone resorption. Osteitis fibrosa cystica, adynamic bone disease, and osteomalacia are the main bone disease groups associated with renal disease [8]. Subclinical changes in bone remodeling begin in early CKD but manifest last with ESRD. The clinical presentation and treatment options vary depending on the dominating metabolic abnormality, the characteristic bone disease, and the severity of the renal impairment.

Milk-Alkali Syndrome

This syndrome consists of hypercalcemia, metabolic alkalosis, and acute kidney injury secondary to increased calcium ingestion along with absorbable alkali. Individuals with mild chronic kidney disease [9], volume depletion, pregnant women [10], and those treated with a thiazide diuretic are particularly at higher risk.

The milk-alkali syndrome can be asymptomatic or present in various ways depending on severity and acuity of hypercalcemia; majority of patients are women on calcium carbonate, usually treated by withdrawing the offending agent. Hypocalcemia may be seen transiently during treatment with furosemide, accompanied by a rebound rise in parathyroid hormone (PTH); this phenomenon is unique to milk-alkali syndrome when removing offending agent [11].

Vitamin D and Vitamin A Toxicity

Vitamin D chronic toxicity can resemble milk-alkali syndrome as the mechanism is the same – see above.

Chronic vitamin A toxicity is usually due to chronic ingestion of excess amount of synthetic vitamin A (more than ten times higher than the Recommended Dietary Allowance (RDA)) [12]. Fasting serum retinyl esters can be used as a marker for chronic hypervitaminosis A when can't rely on serum retinol only [13]. Chronic toxicity can present with fatigue, dry skin, headache, pseudotumor cerebri, irritability, and hyperostosis.

Hyperparathyroidism, Hypoparathyroidism, and Pseudohypoparathyroidism

Discussed in Chaps. 2, 5, and 6.

Hypophosphatemic Osteomalacia

Discussed in Chap. 7.

Paget's Disease of Bone

Discussed in Chap. 8.

Fluorosis and Heavy Metals Toxicity

Fluoride stimulates bone formation in cortical and trabecular bone via osteoblast stimulation. However, its effect on trabecular bone is greater leading to earlier and more pronounced increases in spine density. Despite impressive increases in BMD, overall bone quality is impaired due to osteomalacia. Skeletal fluorosis is the most severe presentation of fluorosis among adults and occurs when more than 10 mg/day of fluoride is consumed for 10 years or longer. It can result in osteosclerosis which can lead to significant long-term disabilities including limited spine mobility, kyphosis, and lower extremity pain [14].

Heavy metal poisoning with lead in children has also been associated with osteosclerosis of the metaphyses and should be distinguished from genetic causes of osteosclerotic metaphyseal dysplasia [15].

Malignancies and Other Secondary Causes

Malignancy of the bone is discussed in Chap. 15.

Diagnosis and Management of Sclerotic Bone Disease

Diagnostic and management options are extremely variable as the etiology can vary from inherited, congenital, metabolic, and acquired causes. Diagnostic and management strategies are discussed briefly in each section above. Diagnosis and management of fibrous and bony dysplasias, hyper-, hypo-, and pseudohypoparathyroidism, hypophosphatemic osteomalacia, and Paget's disease of bone are discussed in detail in the corresponding chapters.

In general, proper and detailed history is of paramount significance including detailed family history of bone disorders and skeletal defects that can give a clue toward genetic and inherited causes of bone disease; obviously majority of those disorders can be seen early in life.

Multiple forms of bony dysplastic disorders are seen and their detailed evaluation is discussed in Chaps. 13 and 14. Detailed history of menstrual history, activity level, falls, and fractures, dietary habits, prescribed and over-the-counter medication use, or herbal use can be of relevance. Personal and family history of malignancies, hematological disorders, and diseases that can potentially cause bone remolding problems such as sickle cell disease, hepatitis, and sarcoidosis is extremely helpful in directing treatment toward the primary etiology.

General and thorough focused physical examination is useful. Any physical deformities can be suggestive or pathognomonic of syndromic disorders especially in younger patients. Dental and skeletal exam looking for deformities, skin exam, and neurological examination are particularly useful.

Laboratory data can be very helpful in evaluating bone mineralization and turn over, looking for secondary causes, and probably reflecting disease chronicity and severity. Basic laboratory tests may include, but not limited to, complete blood counts with differential as needed, calcium, phosphorus, parathyroid hormones, and vitamin D metabolites levels. Renal and liver function tests, bone turn over markers. If history is suggestive; hemoglobin and protein electrophoresis, hepatitis screen, other vitamins and minerals levels (such as vitamin A, and fluoride levels), and FGF 23. In certain cases, genetic testing can be valuable not only in making the diagnosis but to direct follow-up or treatment options if available.

Imaging is the cornerstone in the diagnosis of sclerotic bone disease as increased bone density can be seen on imaging, but also certain radiological features can be characteristic of certain bone disorders and can raise suspicion and direct further evaluation. Imaging includes skeletal plain radiographs, bone mineral density (DXA), trabecular bone score (TBS), HRpQCT, bone scan, computed tomography scans (CT), and magnetic resonance imaging (MRI). Imaging can also identify secondary causes such as malignancies.

Bone biopsy is the gold standard diagnostic procedure in certain sclerotic bone diseases, but it is invasive and expensive so we tend to rely on the above measures most of the times. Treatment options are widely variable depending on the primary etiology; some are discussed under the relevant topic.

Back to Our Case

At the time of her metabolic bone clinic consultation, the patient was clinically feeling well. Her repeat total alkaline phosphatase was 150 U/L. Additional testing yielded a bone alkaline phosphatase (BAP) of 42 mcg/L (premenopausal <14; postmenopausal <22) and the collagen type 1 cross-linked C-telopeptide (CTX) bone turnover marker of 795 pg/mL (premenopausal <573; postmenopausal <1008). The patient had a repeat whole body bone scan (Fig. 12.4), and other than uptake in the area of known orbital surgery and ankle injury, there was no significant change in the diffuse homogenous uptake in the skull and long bones. A radiographic skeletal survey revealed diffuse patchy sclerosis throughout the axial and proximal appendicular skeleton (Figs. 12.5, 12.6, and 12.7). Further evaluation to include vitamin A, hepatitis C serology, serum fluoride, tryptase, heavy metal screen, angiotensin-converting enzyme, and 24-urine calcium and creatinine were obtained and were all normal or negative with the exception of a low urinary calcium level. The patient then had a CT-guided left iliac bone biopsy, and pathology was positive for metastatic adenocarcinoma consistent with breast primary. Subsequent CT scans of the chest, abdomen, and pelvis revealed diffuse lytic and sclerotic densities throughout the intrathoracic bone structures, consistent with metastatic disease.

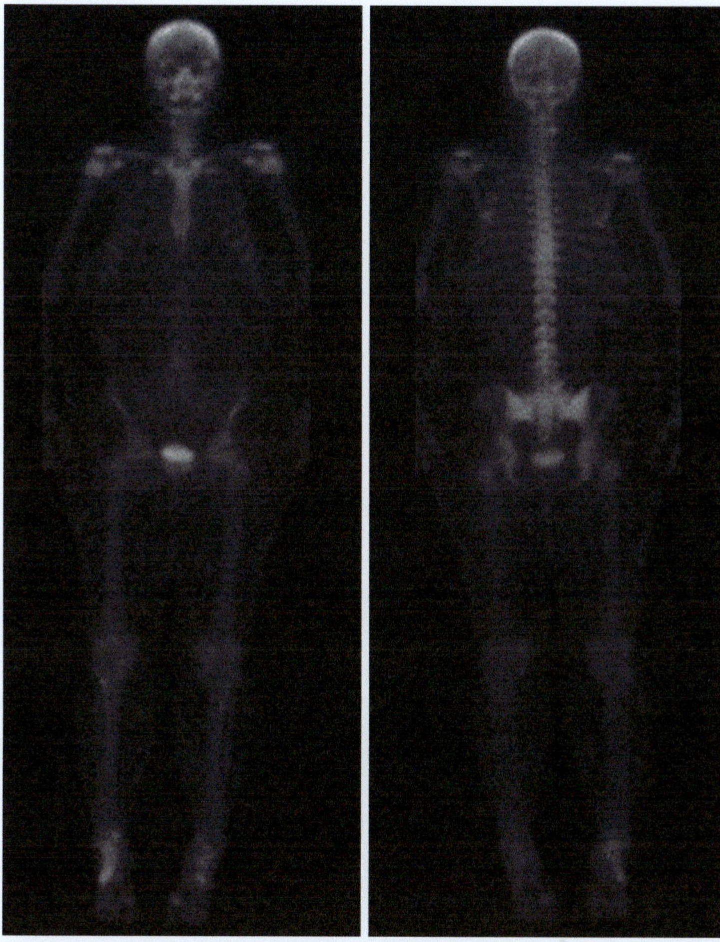

Fig. 12.4 Repeat nuclear medicine (technetium 99m MDP) whole body bone scan; anterior (left) and posterior (right) views. Interpretation: Since prior exam, increased radiotracer uptake in the right foot compatible with recent trauma. Tiny focus of increased uptake about the superolateral left orbit, compatible with history of orbit surgery. No other change since prior exam. Again seen is diffuse homogenous uptake of radiotracer at the superior portion of the calvarium and in the long bones. Degenerative type uptake is seen in the shoulders, cervical and lumbar spine, knees, and left foot. Findings are consistent with a metabolic bone disease

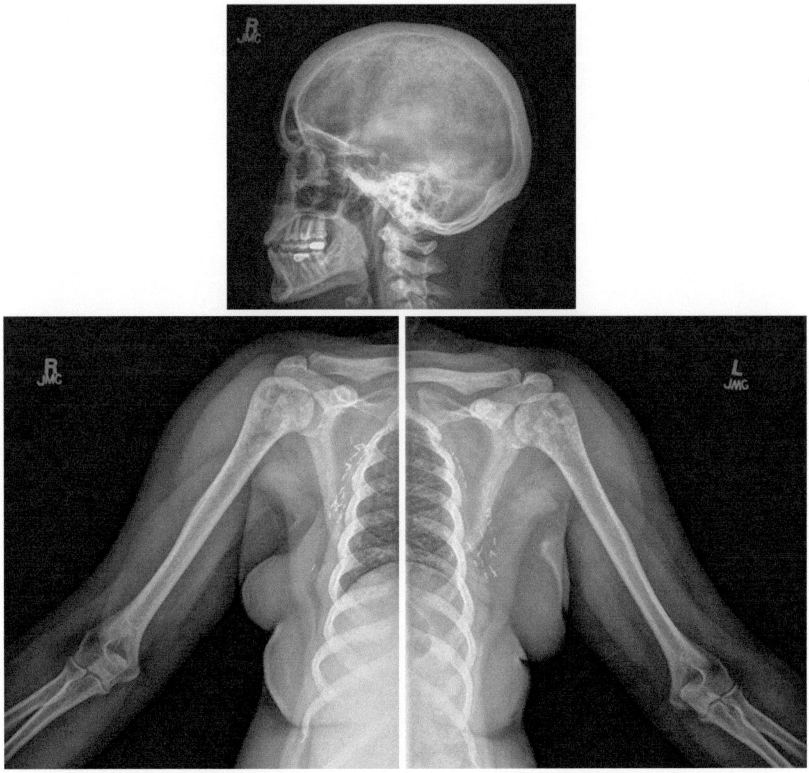

Fig. 12.5 Skeletal radiograph survey; skull and upper body long bones (radius/ulna and hands not shown). Interpretation: Diffuse patchy sclerosis throughout the axial and proximal appendicular skeleton. No periarticular resorption or soft tissue calcifications. Findings are nonspecific; metabolic bone disorder, metastatic disease or mastocytosis cannot be excluded

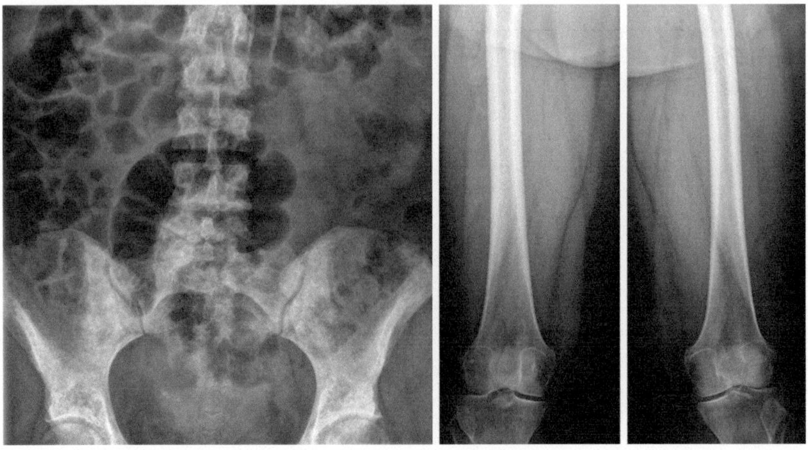

Fig. 12.6 Skeletal radiograph survey; pelvis and lower body long bones (tibia/fibula and feet not shown). Interpretation: Diffuse patchy sclerosis throughout the axial and proximal appendicular skeleton. No periarticular resorption or soft tissue calcifications. Findings are nonspecific; metabolic bone disorder, metastatic disease, or mastocytosis cannot be excluded

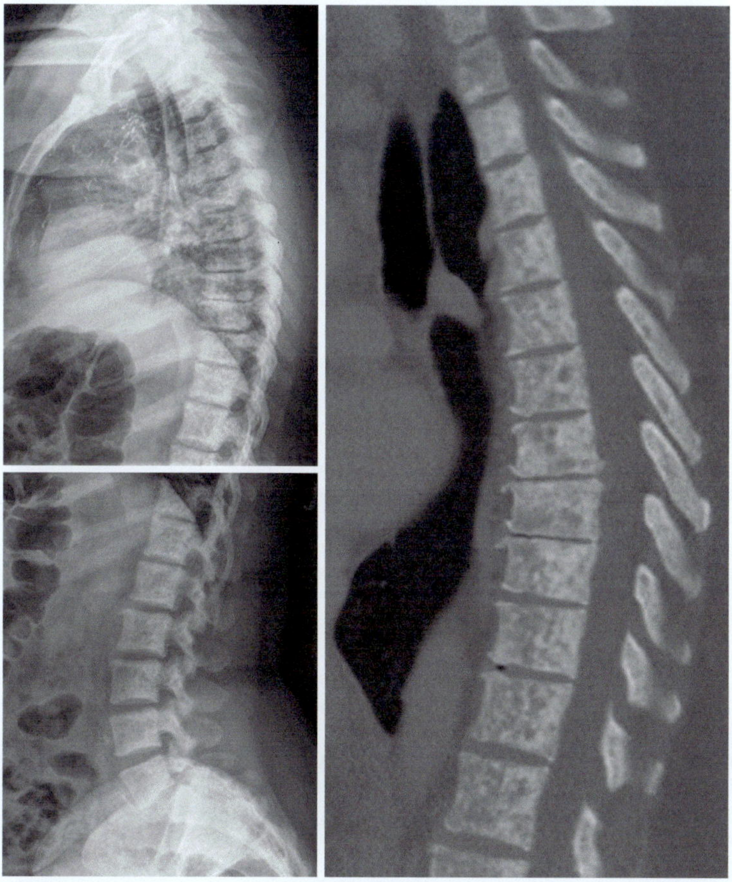

Fig. 12.7 Skeletal radiograph survey of the lateral thoracic/lumbar spine (left), and CT spine (right) (see Figs. 12.5 and 12.6 for interpretation of the skeletal survey). Interpretation of CT spine: Diffuse lytic and sclerotic densities throughout the intrathoracic osseous structures, whereas only a small amount of sclerotic density was present on the previous CT study). Findings are consistent with metastatic carcinoma

Conflict of Interest All authors state that they have no conflicts of interest.

References

1. Whyte MP, McAlister WH, Novack DV, Clements KL, Schoenecker PL, Wenkert D. Bisphosphonate-induced osteopetrosis: novel bone modeling defects, metaphyseal osteopenia, and osteosclerosis fractures after drug exposure ceases. J Bone Miner Res. 2008;23(10):1698–707.
2. Driessen GJ, Gerritsen EJ, Fischer A, Fasth A, Hop WC, Veys P, et al. Long-term outcome of haematopoietic stem cell transplantation in autosomal recessive osteopetrosis: an EBMT report. Bone Marrow Transplant. 2003;32(7):657–63.
3. Sly WS, Hewett-Emmett D, Whyte MP, Yu YS, Tashian RE. Carbonic anhydrase II deficiency identified as the primary defect in the autosomal recessive syndrome of osteopetrosis with renal tubular acidosis and cerebral calcification. Proc Natl Acad Sci U S A. 1983;80(9):2752–6.

4. Olan F, Portela M, Navarro C, Gaxiola M, Silveira LH, Ruiz V, et al. Circulating vascular endothelial growth factor concentrations in a case of pulmonary hypertrophic osteoarthropathy. Correlation with disease activity. J Rheumatol. 2004;31(3):614–6.
5. Uppal S, Diggle CP, Carr IM, Fishwick CW, Ahmed M, Ibrahim GH, et al. Mutations in 15-hydroxyprostaglandin dehydrogenase cause primary hypertrophic osteoarthropathy. Nat Genet. 2008;40(6):789–93.
6. Slobodin G, Rosner I, Feld J, Rimar D, Rozenbaum M, Boulman N, et al. Pamidronate treatment in rheumatology practice: a comprehensive review. Clin Rheumatol. 2009;28(12):1359–64.
7. Moorthi RN, Moe SM. CKD-mineral and bone disorder: core curriculum 2011. Am J Kidney Dis. 2011;58(6):1022–36.
8. Bakkaloglu SA, Wesseling-Perry K, Pereira RC, Gales B, Wang HJ, Elashoff RM, et al. Value of the new bone classification system in pediatric renal osteodystrophy. Clin J Am Soc Nephrol. 2010;5(10):1860–6.
9. Picolos MK, Lavis VR, Orlander PR. Milk-alkali syndrome is a major cause of hypercalcaemia among non-end-stage renal disease (non-ESRD) inpatients. Clin Endocrinol (Oxf). 2005;63(5):566–76.
10. Picolos MK, Sims CR, Mastrobattista JM, Carroll MA, Lavis VR. Milk-alkali syndrome in pregnancy. Obstet Gynecol. 2004;104(5 Pt 2):1201–4.
11. Beall DP, Scofield RH. Milk-alkali syndrome associated with calcium carbonate consumption. Report of 7 patients with parathyroid hormone levels and an estimate of prevalence among patients hospitalized with hypercalcemia. Medicine (Baltimore). 1995;74(2):89–96.
12. Biesalski HK. Comparative assessment of the toxicology of vitamin A and retinoids in man. Toxicology. 1989;57(2):117–61.
13. Penniston KL, Tanumihardjo SA. The acute and chronic toxic effects of vitamin A. Am J Clin Nutr. 2006;83(2):191–201.
14. Sina Jasim DW, Robert A. Wermers. Skeletal fluorosis related to habitual tea consumption: long-term follow up after reduction and discontinuation of tea. AACE Clinical case reports. 2017.
15. Mennel EA, John SD. Osteosclerotic metaphyseal dysplasia: a skeletal dysplasia that my mimic lead poisoning in a child with hypotonia and seizures. Pediatr Radiol. 2003;33:11–4.
16. Whyte MP. Primer on the metabolic bone diseases and disorders of mineral metabolism. 8th edition. 2013

Chapter 13
Fibrous Dysplasia

Anupam Kotwal, Jad G. Sfeir, and Daniel L. Hurley

Abbreviations

BAP	Bone-specific alkaline phosphatase
cAMP	Cyclic adenosine monophosphate
CT	Computed tomography
CTX	Collagen type-1 cross-linked C-telopeptide
FD	Fibrous dysplasia
FGF23	Fibroblast growth factor 23
GNAS	Guanine nucleotide-binding protein, alpha stimulating
IGF-1	Insulin-like growth factor-1
IL-6	Interleukin-6
MAS	McCune-Albright syndrome
MRI	Magnetic resonance imaging
NTX	Collagen type-1 cross-linked N-telopeptide
P1NP	N-terminal propeptides of procollagen type-1
RANKL	Receptor activator of nuclear factor Kappa-B ligand

Case Presentation

A 23-year-old Caucasian man presented to our Metabolic Bone Disease Clinic with recent onset of frontal headache and retrobulbar pain. He reported bilateral testicular enlargement over years but denied precocious puberty or decreased libido. There was no history of clinical fractures. His physical examination revealed large,

A. Kotwal · J. G. Sfeir · D. L. Hurley (✉)
Department of Medicine and Division of Endocrinology, Diabetes, Metabolism and Nutrition, Mayo Clinic College of Medicine, Mayo Clinic, Rochester, MN, USA
e-mail: hurley.daniel@mayo.edu

P. M. Camacho (ed.), *Metabolic Bone Diseases*,
https://doi.org/10.1007/978-3-030-03694-2_13

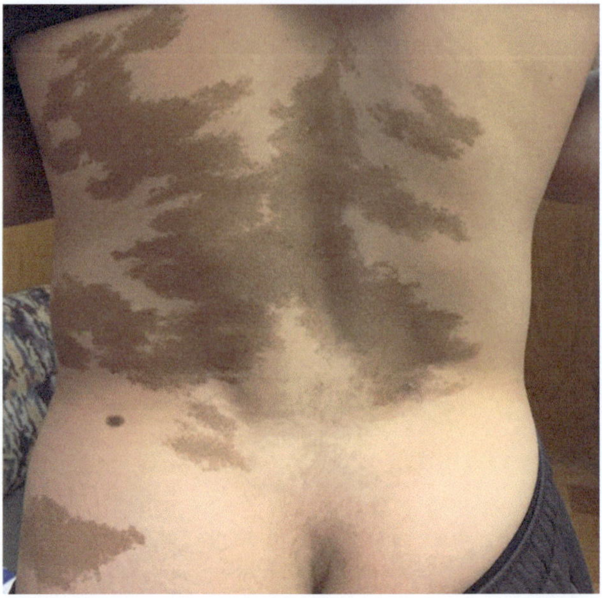

Fig. 13.1 Asymmetric café au lait macules on the back characteristic of McCune-Albright syndrome

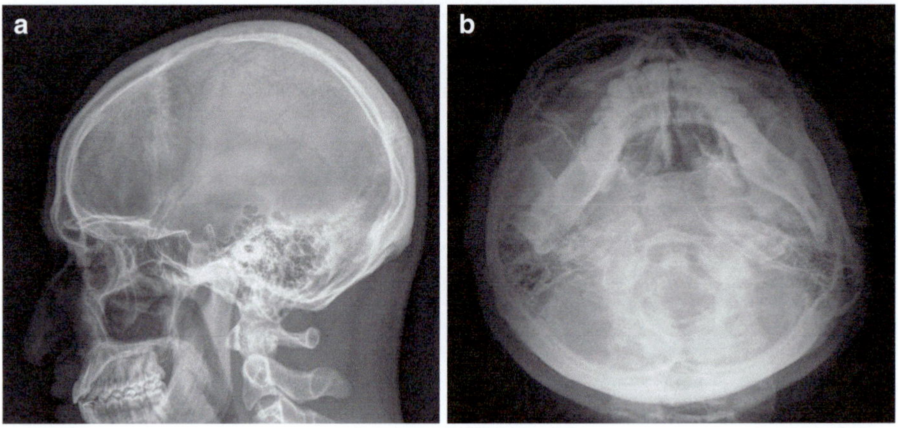

Fig. 13.2 (**a**, **b**) Plain radiographs showing bone changes of fibrous dysplasia involving the mandible on the right, central skull base and clivus, left maxilla, and the left vomer

confluent, asymmetric café au lait macules on the back (Fig. 13.1) and left thigh, which he reported to be present since childhood. He did not have any limb or facial deformities, and his visual field testing was unremarkable.

Plain radiographs (Fig. 13.2a, b) and a low enhancement computed tomography (CT) scan (Fig. 13.3) demonstrated areas of "ground glass" attenuation in the central skull base, clivus, body of the sphenoid bone, left orbital floor, left maxillary bone, right mandibular condyle extending to the temporomandibular joint, left max-

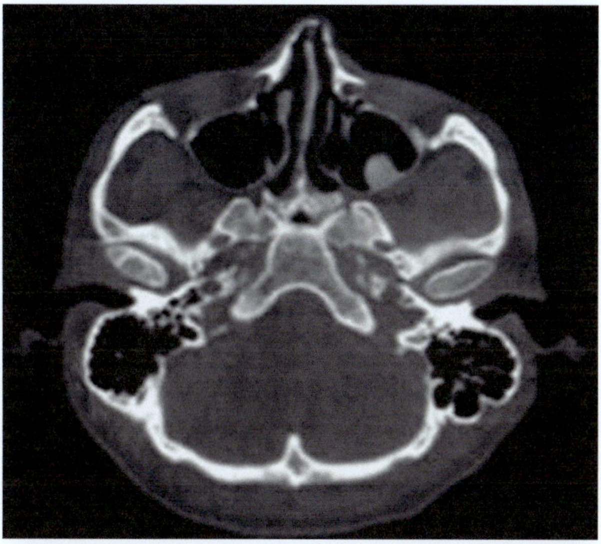

Fig. 13.3 CT scan showing "ground glass" attenuation (arrow) of the skull base

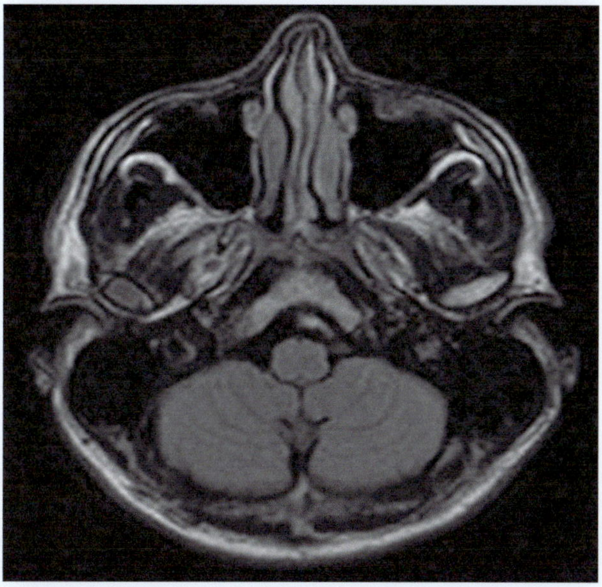

Fig. 13.4 MRI showing replacement of normal bone marrow signal in the skull base

illa, and right mandibular region. Magnetic resonance imaging (MRI) of his brain (Fig. 13.4) revealed replacement of normal marrow signal and bony expansion in these areas, with the enhancement of the clivus measuring 1.8 cm. These areas had increased radiotracer uptake with technetium whole body bone scan (Fig. 13.5a, b). Biochemical testing was normal for serum calcium, phosphorous, insulin-like growth factor-1 (IGF-1), and thyroid function tests. The total serum 25-hydroxyvitamin D level was 72 ng/mL (Institutes of Medicine reference range

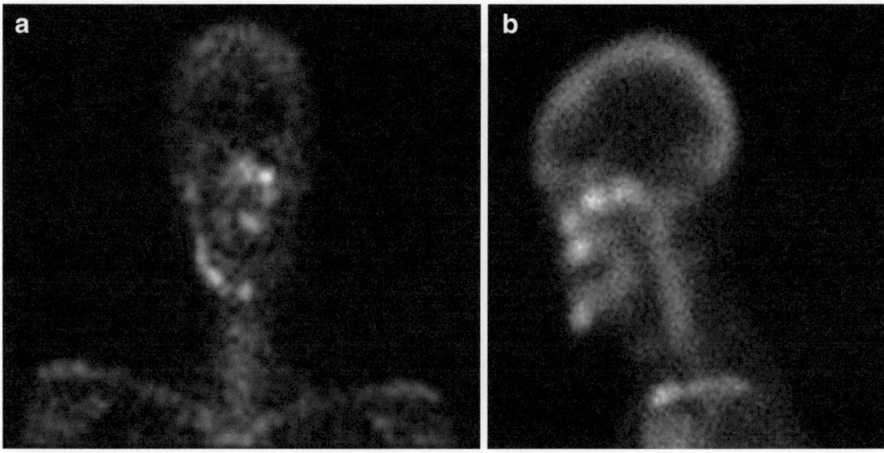

Fig. 13.5 (**a**, **b**) Technetium whole body scan showing increased uptake in the involved craniofacial bones and the skull base

20–50), collagen type-1 cross-linked C-telopeptide (CTX) elevated at 933 pg/mL (reference range 155–873 for 18–39 years of age), and bone-specific alkaline phosphatase (BAP) normal at 15 mcg/L (reference range 0–20).

Assessment and Diagnosis

Fibrous dysplasia (FD) is an uncommon nonneoplastic skeletal condition characterized by replacement of medullary bone and bone marrow by fibrous tissue, involving one (monostotic) or more (polyostotic) bones. Its manifestations can vary widely, ranging from asymptomatic incidental radiographic skeletal findings to disabling disease with fractures, bone deformities, and significant pain. FD accounts for 7% of all benign bone tumors; 5–12% of patients have one or more extra-skeletal manifestations, especially café au lait skin pigmentation. The latter is part of the McCune-Albright syndrome (MAS) [1] that is prevalent in 1 out of every 1,000,000 individuals worldwide and includes, in addition to FD bone lesions and café au lait spots, endocrine dysfunction such as precocious puberty, acromegaly, Cushing's syndrome, or hyperthyroidism. Café au lait skin macules have characteristic features; those with jagged, irregular borders are often referred to as "coast of Maine" lesions in contrast to the smooth-bordered "coast of California" lesions seen in neurofibromatosis [2]. Interestingly, similar to the bone lesions, the skin lesions tend to not cross the body midline; rather, they follow the developmental lines of Blaschko, which reflect patterns of embryonic cell migration.

Clinically, the sites of skeletal involvement are established early and do not seem to correlate with the extent of the skin lesions. Bones are most affected during rapid bone growth, and hence the disease commonly presents with the most symptoms and highest fracture rates in childhood or early adolescence. Most craniofacial lesions occur by 5 years of age, and other clinically significant bone lesions appear by 15 years of age, after which new lesions rarely develop and existing lesions become less active, likely due to apoptosis of the mutation-bearing cells [3]. Nonetheless, FD can proceed unrecognized until adulthood when symptoms first appear, such as the patient in this clinical vignette. While there is generally a central to peripheral gradient of bone involvement, any combination of skeletal sites may occur. FD frequently involves the skull base and proximal femur, with other common sites to include the spine and ribs.

The skeletal map is determined early, and lesions usually become less active with age, especially in adulthood. Symptoms depend on the location of FD bone lesions, and the most common presenting symptoms are bone pain in the areas of involvement, a limp, or a fracture, the latter usually peaking in the first decade of life with a decreased incidence thereafter. Based on the site of involvement, neuropathies may also occur due to nerve impingement. Craniofacial FD can present as facial "bump" or asymmetry or nerve impingement leading to pain and neurological deficits. Visual and hearing losses are uncommon and more likely to occur with IGF-1 excess in the presence of MAS. Vertebral involvement rarely causes pain until associated with progressive scoliosis or a pathological fracture. Limb lesions may also lead to pathologic fractures and deformities, particularly in the proximal femur. Recurrent fractures and progressive deformities may affect ambulation and overall mobility.

The prognosis of FD depends mainly on the location of skeletal lesions and the severity and extent of disease involvement. Active FD lesions can produce excess fibroblast growth factor-23 (FGF23) resulting in phosphaturia [5, 6] that can occasionally lead to hypophosphatemia with additional subsequent bone pain and increased fracture risk due to rickets in children or osteomalacia in adults [7]. Polyostotic FD has been associated with a higher risk of fractures [1, 7], and the FRANCEDYS study reported that both polyostotic disease and bisphosphonate use were significant predictors of fracture risk [1]. Malignant transformation of FD lesions is extremely rare and has been associated with previous radiation treatment or acromegaly [4, 5]. In a review of FD patients seen at the Mayo Clinic [4], 28 of 1122 patients (2.5%) developed malignant transformation, 46% of these had previously received radiation therapy, and the most common malignancy was osteosarcoma. Rapidly expanding FD lesions and disruption of the cortex are worrisome signs of malignant transformation. The clinical course of malignancy is usually aggressive, and surgery is the primary treatment.

Initial assessment of patients with FD aims at determining the extent of skeletal involvement and associated endocrine and/or other organ involvement. Radiographs aid the clinical evaluation but there are similarities with other skeletal disorders. Genetic mutation analysis is rarely needed but may be helpful in cases of equivocal clinical and/or radiographic findings to distinguish FD from other fibro-osseous conditions, such as osteofibrous dysplasia and ossifying fibromas. It is important to note that since FD is not a hereditary condition, genetic testing should only be done if needed for diagnosis, and screening family members of an affected individual is not necessary.

The radiographic appearance of FD varies according to its skeletal location and age of the lesion. Craniofacial lesions are typically expansive with a homogenous "ground glass" appearance on CT scan. Lesions involving the appendicular skeleton are usually expansive with endosteal scalloping, cortical thinning, and also a "ground glass" appearance. With aging, FD lesions can develop a "mosaic" radiographic appearance (i.e., both sclerotic and cystic features); appendicular lesions tend to become sclerotic (corresponding to decreased disease activity), while craniofacial lesions develop a cystic appearance. Total body bone scintigraphy should be used to identify and determine the extent of skeletal FD. The majority of clinically significant osseous lesions will have increased tracer uptake early in the course of the disease. MRI is not required for diagnosis but may be helpful in the longitudinal follow-up of craniofacial lesions as normal bone marrow is replaced by fibrosis. *In our patient, (a) the "ground glass" expansile lesions seen in the skull base, clivus, and facial bones on plain radiographs and CT scan, (b) corresponding replacement of normal marrow signal on MRI, and (c) hypermetabolic activity on PET scan all support the diagnosis of FD.* FD involvement of the clivus present in this patient is a reportedly rare occurrence [6].

Laboratory markers of bone turnover are usually elevated with greater increases in markers of bone resorption (serum CTX and urine collagen type-1 cross-linked N-telopeptide [NTX]) than markers of bone formation (BAP and N-terminal propeptides of procollagen type-1 [P1NP]), in line with increased osteoclastogenesis. With the exception of hypophosphatemia due to excess production of FGF23, serum minerals and electrolytes are typically normal. *In our patient, the serum CTX was elevated and BAP was normal. Serum electrolytes and minerals, including phosphorous, were normal.*

Etiology

FD is a rare genetic disease resulting from somatic activating mutation of the guanine nucleotide-binding protein, alpha stimulating *(GNAS)* gene encoding the alpha subunit of the stimulatory G-protein early in embryogenesis with a mosaic distribution [7]. This leads to increased stimulation of adenylyl cyclase and overproduction of cyclic adenosine monophosphate (cAMP) and c-fos protein [8]. The result is proliferation of undifferentiated stromal cells causing bone marrow fibrosis (that replaces the medullary bone), unmineralized osteoid deposition, and increased osteoclastogenesis [9]. Most of the histopathological features of FD are due to the osteogenic nature of the lesions. Osteoclastogenesis in FD lesions is dependent on the secretion of interleukin-6 (IL-6) by osteogenic cells and the upregulation of receptor activator of nuclear factor kappa-B ligand (RANKL) caused by the *GNAS* mutation. The unmineralized osteoid deposition (i.e., osteomalacia) [10] is most likely due to the excess production of FGF23 by the osteogenic FD tissue [11, 12].

Alpha subunit of the stimulatory G protein is ubiquitous, which explains involvement of non-skeletal organs in FD, such as skin and other endocrine organs. FD, MAS, and non-skeletal isolated endocrine lesions associated with *GNAS1* mutations represent a spectrum of phenotypic expressions likely reflecting different patterns of somatic mosaicism of the same basic disorder. A spectrum of bone lesions associated with such mutations was identified and recognized as three distinct histopathologic patterns, defined as Chinese writing type, sclerotic pagetoid type, and sclerotic hypercellular type, which are characteristically associated with the axial/appendicular skeleton, cranial bones, or gnathic bones, respectively [13].

Management

FD is a skeletal disorder that can involve endocrine organs and affect children as well as adults and, hence, requires a multidisciplinary approach to patient care. After establishing a diagnosis of FD, efforts should be made to evaluate the presence of extra-skeletal disease in order to identify patients with MAS. Pituitary, adrenal, thyroid, parathyroid, and gonadal function should be evaluated, and any endocrine dysfunction treated appropriately and monitored.

Non-gonadotropin-mediated precocious puberty in FD/MAS is much more common in girls where it occurs due to recurrent ovarian cysts with excess estrogen production, and treatment usually includes aromatase inhibitor (letrozole) and/or selective estrogen receptor modulator (tamoxifen). In contrast, precocious puberty is much rarer in boys, occurs due to testicular enlargement with excess testosterone production, and can be managed with combination of androgen receptor blocker and aromatase inhibitor (letrozole). If these children subsequently develop central precocious puberty, then leuprolide therapy may be effective. Thyroid disease usually occurs as nonfunctioning goiter or as autoimmune hyperthyroidism, although both might occur simultaneously in which case the best course of action may be a total thyroidectomy. Radioiodine ablation should be avoided in these cases due to concern for uptake of radioiodine by mutation-bearing tissue which may lead to increased risk of malignancy in the remaining gland. FGF23-mediated phosphaturia can lead to hypophosphatemia necessitating oral phosphorous and calcitriol supplementation. Unlike other disorders of FGF23 excess, bone turnover markers are usually constitutively elevated in FD and do not help in guiding response to therapy. Acromegaly due to autonomous growth hormone secretion from anterior pituitary tumors can lead to growth of FD bone lesions due to excess IGF-1, necessitating timely diagnosis and management. Medical therapy with octreotide and/or growth hormone receptor antagonist (pegvisomant) is recommended initial management because pituitary tumor resection is usually fraught with technical difficulties and complications in cases of craniofacial FD. Growth hormone excess is usually accompanied by hyperprolactinemia (due to co-secretion) which can be managed with dopamine agonists (bromocriptine and cabergoline). Hypercortisolism has been rarely reported in FD/MAS and if present, it usually presents in the neonatal period [14]. Definitive treatment includes surgical adrenalectomy but medical therapy with metyrapone can also be used. Some cases have shown spontaneous remission [14], likely due to fetal adrenal involution.

There is currently no medical therapy that will alter the disease course of FD, particularly pertaining to skeletal lesions. Treatment should take into account the age of the patient and the site of skeletal involvement for impending fractures or nerve impingement. As previously noted, craniofacial disease can be aggressive, causing pain and compression of vital cranial nerves and other neurological structures. Surgery is usually reserved for lesions in bones with impending fracture such as the proximal femur, in which case insertion of an intramedullary nail is the preferred intervention. Surgical measures are also used to treat limb length discrepancy and spine deformity. For craniofacial involvement, surgery may be required if there is impending loss of vision or hearing. The risk of FD recurrence into the grafted bone needs to be kept in mind [14]. For this reason, cosmetic surgery should be approached cautiously and only after thoroughly discussing the risk of disease recurrence with the patient. Prophylactic surgery to guard against vision loss is usually not advocated given its high failure rate and the risk of graft resorption [15]. Surgery could be considered for rapidly expanding aneurysmal fluid-filled bone cysts that form within highly vascular lesions of FD associated with visual loss in <5% of patients [16].

Medical therapy for FD is focused on symptomatic pain management. Pain control and physical therapy are a major part of long-term management of patients. There is anecdotal evidence of bisphosphonates decreasing bone pain and biochemical markers of bone turnover and in a number of cases improving the radiographic features of FD [17]. Both pamidronate and zoledronic acid have been used to treat FD involving craniofacial bones or the proximal femur [18]. Chapurlat et al. [18] suggested superiority of zoledronic acid (at a dose of 4 mg every 6 months) over pamidronate in reducing pain and bone turnover markers after patients with FD were switched from pamidronate therapy. Oral alendronate therapy has been shown to reduce the NTX bone resorption marker, but improvement in pain was only modest when compared to pamidronate in a series of six adults [18, 19]. Boyce et al. similarly showed in a randomized clinical trial a reduction in NTX and improvement in areal BMD but no significant change in pain or functional parameters with alendronate therapy [20]. With the currently available data, we can infer that intravenous zoledronic acid appears to be the most effective bisphosphonate for pain control as well as reducing bone resorption in patients with FD. Bone histopathology examination can show changes related to vitamin D deficiency and hyperparathyroidism [21]; hence, it is important to screen for vitamin D insufficiency/deficiency and ensure adequate provision of calcium and vitamin D. Phosphorous supplementation is only necessary in patients with significant hypophosphatemia. If acromegaly is present, its management is essential to prevent the effect of excess IGF-1 on the growth of FD bone lesions.

Presently available medical therapies have been largely ineffective in altering the disease course of FD. Osteoclastogenesis observed in FD lesions is dependent on the secretion of IL-6 by osteogenic cells and the upregulation of RANKL caused by the *GNAS* mutation. Tocilizumab is an antagonist of IL-6 approved for the treatment of rheumatoid arthritis, and denosumab is a monoclonal antibody against RANKL approved for treatment of osteoporosis and cancer-related bone metastases. Boyce et al. [22] described the case of a 9-year-old boy with severe FD involving a rapidly expanding femoral lesion and marked RANKL expression on pretreatment bone biopsy, who was treated with monthly denosumab injections for 7 months leading to a marked reduction in pain, bone turnover markers, and tumor growth rate. Studies to explore potential new therapies for FD are indeed needed.

Case Management

The patient in this clinical vignette had (a) "ground glass" expansile lesions in the skull base, clivus, and facial bones on plain radiographs and CT scan, (b) corresponding replacement of normal marrow signal seen with MRI, and (c) hypermetabolic activity on PET scan all highly suggestive of the diagnosis of FD. Although the involvement of the clivus, skull base, and maxilla did not produce any cosmetic abnormality, it contributed to the patient's headaches and retrobulbar pain. The elevated CTX and normal BAP suggested uncoupled bone remodeling (i.e., an increase in bone resorption out of proportion to bone formation) and supports increased osteoclastogenesis that occurs in FD lesions. There were no serum phosphate or other laboratory mineral abnormalities noted. The patient was treated with 5 mg intravenous zoledronic acid, which led to significant symptomatic improvement within a few weeks. A second 5 mg dose of zoledronic acid 6 months later resulted in complete resolution of his symptoms.

References

1. Benhamou J, Gensburger D, Messiaen C, Chapurlat R. Prognostic factors from an epidemiologic evaluation of fibrous dysplasia of bone in a modern cohort: the FRANCEDYS study. J Bone Miner Res Off J Am Soc Bone Miner Res. 2016;31(12):2167–72.
2. Volkl TM, Dorr HG. McCune-Albright syndrome: clinical picture and natural history in children and adolescents. J Pediatr Endocrinol Metab. 2006;19(Suppl 2):551–9.
3. Kuznetsov SA, Cherman N, Riminucci M, Collins MT, Robey PG, Bianco P. Age-dependent demise of GNAS-mutated skeletal stem cells and "normalization" of fibrous dysplasia of bone. J Bone Miner Res Off J Am Soc Bone Miner Res. 2008;23(11):1731–40.
4. Ruggieri P, Sim FH, Bond JR, Unni KK. Malignancies in fibrous dysplasia. Cancer. 1994;73(5):1411–24.
5. Salenave S, Boyce AM, Collins MT, Chanson P. Acromegaly and McCune-Albright syndrome. J Clin Endocrinol Metab. 2014;99(6):1955–69.
6. Adada B, Al-Mefty O. Fibrous dysplasia of the clivus. Neurosurgery. 2003;52(2):318–22. discussion 23
7. Weinstein LS, Shenker A, Gejman PV, Merino MJ, Friedman E, Spiegel AM. Activating mutations of the stimulatory G protein in the McCune-Albright syndrome. N Engl J Med. 1991;325(24):1688–95.

8. Candeliere GA, Glorieux FH, Prud'homme J, St-Arnaud R. Increased expression of the c-fos proto-oncogene in bone from patients with fibrous dysplasia. N Engl J Med. 1995;332(23):1546–51.
9. Riminucci M, Fisher LW, Shenker A, Spiegel AM, Bianco P, Gehron Robey P. Fibrous dysplasia of bone in the McCune-Albright syndrome: abnormalities in bone formation. Am J Pathol. 1997;151(6):1587–600.
10. Bianco P, Riminucci M, Majolagbe A, Kuznetsov SA, Collins MT, Mankani MH, et al. Mutations of the GNAS1 gene, stromal cell dysfunction, and osteomalacic changes in non-McCune-Albright fibrous dysplasia of bone. J Bone Miner Res Off J Am Soc Bone Miner Res. 2000;15(1):120–8.
11. Collins MT, Chebli C, Jones J, Kushner H, Consugar M, Rinaldo P, et al. Renal phosphate wasting in fibrous dysplasia of bone is part of a generalized renal tubular dysfunction similar to that seen in tumor-induced osteomalacia. J Bone Miner Res Off J Am Soc Bone Miner Res. 2001;16(5):806–13.
12. Riminucci M, Collins MT, Fedarko NS, Cherman N, Corsi A, White KE, et al. FGF-23 in fibrous dysplasia of bone and its relationship to renal phosphate wasting. J Clin Invest. 2003;112(5):683–92.
13. Riminucci M, Liu B, Corsi A, Shenker A, Spiegel AM, Robey PG, et al. The histopathology of fibrous dysplasia of bone in patients with activating mutations of the Gs alpha gene: site-specific patterns and recurrent histological hallmarks. J Pathol. 1999;187(2):249–58.
14. Brown RJ, Kelly MH, Collins MT. Cushing syndrome in the McCune-Albright syndrome. J Clin Endocrinol Metab. 2010;95(4):1508–15.
15. Lee JS, FitzGibbon EJ, Chen YR, Kim HJ, Lustig LR, Akintoye SO, et al. Clinical guidelines for the management of craniofacial fibrous dysplasia. Orphanet J Rare Dis. 2012;7(Suppl 1):S2.
16. Manjila S, Zender CA, Weaver J, Rodgers M, Cohen AR. Aneurysmal bone cyst within fibrous dysplasia of the anterior skull base: continued intracranial extension after endoscopic resections requiring craniofacial approach with free tissue transfer reconstruction. Child's Nerv Syst. 2013;29(7):1183–92.
17. Mansoori LS, Catel CP, Rothman MS. Bisphosphonate treatment in polyostotic fibrous dysplasia of the cranium: case report and literature review. Endocr Pract. 2010;16(5):851–4.
18. Chapurlat RD. Medical therapy in adults with fibrous dysplasia of bone. J Bone Miner Res Off J Am Soc Bone Miner Res. 2006;21(Suppl 2):P114–9.
19. Lane JM, Khan SN, O'Connor WJ, Nydick M, Hommen JP, Schneider R, et al. Bisphosphonate therapy in fibrous dysplasia. Clin Orthop Relat Res. 2001;382:6–12.
20. Boyce AM, Kelly MH, Brillante BA, Kushner H, Wientroub S, Riminucci M, et al. A randomized, double blind, placebo-controlled trial of alendronate treatment for fibrous dysplasia of bone. J Clin Endocrinol Metab. 2014;99(11):4133–40.
21. Corsi A, Collins MT, Riminucci M, Howell PG, Boyde A, Robey PG, et al. Osteomalacic and hyperparathyroid changes in fibrous dysplasia of bone: core biopsy studies and clinical correlations. J Bone Miner Res Off J Am Soc Bone Miner Res. 2003;18(7):1235–46.
22. Boyce AM, Chong WH, Yao J, Gafni RI, Kelly MH, Chamberlain CE, et al. Denosumab treatment for fibrous dysplasia. J Bone Miner Res. 2012;27(7):1462–70.

Chapter 14
Osteochondrodysplasias

Jad G. Sfeir, Anupam Kotwal, and Daniel L. Hurley

Abbreviations

AHO Albright hereditary osteodystrophy
FOP Fibrodysplasia ossificans progressiva
MCTO Multicentric carpotarsal osteolysis syndrome
PHP Pseudohypoparathyroidism
PPHP Pseudopseudohypoparathyroidism
SEDC Spondyloepiphyseal dysplasia congenita

Case Presentation

A 21-year-old Caucasian woman presented for musculoskeletal evaluation. She first noted deformities of her fingers and difficulty extending her wrists in her childhood years. She had gradual progressive flexure deformity of her fingers limiting extension. In addition, she became unable to flex her toes and fully extend her elbows and ankles. Her past history was remarkable for several teeth pulled with a graft to her lower gingiva at age 14 and a history of papilledema treated with acetazolamide. She denied a history of fractures. Physical examination was notable for mild proptosis, small ears, a small and slim nose, and joint range-of-motion limitations consistent with her history. Her mother, 9-year-old brother, maternal uncle, and maternal grandfather have a similar but milder phenotype. Her grandfather has kidney disease of unknown etiology.

Radiographs of her hands and feet (Fig. 14.1) revealed the absence of the majority of carpal bones. There was also a focal absence of multiple metacarpals and proximal phalangeal heads as well as an absence of the distal phalanges of the left third, right fourth, and both fifth toes. Axial bone mineral density measurements

J. G. Sfeir · A. Kotwal · D. L. Hurley (✉)
Department of Medicine and Division of Endocrinology, Diabetes, Metabolism and Nutrition, Mayo Clinic College of Medicine, Mayo Clinic, Rochester, MN, USA
e-mail: hurley.daniel@mayo.edu

P. M. Camacho (ed.), *Metabolic Bone Diseases*,
https://doi.org/10.1007/978-3-030-03694-2_14

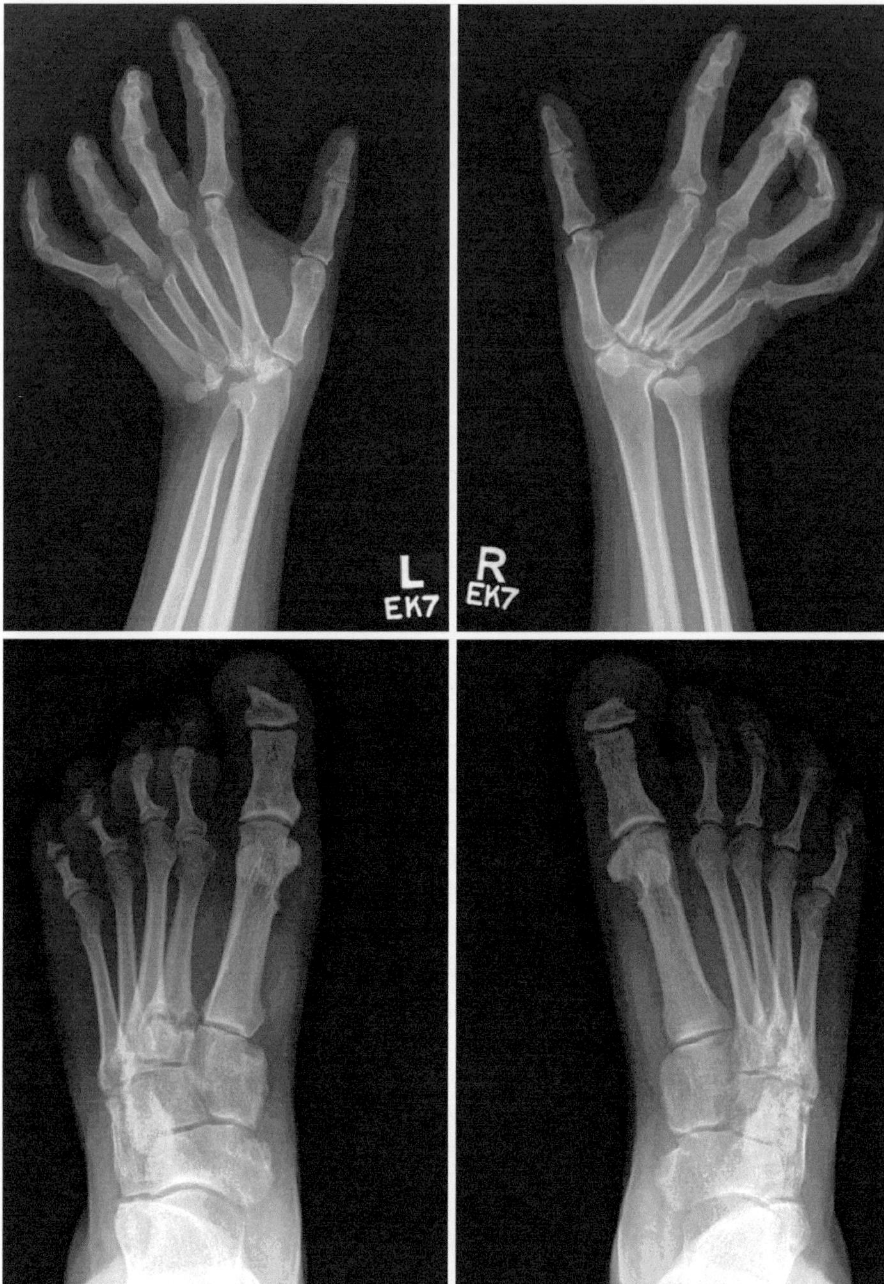

Fig. 14.1 Radiographs of patient's hand and feet: absence of the majority of carpal bones with focal absence of multiple metacarpal and proximal phalangeal heads as well as absence of the distal phalanges of the left third, right fourth, and both fifth toes

were normal (Z scores of +0.1, +0.6, and +1.9 at the left femoral neck, left total hip, and lumbar spine, respectively). Chemistries to include electrolytes, creatinine, minerals, parathyroid hormone, and urinary protein were normal.

Introduction

Skeletal dysplasias are a heterogeneous group of over 430 heritable disorders that, even though individually rare, collectively culminate to an incidence of about 1 in every 5000 live births [1].

As the name osteochondrodysplasia indicates, they affect the bone (osteo) and/or cartilage (chondro) leading to deformities in the limbs and/or the axial skeleton that commonly result in short stature. There is, however, significant heterogeneity in the clinical presentation, radiographic features, genetic basis, and mode of inheritance of these disorders. Disease severity and age of presentation also vary widely; some dysplasias are lethal prenatally or at birth, whereas others can be asymptomatic and discovered incidentally in adulthood. Improvement in diagnostic imaging as well as a better understanding of these disorders allow for a number of them to be diagnosed in utero [2].

Over the years, there have been significant efforts to classify the numerous osteochondrodysplasia disorders. Although initially categorized by phenotypic and radiographic description, the classification system has increasingly recognized subgroups of genetically related disorders through genetic mapping and molecular diagnostics that complement the wide range of clinical presentations [3]. The most recent 2015 revision of the nosology and classification of genetic skeletal disorders is included in Table 14.1 for a complete list of disorders. It identifies 42 groups of diseases as follows:

- Groups 1–8 based on a common gene defect or pathophysiologic pathway
- Groups 9–17 based on radiographic changes localized to particular bone structures (vertebrae, epiphyses, metaphyses, etc.) or segment
- Groups 18–20 based on macroscopic radiographic and clinical features
- Groups 21–26 and 28 based on defects in bone mineralization
- Group 27 based on skeletal involvement in lysosomal storage diseases
- Group 29 based on developmental disorganization of skeletal components
- Group 30 based on overgrowth syndromes
- Group 31 based on skeletal involvement in inflammatory diseases
- Groups 32–42 based on the various dysostoses

The following text describes only a few of these disorders that are more commonly encountered clinically. We then discuss the approach to patients with skeletal dysplasias.

Table 14.1 2015 Nosology and classification of genetic skeletal disorders

Group/name of disorder	Inheritance	MIM No.	Locus or gene	Protein	Notes
1. FGFR3 chondrodysplasia group					
Thanatophoric dysplasia type 1 (TD1)	AD	187600	*FGFR3*	FGFR3	Includes previous San Diego type
Thanatophoric dysplasia type 2 (TD2)	AD	187601	*FGFR3*	FGFR3	
Severe achondroplasia with developmental delay and acanthosis nigricans (SADDAN)	AD	187600	*FGFR3*	FGFR3	
Achondroplasia	AD	100800	*FGFR3*	FGFR3	
Hypochondroplasia	AD	146000	*FGFR3*	FGFR3	
Camptodactyly, tall stature, scoliosis, and hearing loss syndrome (CATSHL)	AD	610474	*FGFR3*	FGFR3	Inactivating mutation
Hypochondroplasia-like dysplasia(s)	AD, SP				Similar to hypochondroplasia but unlinked to FGFR3, probably heterogeneous; uncertain diagnostic criteria
See also group 33 for craniosynostoses syndromes linked to FGFR3 mutations, as well as LADD syndrome in group 41 for another FGFR3-related phenotype					
2. Type 2 collagen group					
Achondrogenesis type 2 (ACG2; Langer–Saldino)	AD	200610	COL2A1	Type 2 collagen	
Platyspondylic dysplasia, Torrance type	AD	151210	COL2A1	Type 2 collagen	See also severe spondylodysplastic dysplasias (group 14)
Hypochondrogenesis	AD	200610	COL2A1	Type 2 collagen	
Spondyloepiphyseal dysplasia congenita (SEDC)	AD	183900	COL2A1	Type 2 collagen	

Spondyloepimetaphyseal dysplasia (SEMD) Strudwick type	AD	184250	COL2A1	Type 2 collagen	Includes previous SMD Algerian type, Dysspondyloenchondromatosis and former SMD with severe genu valgum
Kniest dysplasia	AD	156550	COL2A1	Type 2 collagen	
Spondyloperipheral dysplasia	AD	271700	COL2A1	Type 2 collagen	
Mild SED with premature onset arthrosis	AD		COL2A1	Type 2 collagen	
SED with metatarsal shortening (formerly Czech dysplasia)	AD	609162	COL2A1	Type 2 collagen	
Stickler syndrome type 1	AD	108300	COL2A1	Type 2 collagen	See also COL11A1, COL11A2, and COL9A1
3. Type 11 collagen group					
Stickler syndrome type 2	AD	604841	COL11A1	Type 11 collagen alpha-1 chain	
Marshall syndrome	AD	154780	COL11A1	Type 11 collagen alpha-1 chain	
Stickler syndrome type 3 (non-ocular)	AD	184840	COL11A2	Type 11 collagen alpha-2 chain	
Fibrochondrogenesis	AR	228520	COL11A1	Type 11 collagen alpha-1 chain	
	AR, AD	614524	COL11A2	Type 11 collagen alpha-2 chain	
Oto-spondylo-mega-epiphyseal dysplasia (OSMED), recessive type	AR	215150	COL11A2	Type 11 collagen alpha-2 chain	
Oto-spondylo-mega-epiphyseal dysplasia (OSMED), dominant type (Weissenbacher–Zweymüller syndrome, Stickler syndrome type 3)	AD	277610	COL11A2	Type 11 collagen alpha-2 chain	
See also Stickler syndrome type 1 in group 2					

(continued)

Table 14.1 (continued)

Group/name of disorder	Inheritance	MIM No.	Locus or gene	Protein	Notes
4. Sulfation disorders group					
Achondrogenesis type 1B (ACG1B)	AR	600972	DTDST	SLC26A2 sulfate transporter	Formerly known as Fraccaro type achondrogenesis
Atelosteogenesis type 2 (AO2)	AR	256050	DTDST	SLC26A2 sulfate transporter	Includes de la Chapelle dysplasia, McAlister dysplasia, and "neonatal osseous dysplasia"
Diastrophic dysplasia (DTD)	AR	222600	DTDST	SLC26A2 sulfate transporter	
MED, autosomal recessive type (rMED; EDM4)	AR	226900	DTDST	SLC26A2 sulfate transporter	See also multiple epiphyseal dysplasias and pseudoachondroplasia group (group 9)
SEMD, PAPSS2 type	AR	612847	PAPSS2	PAPS synthetase 2	Formerly "Pakistani type." See also SEMD group (group 13)
Brachyolmia, recessive type	AR	612847	PAPSS2	PAPS synthetase 2	Probably includes Toledo and Hobaek types of brachyolmia
Chondrodysplasia gPAPP type (includes Catel–Manzke-like syndrome)	AR	614078	IMPAD1	Golgi 3-prime phosphoadenosine 5-prime phosphate 3-prime phosphatase	
Chondrodysplasia with congenital joint dislocations, CHST3 type (recessive Larsen syndrome)	AR	608637	CHST3	Carbohydrate sulfotransferase 3, chondroitin 6-sulfotransferase	Includes recessive Larsen syndrome, Humero–Spinal Dysostosis, and SED Omani type
Ehlers–Danlos syndrome, CHST14 type ("musculoskeletal variant")	AR	601776	CHST14	Carbohydrate sulfotransferase 14, dermatan 4-sulfotransferase	Includes Adducted Thumb–Clubfoot syndrome
See also group 7 and group 20 for other conditions with multiple dislocations					

5. Perlecan group					
Dyssegmental dysplasia, Silverman–Handmaker type	AR	224410	PLC (HSPG2)	Perlecan	
Dyssegmental dysplasia, Rolland–Desbuquois type	AR	224400	PLC (HSPG2)	Perlecan	
Schwartz–Jampel syndrome (myotonic chondrodystrophy)	AR	255800	PLC (HSPG2)	Perlecan	Mild and severe forms, includes previous Burton dysplasia
6. Aggrecan group					
SED, Kimberley type	AD	608361	AGC1	Aggrecan	
SEMD, Aggrecan type	AR	612813	AGC1	Aggrecan	
Familial osteochondritis dissecans	AD	165800	AGC1	Aggrecan	
7. Filamin group and related disorders					
Frontometaphyseal dysplasia	XLD	305620	FLNA	Filamin A	Some cases lack FLNA mutations
Osteodysplasty, Melnick–Needles	XLD	309350	FLNA	Filamin A	
Otopalatodigital syndrome type 1 (OPD1)	XLD	311300	FLNA	Filamin A	
Otopalatodigital syndrome type 2 (OPD2)	XLD	304120	FLNA	Filamin A	
Terminal osseous dysplasia with pigmentary defects (TODPD)	XLD	300244	FLNA	Filamin A	
Atelosteogenesis type 1 (AO1)	AD	108720	FLNB	Filamin B	Includes Boomerang dysplasia, Piepkorn dysplasia, and spondylohumerofemoral (giant cell) dysplasia
Atelosteogenesis type 3 (AO3)	AD	108721	FLNB	Filamin B	
Larsen syndrome (dominant)	AD	150250	FLNB	Filamin B	

(continued)

Table 14.1 (continued)

Group/name of disorder	Inheritance	MIM No.	Locus or gene	Protein	Notes
Spondylo-carpal-tarsal dysplasia	AR	272460	FLNB	Filamin B	Some cases unlinked to FLNB
Frank-ter Haar syndrome	AR	249420	SH3PXD2B	TKS4	
See also group 4 for recessive Larsen syndrome and group 20 for conditions with multiple dislocations					
8. TRPV4 group					
Metatropic dysplasia	AD	156530	TRPV4	Transient receptor potential cation channel, subfamily V, member 4	Includes "hyperplastic," lethal and nonlethal forms
Spondyloepimetaphyseal dysplasia, Maroteaux type (pseudo-Morquio syndrome type 2)	AD	184095	TRPV4	Transient receptor potential cation channel, subfamily V, member 4	Includes parastremmatic (MIM 168400)
Spondylometaphyseal dysplasia, Kozlowski type	AD	184252	TRPV4	Transient receptor potential cation channel, subfamily V, member 4	
Brachyolmia, autosomal dominant type	AD	113500	TRPV4	Transient receptor potential cation channel, subfamily V, member 4	
Familial digital arthropathy with brachydactyly	AD	606835	TRPV4	Transient receptor potential cation channel, subfamily V, member 4	
9. Ciliopathies with major skeletal involvement					
Chondroectodermal dysplasia (Ellis-van Creveld)	AR	225500	EVC1	EVC gene 1	See also Weyers acrofacial (acrodental) dysostosis in group 34
			EVC2	EVC gene 2	
Short rib polydactyly syndrome (SRPS) type 1/3 (Saldino–Noonan/Verma–Naumoff)	AR	208500	DYNC2H1	Dynein, cytoplasmic 2, heavy chain 1	There is significant clinical and radiological overlap between SRP1/3 and ATD. Some forms of both remain unlinked to the known genes
		613091	IFT80	Intraflagellar transport 80 (homolog of)	

			WDR34	WD repeat-containing protein 34	
Asphyxiating thoracic dysplasia (ATD, Jeune)	AR	263510	DYNC2H1	Dynein, cytoplasmic 2, heavy chain 1	
			IFT80	Intraflagellar transport 80 (homolog of)	
			WDR34	WD repeat-containing protein 34	
			TTC21B	Tetratricopeptide repeat domain-containing protein 21B	
			WDR19	WD repeat-containing protein 19	
			IFT172	Intraflagellar transport 172	
			IFT140	Intraflagellar transport 140	
SRPS type 2 (Majewski)	AR	263520	DYNC2H1	Dynein, cytoplasmic 2, heavy chain 1	
			NEK1	Never in mitosis gene a-related kinase 1	
SRPS type 4 (Beemer)	AR	269860			Not yet proven ciliopathy
SRPS type 5	AR	614091	WDR35	WD repeat-containing protein 19	
Oral-facial-digital syndrome type 4 (Mohr–Majewski)	AR	258860	TCTN3	Tectonic family, member 3	
Cranioectodermal dysplasia (Levin–Sensenbrenner) type 1, 2	AR	218330	IFT122	Intraflagellar transport 122	
		613610	WDR35	WD repeat-containing protein 35	
		614099	WDR19	WD repeat-containing protein 19	
			IFT43	Intraflagellar transport 43	
Thoracolaryngopelvic dysplasia (Barnes)	AD	187760			
See also paternal UPD14 and cerebro-costo-mandibular syndrome					

(continued)

Table 14.1 (continued)

Group/name of disorder	Inheritance	MIM No.	Locus or gene	Protein	Notes
10. Multiple epiphyseal dysplasia and pseudoachondroplasia group					
Pseudoachondroplasia (PSACH)	AD	177170	COMP	COMP	
Multiple epiphyseal dysplasia (MED) type 1 (EDM1)	AD	132400	COMP	COMP	
Multiple epiphyseal dysplasia (MED) type 2 (EDM2)	AD	600204	COL9A2	Collagen 9 alpha-2 chain	
Multiple epiphyseal dysplasia (MED) type 3 (EDM3)	AD	600969	COL9A3	Collagen 9 alpha-3 chain	
Multiple epiphyseal dysplasia (MED) type 5 (EDM5)	AD	607078	MATN3	Matrilin 3	
Multiple epiphyseal dysplasia (MED) type 6 (EDM6)	AD	120210	COL9A1	Collagen 9 alpha-1 chain	
Multiple epiphyseal dysplasia (MED), other types					Some MED-like cases unlinked to known genes
Stickler syndrome, recessive type	AR	120210	COL9A1	Collagen 9 alpha-1 chain	See also groups 2 and 3
Familial hip dysplasia (Beukes)	AD	142669	4q35		
Multiple epiphyseal dysplasia with microcephaly and nystagmus (Lowry–Wood)	AR	226960		Collagen 10 alpha-1 chain	
See also multiple epiphyseal dysplasia, recessive type (rMED; EDM4) in sulfation disorders (group 4), familial osteochondritis dissecans in the aggrecan group, as well as ASPED in the acromelic group					
11. Metaphyseal dysplasias					
Metaphyseal dysplasia, Schmid type (MCS) AD 156500 COL10A1					
Cartilage-hair hypoplasia (CHH; metaphyseal dysplasia, McKusick type)	AR	250250	RMRP	RNA component of RNAse H	Includes anauxetic dysplasia

Metaphyseal dysplasia, CHH-like, POP1 type	AR		POP1	Processing of precursor RNA	
Metaphyseal dysplasia, Jansen type	AD	156400	PTHR1	PTH/PTHrP receptor 1	Activating mutations; see also Blomstrand dysplasia (group 23)
Eiken dysplasia	AR	600002	PTHR1	PTH/PTHrP receptor 1	Activating mutations; see also Blomstrand dysplasia (group 23)
Metaphyseal dysplasia with pancreatic insufficiency and cyclic neutropenia (Shwachman–Bodian–Diamond syndrome, SBDS)	AR	260400	SBDS	SBDS protein	
Metaphyseal anadysplasia type 1	AD, AR	602111	MMP13	Matrix metalloproteinase 13	Includes SEMD Missouri type
Metaphyseal anadysplasia type 2	AR	613073	MMP9	Matrix metalloproteinase 9	
Metaphyseal dysplasia, Spahr type	AR	250400	MMP13	Matrix metalloproteinase 13	Includes autosomal recessive anadysplasia
Metaphyseal dysplasia with maxillary hypoplasia	AD	156510	RUNX2	Runt-related transcription factor 2	
12. Spondylometaphyseal dysplasias (SMD)					
Spondyloenchondrodysplasia (SPENCD)	AR	271550	ACP5	Tartrate-resistant acid phosphatase (TRAP)	Includes combined immunodeficiency with autoimmunity and spondylometaphyseal dysplasia (MIM 607944)
Odontochondrodysplasia (ODCD)	AR	184260			
SMD, Sutcliffe type or corner fracture type	AD	184255			Some cases are linked to COL2A1 but not the original family

(continued)

Table 14.1 (continued)

Group/name of disorder	Inheritance	MIM No.	Locus or gene	Protein	Notes
SMD with cone-rod dystrophy	AR	608940	PCYT1A	Phosphate cytidylyltransferase 1	
SMD with retinal degeneration, axial type	AR	602271			
See also SMD Kozlowski (group TRPV4) as well as SMD Sedaghatian type in group 14; there are many individual reports of SMD variants					
13. Spondylo-epi-(meta)-physeal dysplasias (SE(M)D)					
Dyggve–Melchior–Clausen dysplasia (DMC)	AR	223800	DYM	Dymeclin	Includes Smith–McCort dysplasia (MIM 615222 RAB33B RAS-associated protein rab33b 607326)
Immuno-osseous dysplasia (Schimke)	AR	242900	SMARCAL1	SWI/SNF-related regulator of chromatin subfamily A-like protein 1	
SED, Wolcott–Rallison type	AR	226980	EIF2AK3	Translation initiation factor 2-alpha kinase-3	
SEMD, matrilin type	AR	608728	MATN3	Matrilin 3	See also matrilin-related MED in group 10
SEMD, short limb-abnormal calcification type	AR	271665	DDR2	Discoidin domain receptor family, member 2	See also other dysplasias with stippling in group 21
SED tarda, X-linked (SED-XL)	XLR	313400	SEDL	Sedlin	
Spondylodysplastic Ehlers–Danlos syndrome	AR	612350	SLC39A13	Zinc transporter ZIP13	
SPONASTRIME dysplasia	AR	271510			
Platyspondyly (brachyolmia) with amelogenesis imperfecta	AR	601216			
CODAS syndrome	AR	600373	LONP1	LON peptidase 1	
See also opsismodysplasia (group 14), mucopolysaccharidosis type 4 (Morquio syndrome), and other conditions in group 27, as well as PPRD (SED with progressive arthropathy) in group 31					
14. Severe spondylodysplastic dysplasias					
Achondrogenesis type 1A (ACG1A)	AR	200600	TRIP11	Golgi-microtubule-associated protein, 210-KD; GMAP210	

Schneckenbecken dysplasia	AR	269250	SLC35D1	solute carrier family 35 member D1; UDP-glucuronic acid/UDP-Nacetylgalactosamine dual transporter	
Spondylometaphyseal dysplasia, Sedaghatian type	AR	250220	GPX4	Glutathione peroxidase 4	
Severe spondylometaphyseal dysplasia (SMD Sedaghatian like)	AR		SBDS	SBDS gene, function still unclear	
Opsismodysplasia	AR	258480	INPPL1	Inositol polyphosphate phosphatase-like 1	Includes lethal and milder cases
MAGMAS related skeletal dysplasia	AR		MAGMAS	Presequence translocaseassociated motor 16	
See also thanatophoric dysplasia types 1 and 2 (group 1), ACG2 and Torrance dysplasia (group 2), fibrochondrogenesis (group 3), achondrogenesis type 1B (group 4), and metatropic dysplasia (group 8)					
15. Acromelic dysplasias					
Trichorhinophalangeal dysplasia types 1/3	AD	190350	TRPS1	Zinc finger transcription factor	
Trichorhinophalangeal dysplasia type 2 (Langer–Giedion)	AD	150230	TRPS1 and EXT1	Zinc finger transcription factor and Exostosin 1 Microdeletion syndrome	see also multiple cartilaginous exostoses in group 28
Acrocapitofemoral dysplasia	AR	607778	IHH	Indian hedgehog	
Geleophysic dysplasia	AR	231050	ADAMTSL2	ADAMTS-like protein 2	Some forms unlinked to either gene
	AD	614185	FBN1	Fibrillin 1	
Acromicric dysplasia	AD	102370	FBN1	Fibrillin 1	Includes acrolaryngeal dysplasia, previously known as Fantasy Island dysplasia or Tattoo dysplasia
Weill–Marchesani	AD		FBN1	Fibrillin 1	

(continued)

Table 14.1 (continued)

Group/name of disorder	Inheritance	MIM No.	Locus or gene	Protein	Notes
	AR		ADAMTS10	A disintegrin-like and metalloproteinase with thrombospondin type 1 motif, 10,17	
			ADAMTS17		
			LTBP2	Latent transforming growth factor beta-binding protein 2	
Myhre dysplasia	AD	139210	SMAD4	Mothers against decapentaplegic, drosophila, homolog of, 4	
Acrodysostosis	AD	101800	PDE4D	Phosphodiesterase 4D, camp specific	Includes some cases of acroscyphodysostosis
			PRKAR1A	Protein kinase, camp-dependent, regulatory, type 1, alpha	
Angel-shaped phalango-epiphyseal dysplasia (ASPED)	AD	105835			Possibly related or allelic to Brachydactyly type C
Albright hereditary osteodystrophy	AD	103580	GNAS	Guanine nucleotide-binding protein, alpha-stimulating activity polypeptide 1	Includes some cases of acroscyphodysostosis
See also brachydactyly group (group 37)					
16. Acromesomelic dysplasias					
Acromesomelic dysplasia, Maroteaux type (AMDM)	AR	602875	NPR2	Natriuretic peptide receptor 2	
Grebe dysplasia	AR	200700	GDF5	Growth and differentiation factor 5	Includes acromesomelic dysplasia Hunter–Thompson type; see also brachydactylies (group 34)
Fibular hypoplasia and complex brachydactyly (Du Pan)	AR	228900	GDF5	Growth and differentiation factor 5	See also brachydactylies (group 34)
Acromesomelic dysplasia with genital anomalies	AR	609441	BMPR1B	Bone morphogenetic protein receptor 1B	

Acromesomelic dysplasia, Osebold–Remondini type	AD	112910			
17. Mesomelic and rhizo-mesomelic dysplasias					
Dyschondrosteosis (Leri–Weill)	Pseudo-AD	127300	SHOX	Short stature homeobox gene	Includes Reinhardt–Pfeiffer dysplasia, MIM 191400
Langer type (homozygous dyschondrosteosis)	Pseudo-AR	249700	SHOX	Short stature homeobox gene	
Omodysplasia	AR	258315	GPC6	Glypican-6	
Omodysplasia, dominant	AD	164745	FZD2	Frizzled 2	
Robinow syndrome, recessive type	AR	268310	ROR2	Receptor tyrosine kinase-like orphan receptor 2	Includes previous COVESDEM (costovertebral segmentation defect with mesomelia); see also brachydactyly type B
Robinow syndrome, dominant type	AD	180700	WNT5A	Wingless-type mmtv integration site family, member 5a	
		601365	DVL1	Disheveled 1	
Mesomelic dysplasia, Kantaputra type	AD	156232		Duplications in HOXD gene cluster	Includes mesomelic dysplasia, Korean type
Mesomelic dysplasia, Nievergelt type	AD	163400			
Mesomelic dysplasia, Kozlowski–Reardon type	AR	249710			
Mesomelic dysplasia with acral synostoses (Verloes–David – Pfeiffer type)	AD	600383	SULF1 and SLCO5A1	Heparan sulfate 6-Oendosulfatase 1 and solute carrier organic anion transporter family member 5A1	Microdeletion syndrome involving two adjacent genes
Mesomelic dysplasia, Savarirayan type (triangular tibia – fibular aplasia)	SP	605274		6p22.3 deletions	Possibly related to Nievergelt dysplasia

(continued)

Table 14.1 (continued)

Group/name of disorder	Inheritance	MIM No.	Locus or gene	Protein	Notes
18. Campomelic dysplasia and related disorders					
Campomelic dysplasia (CD)	AD	114290	SOX9	SRY-box 9	Includes acampomelic campomelic dysplasia (ACD), mild campomelic dysplasia (MIM 602196), and isolated Pierre–Robin
Stüve–Wiedemann dysplasia	AR	601559	LIFR	Leukemia inhibitory factor receptor	Includes former neonatal Schwartz–Jampel syndrome or SJS type 2
Kyphomelic dysplasia, several forms		211350		Probably heterogeneous	
See also group 33 for craniosynostoses syndromes linked to FGFR2					
19. Slender bone dysplasia group					
3-M syndrome	AR	273750	CUL7	Cullin 7	Includes dolichospondylic dysplasia and Yakut short stature syndrome
		612921 Obscurin-like 1	OBSL1		
		614205	CCDC8	Coiled-coil domain-containing protein 8	
Kenny–Caffey dysplasia	AR	244460	TBCE	Tubulin-specific chaperone E	Referred to in OMIM as type 1 but does not correspond to the disorder described by Kenny and Caffey which is the dominant form
Kenny–Caffey dysplasia	AD	127000	FAM111A	Family with sequence similarity 111, member A	
Osteocraniostenosis	AD	602361	FAM111A	Family with sequence similarity 111, member A	

Microcephalic osteodysplastic primordial dwarfism type 1/3 (MOPD1)	AR	210710	RNU4ATAC	RNA, U4ATAC small nuclear	Includes Taybi–Linder cephaloskeletal dysplasia
Microcephalic osteodysplastic primordial dwarfism type 2 (MOPD2; Majewski type)	AR	210720	PCNT2	Pericentrin 2	
IMAGe syndrome (intrauterine growth retardation, metaphyseal dysplasia, adrenal hypoplasia, and genital anomalies)	AD	614732	CDKN1C	Cyclin-dependent kinase inhibitor 1C	Possibly heterogeneous
Hallermann–Streiff syndrome	AR	234100			Mutations in GJA1 reported in one case only
See also cerebro-arthro-digital dysplasia					
20. Dysplasias with multiple joint dislocations					
Desbuquois dysplasia (with accessory ossification center in digit 2) AR 251450 CANT1 calcium-activated nucleotidase 1					Other variants with or without accessory ossification centers unlinked to CANT1
Desbuquois dysplasia with short metacarpals and elongated phalanges (Kim type)	AR	251450	CANT1	Calcium-activated nucleotidase 1	
Desbuquois dysplasia type 2	AR	615777	XYLT1	Xylosyltransferase 1	
Pseudodiastrophic dysplasia	AR	264180			
SEMD with joint laxity (SEMD-JL) leptodactylic or Hall type	AD	603546	KIF22	Kinesin family member 22	

(continued)

Table 14.1 (continued)

Group/name of disorder	Inheritance	MIM No.	Locus or gene	Protein	Notes
SEMD with joint laxity (SEMD-JL) Beighton type	AR	271640	B3GALT6	Beta-1,3-galactosyltransferase polypeptide 6	
See also SED with congenital dislocations, CHST3 type (group 4); atelosteogenesis type 3 and Larsen syndrome (group 7)					
21. Chondrodysplasia punctata (CDP) group					
CDP, X-linked dominant, Conradi–Hünermann type (CDPX2)	XLD	302960	EBP	Emopamil binding protein	
CDP, X-linked recessive, brachytelephalangic type (CDPX1)	XLR	302950	ARSE	Arylsulfatase E	
CHILD (congenital hemidysplasia, ichthyosis, limb defects)	XLD	308050	NSDHL	NAD(P)H steroid dehydrogenase-like protein	
Keutel syndrome	AR	245150	MGP	Matrix gamma-carboxyglutamic acid	
Greenberg dysplasia	AR	215140	LBR	Lamin B receptor, 3-beta-hydroxysterol delta (14)- reductase	Includes hydrops-ectopic calcification moth-eaten appearance dysplasia (HEM) and dappled diaphyseal dysplasia
Rhizomelic CDP type 1	AR	215100	PEX7	Peroxisomal PTS2 receptor	
Rhizomelic CDP type 2	AR	222765	DHPAT	Dihydroxyacetonephosphate acyltransferase (DHAPAT)	
Rhizomelic CDP type 3	AR	600121	AGPS	Alkylglycerone phosphate synthase (AGPS)	
CDP tibial-metacarpal type	AD/AR	118651			Nosologic status uncertain
Astley–Kendall dysplasia	AR				Relationship to OI and to Greenberg dysplasia unclear
Note that stippling can occur in maternal autoimmune disease and several syndromes such as Zellweger, Smith–Lemli–Opitz, and others *See also desmosterolosis as well as SEMD short limb-abnormal calcification type in group 13*					

22. Neonatal osteosclerotic dysplasias					
Blomstrand dysplasia	AR	215045	PTHR1	PTH/PTHrP receptor 1	Caused by recessive inactivating mutations; see also Eiken dysplasia and Jansen dysplasia
Desmosterolosis	AR	602398	DHCR24	3-beta-hydroxysterol delta-24-reductase	See also other sterol metabolism related conditions
Caffey disease (including prenatal, infantile, and attenuated forms)	AD	114000	COL1A1	Collagen 1, alpha-1 chain	See also osteogenesis imperfecta related to collagen 1 genes (group 24)
Caffey dysplasia (severe variants with prenatal onset)	AR	114000			
Raine dysplasia (lethal and nonlethal forms)	AR	259775	FAM20C	Dentin matrix protein 4	Includes lethal and nonlethal cases
See also Astley–Kendall dysplasia and CDPs in group 21					
23. Osteopetrosis and related disorders					
Osteopetrosis, severe neonatal, or infantile forms (OPTB1)	AR	259700	TCIRG1	Subunit of ATPase proton pump	
Osteopetrosis, severe neonatal, or infantile forms (OPTB4)	AR	611490	CLCN7	Chloride channel 7	
Osteopetrosis, severe neonatal, or infantile forms (OPTB8)	AR	615085	SNX10	Sorting nexin 10	
Osteopetrosis, infantile form, with nervous system involvement (OPTB5)	AR	259720	OSTM1	Gray lethal/osteopetrosis-associated transmembrane protein	Includes former osteopetrosis with infantile neuraxonal dysplasia
Osteopetrosis, intermediate form, osteoclast-poor (OPTB2)	AR	259710	RANKL (TNFSF11)	Receptor activator of NF-kappa-B ligand (tumor necrosis factor ligand superfamily, member 11)	

(continued)

Table 14.1 (continued)

Group/name of disorder	Inheritance	MIM No.	Locus or gene	Protein	Notes
Osteopetrosis, infantile form, osteoclast- poor with immunoglobulin deficiency (OPTB7)	AR	612302	RANK (TNFRSF11A)	Receptor activator of NF-kappa-B	See also familial expansile osteolysis in osteolysis group (group 28)
Osteopetrosis, intermediate form (OPTB6)	AR	611497	PLEKHM1	Pleckstrin homology domain-containing protein, family M, member 1	
Osteopetrosis, intermediate form (OPTA2)	AR	259710	CLCN7	Chloride channel pump	
Osteopetrosis with renal tubular acidosis (OPTB3)	AR	259730	CA2	Carbonic anhydrase 2	
Osteopetrosis, late-onset form type 1 (OPTA1)	AD	607634	LRP5	Low density lipoprotein receptor-related protein 5	Includes Worth type osteosclerosis (MIM 144750)
Osteopetrosis, late-onset form type 2 (OPTA2)	AD	166600	CLCN7	Chloride channel 7	
Osteopetrosis with ectodermal dysplasia and immune defect (OLEDAID)	XL	300301	IKBKG (NEMO)	Inhibitor of kappa light polypeptide gene enhancer, kinase of	
Osteopetrosis, moderate form with defective leucocyte adhesion (LAD3)	AR	612840	FERMT3 (KIND3)	Fermitin 3 (Kindlin 3)	
Osteopetrosis, moderate form with defective leucocyte adhesion	AR	612840	RASGRP2 (CalDAGGEF1)	Ras guanyl nucleotide-releasing protein 2	
Pyknodysostosis	AR	265800	CTSK	Cathepsin K	
Osteopoikilosis	AD	155950	LEMD3	LEM domain-containing 3	Includes Buschke–Ollendorff syndrome (MIM 166700)
Melorheostosis with osteopoikilosis	AD	155950	LEMD3	LEM domain-containing 3	Includes mixed sclerosing bone dysplasia

Osteopathia striata with cranial sclerosis (OSCS)	XLD	300373	WTX	FAM123B	
Melorheostosis	SP				No germ line LEMD3 mutations identified so far
Dysosteosclerosis	AR	224300	SLC29A3	Solute carrier family 29 (nucleoside transporter)	
Note: Osteomesopyknosis may represent a form of osteopetrosis					
24. Other sclerosing bone disorders					
Craniometaphyseal dysplasia, autosomal dominant type	AD	123000	ANKH	Homolog of mouse ANK (ankylosis) gene	Gain of function mutations
Diaphyseal dysplasia Camurati–Engelmann	AD	131300	TGFB1	Transforming growth factor beta 1	
Hematodiaphyseal dysplasia, Ghosal	AR	231095	TBXAS1	Thromboxane A synthase 1	
Hypertrophic osteoarthropathy	AR	259100	HPGD	15-alpha-hydroxyprostaglandin dehydrogenase	Includes cranio-osteoarthropathy and cases of recessive pachydermoperiostosis
Pachydermoperiostosis (hypertrophic osteoarthropathy, primary, autosomal dominant)	AD	167100			Relationship to recessive form (MIM 259100, HPGD deficiency) unclear
Oculo-dento-osseous dysplasia (ODOD) mild type	AD	164200	GJA1	Gap junction protein alpha-1	
Oculo-dento-osseous dysplasia (ODOD) severe type	AR	257850	GJA1	Gap junction protein alpha-1	Possibly homozygous form of mild ODOD
Osteoectasia with hyperphosphatasia (juvenile Paget disease)	AR	239000	OPG	Osteoprotegerin	
Sclerosteosis	AR, AD	269500	SOST	Sclerostin	

(continued)

Table 14.1 (continued)

Group/name of disorder	Inheritance	MIM No.	Locus or gene	Protein	Notes
		614305	LRP4	Low-density lipoprotein receptor-related protein 4	
Endosteal hyperostosis, van Buchem type	AR	239100	SOST	Sclerostin	Specific 52 kb deletion downstream of SOST
Trichodentoosseous dysplasia	AD	190320	DLX3	Distal-less homeobox 3	
Craniometaphyseal dysplasia, autosomal recessive type	AR	218400	GJA1	Gap junction protein alpha-1	
Diaphyseal medullary stenosis with malignant fibrous histiocytoma	AD	112250			Also known as Hardcastle
Craniodiaphyseal dysplasia	AD	122860	SOST	Sclerostin	Dominant negative
Craniometaphyseal dysplasia, Wormian bone type	AR	615118			Also known as Schwartz–Lelek dysplasia
Endosteal sclerosis with cerebellar hypoplasia	AR	213002			
Lenz-Majewski hyperostotic dysplasia	SP	151050	PTDSS1	Phosphatidylserine synthase 1	
Metaphyseal dysplasia, Braun–Tinschert type	AD	605946			
Pyle disease	AR	265900			
25. Osteogenesis imperfecta and decreased bone density group					
Osteogenesis imperfecta, non-deforming form (OI type 1)	AD		COL1A1	Collagen 1 alpha-1 chain	Form with persistently blue sclerae
			COL1A2	Collagen 1 alpha-2 chain	
Osteogenesis imperfecta, perinatal lethal form (OI type 2)	AD, AR		COL1A1 COL1A2		
			CRTAP	Cartilage-associated protein	See also Bruck syndrome (below)

			LEPRE1	Leucine proline-enriched proteoglycan (leprecan) 1	
			PPIB	Peptidylprolyl isomerase B (cyclophilin B)	
Osteogenesis imperfecta, progressively deforming type (OI type 3)	AD, AR		COL1A1		
			COL1A2		
			CRTAP		
			LEPRE1		
			PPIB		
			SERPINH1	Serpin peptidase inhibitor, clade H, member 1	
			BMP1	Bone morphogenetic protein 1	
			FKBP10	FK506-binding protein 10	
			PLOD2	Procollagen lysyl hydroxylase 2	
			SERPINF1	Serpin peptidase inhibitor, clade F, member 1	
			SP7	Transcription factor (Osterix)	
			WNT1	Wingless-type MMTV integration site family, member	
			TMEM38B	Transmembrane protein 38B	
			CREB3L1	OASIS	
			SEC24D	SEC24-related gene family, member D	
Osteogenesis imperfecta, moderate form (OI type 4)	AD, AR		COL1A1		

(continued)

Table 14.1 (continued)

Group/name of disorder	Inheritance	MIM No.	Locus or gene	Protein	Notes
			COL1A2		Sclerae generally normal
			CRTAP		
			PPIB		
			FKBP10		
			SERPINF1		
			WNT1		
			SP7		
Osteogenesis imperfecta with calcification of the interosseous membranes and/or hypertrophic callus (OI type 5)	AD	610967	IFITM5	Interferon-Induced Transmembrane Protein 5	
X-linked osteoporosis	XL	300910	PLS3	Plastin 3	May be the same as Juvenile idiopathic osteoporosis (MIM259750)
Bruck syndrome type 1 (BS1)	AR	259450	FKBP10	FK506-binding protein 10	See autosomal recessive OI, above; intrafamilial variability between OI3 and BS1 documented
Bruck syndrome type 2 (BS2)	AR	609220	PLOD2	Procollagen lysyl hydroxylase 2	
Osteoporosis-pseudoglioma syndrome	AR	259770	LRP5	LDL-receptor related protein 5	May mimic OI types 3 and 4
LRP5 primary osteoporosis	AD		LRP5		
Calvarial doughnut lesions with bone fragility	AD	126550			
Idiopathic juvenile osteoporosis	SP	259750			Some patients reported with heterozygous mutations in the LRP5 gene and perhaps X-linked osteoporosis

Cole-Carpenter dysplasia (bone fragility with craniosynostosis)	AD	112240	P4HB	Prolyl 4-hydroxylase, beta-subunit	See also craniosynostosis syndromes in group 30
Spondylo-ocular dysplasia	AR	605822	XYLT2	Xylosyltransferase 2 probably heterogeneous	
Osteopenia with radiolucent lesions of the mandible	AD	166260			
Ehlers–Danlos syndrome, progeroid form	AR	130070	B4GALT7	Xylosylprotein 4-betagalactosyltransferase deficiency	
Geroderma osteodysplasticum	AR	231070	GORAB	SCYL1 binding protein 1	
Cutis laxa, autosomal recessive form, type 2B (ARCL2B)	AR	612940	PYCR1	Pyrroline-5-carboxylate reductase 1	Skeletal features overlapping with progeroid EDS and geroderma osteodysplasticum
Cutis laxa, autosomal recessive form, type 2A (ARCL2A) (Wrinkly skin syndrome)	AR	278250 219200	ATP6VOA2	ATPase, Hþ transporting, lysosomal, V0 subunit A2	Skeletal features overlapping with progeroid EDS and geroderma osteodysplasticum
Singleton–Merten dysplasia	AD	182250			
26. Abnormal mineralization group					
Hypophosphatasia, perinatal lethal, infantile, and juvenile forms	AR	241500	ALPL	Alkaline phosphatase, tissue nonspecific (TNSALP)	Intrafamilial variability
Hypophosphatasia, juvenile, and adult forms	AD	146300	ALPL	Alkaline phosphatase, tissue nonspecific (TNSALP)	Includes odontohypophosphatasia
Hypophosphatemic rickets, X-linked dominant	XLD	307800	PHEX	X-linked hypophosphatemia membrane protease	
Hypophosphatemic rickets, autosomal dominant	AD	193100	FGF23	Fibroblast growth factor 23	

(continued)

Table 14.1 (continued)

Group/name of disorder	Inheritance	MIM No.	Locus or gene	Protein	Notes
Hypophosphatemic rickets, autosomal recessive, type 1 (ARHR1)	AR	241520	DMP1	Dentin matrix acidic phosphoprotein 1	
Hypophosphatemic rickets, autosomal recessive, type 2 (ARHR2)	AR	613312	ENPP1	Ectonucleotide pyrophosphatase/ phosphodiesterase 1	
Hypophosphatemic rickets with hypercalciuria, X-linked recessive	XLR	300554	ClCN5	Chloride channel 5	Part of Dent's disease complex
Hereditary hypophosphatemic rickets with hypercalciuria, autosomal recessive (HHRH)	AR	241530	SLC34A3	Sodium-phosphate cotransporter	
Neonatal hyperparathyroidism, severe form	AR	239200	CASR	Calcium-sensing receptor	
Familial hypocalciuric hypercalcemia with transient neonatal hyperparathyroidism	AD	145980	CASR	Calcium-sensing receptor	
Calcium pyrophosphate deposition disease (familial chondrocalcinosis) type 2	AD	118600	ANKH	Homolog of mouse ANK (ankylosis) gene	Loss of function mutations (see craniometaphyseal dysplasia in group 24)
See also Jansen dysplasia and Eiken dysplasia					
27. Lysosomal storage diseases with skeletal involvement (dysostosis multiplex group)					
Mucopolysaccharidosis type 1H/1S (Hurler, Hurler–Scheie, Scheie)	AR	607014	IDA	Alpha-1-iduronidase	
Mucopolysaccharidosis type 2 (Hunter)	XLR	309900	IDS	Iduronate-2-sulfatase	
Mucopolysaccharidosis type 3A (Sanfilippo A)	AR	252900	HSS	Heparan sulfate sulfatase	

Mucopolysaccharidosis type 3B (Sanfilippo B)	AR	252920	NAGLU	N-Ac-beta-D-glucosaminidase	
Mucopolysaccharidosis type 3C (Sanfilippo C)	AR	252930	HSGNAT	Ac-CoA: alpha-glucosaminide Nacetyltransferase	
Mucopolysaccharidosis type 3D (Sanfilippo D)	AR	252940	GNS	N-acetylglucosamine-6-sulfatase	
Mucopolysaccharidosis type 4A (Morquio A)	AR	253000	GALNS	Galactosamine-6-sulfate sulfatase	
Mucopolysaccharidosis type 4B (Morquio B)	AR	253010	GLBI	Beta-galactosidase	
Mucopolysaccharidosis type 6 (Maroteaux–Lamy)	AR	253200	ARSB	Arylsulfatase B	
Mucopolysaccharidosis type 7 (Sly)	AR	253220	GUSB	Beta-glucuronidase	
Fucosidosis	AR	230000	FUCA	Alpha-fucosidase	
Alpha-mannosidosis	AR	248500	MANA	Alpha-mannosidase	
Beta-mannosidosis	AR	248510	MANB	Beta-mannosidase	
Aspartylglucosaminuria	AR	208400	AGA	Aspartyl-glucosaminidase	
GM1 gangliosidosis, several forms	AR	230500	GLB1	Beta-galactosidase	
Sialidosis, several forms	AR	256550	NEU1	Neuraminidase (sialidase)	
Infantile sialic acid storage disease (ISSD)	AR	269920	SLC17A5	Sialin (sialic acid transporter)	
Galactosialidosis, several forms	AR	256540	PPGB	Beta-galactosidase protective protein	
Multiple sulfatase deficiency	AR	272200	SUMF1	Sulfatase-modifying factor-1	
Mucolipidosis II (I-cell disease), alpha/beta type	AR	252500	GNPTAB	N-acetylglucosamine-1-phosphotransferase, alpha/beta subunits	

(continued)

Table 14.1 (continued)

Group/name of disorder	Inheritance	MIM No.	Locus or gene	Protein	Notes
Mucolipidosis III (Pseudo–Hurler polydystrophy), alpha/ beta type	AR	252600	GNPTAB	N-acetylglucosamine-1-phosphotransferase, alpha/beta subunits	
Mucolipidosis III (Pseudo–Hurler polydystrophy), gamma type	AR	252605	GNPTG	N-acetylglucosamine-1-phosphotransferase, gamma subunit	
Other conditions resembling storage diseases: congenital disorders of glycosylation and geleophysic					
28. Osteolysis group					
Familial expansile osteolysis	AD	174810	RANK	(TNFRSF11A)	Includes expansile skeletal hyperphosphatasia (MIM 602080)
Mandibuloacral dysplasia type A	AD	248370	LMNA	Lamin A/C	
Mandibuloacral dysplasia type B	AR	608612	ZMPSTE24	Zinc metalloproteinase	
Progeria, Hutchinson–Gilford type	AD	176670	LMNA	Lamin A/C	
Torg–Winchester syndrome	AR	259600	MMP2	Matrix metalloproteinase 2	Includes nodulosis–arthropathy–osteolysis syndrome (MIM 605156)
Hajdu–Cheney syndrome	AD	102500	NOTCH2	NOTCH2	Includes serpentine fibula-polycystic kidney syndrome
Multicentric carpal-tarsal osteolysis with and without nephropathy	AD	166300	MAFB	V-maf musculoaponeurotic fibrosarcoma oncogene family, protein b	
See also pycnodysostosis, cleidocranial dysplasia, and Keutel and Singleton–Merten syndrome. Note: Several neurologic conditions may cause acroosteolysis					
29. Disorganized development of skeletal components group					
Multiple cartilaginous exostoses 1	AD	133700	EXT1	Exostosin-1	
Multiple cartilaginous exostoses 2	AD	133701	EXT2	Exostosin-2	
Multiple cartilaginous exostoses 3	AD	600209			Unclear if other genes/loci
Cherubism	AD	118400	SH3BP2	SH3 domain-binding protein 2	

Fibrous dysplasia, polyostotic form (McCune–Albright)	SP	174800	GNAS	Guanine nucleotide-binding protein, alpha-stimulating activity subunit 1	Somatic mosaicism and imprinting phenomena
Progressive osseous heteroplasia	AD	166350	GNAS	Guanine nucleotide-binding protein, alpha-stimulating activity subunit 1	Gene subject to imprinting
Gnathodiaphyseal dysplasia	AD	166260	TMEM16E	Transmembrane protein 16E	
Metachondromatosis	AD	156250	PTPN11	Protein tyrosine phosphatase nonreceptor-type 11	
Osteoglophonic dysplasia	AD	166250	FGFR1	Fibroblast growth factor receptor 1	See also craniosynostosis syndromes in group 30
Fibrodysplasia ossificans progressiva (FOP)	AD, SP	135100	ACVR1	Activin A (BMP type 1) receptor	
Neurofibromatosis type 1 (NF1)	AD	162200	NF1	Neurofibromin	
Carpotarsal osteochondromatosis	AD	127820			
Cherubism with gingival fibromatosis (Ramon syndrome)	AR	266270			
Dysplasia epiphysealis hemimelica (Trevor)	SP	127800			
Lipomembranous osteodystrophy with leukoencephalopathy (presenile dementia with bone cysts; Nasu–Hakola)	AR	221770	TREM2, TYROBP	Triggering receptor expressed on myeloid cells 2, TYRO protein tyrosine kinase-binding protein	
Enchondromatosis (Ollier) and enchondromatosis with hemangiomata (Maffucci)	SP	166000	IDH1, IDH2	Isocitrate dehydrogenase 1, 2	PTHR1 mutations found in a few cases only, role still unclear
Metaphyseal chondromatosis with D-2-hydroxyglutaric aciduria	SP	614875	IDH1, IDH2	Isocitrate dehydrogenase 1, 2	
Genochondromatosis	SP/AD	137360			
Gorham–Stout					
See also Proteus syndrome in group 30 and spondyloenchondrodysplasia in group 12					

(continued)

Table 14.1 (continued)

Group/name of disorder	Inheritance	MIM No.	Locus or gene	Protein	Notes
30. Overgrowth (tall stature) syndromes with skeletal involvement					
Weaver syndrome	SP/AD	277590	EZH2	Enhancer of zeste, drosophila, homolog 2	Some cases reported with NSD1 mutations (see Sotos syndrome)
Sotos syndrome	AD	117550	NSD1	Nuclear receptor-binding su-var, enhancer of zeste, and trithorax domain protein 1	Some cases may have NFIX mutations (see Marshall–Smith syndrome)
Sotos-like syndrome	AD		SETD2	Set domain-containing protein 2	
Marshall–Smith syndrome	SP	602535	NFIX	nuclear factor I/X	Some clinical overlap with Sotos syndrome (see above)
Proteus syndrome	SP	176920	AKT1	V-akt murine thymoma viral oncogene homolog 1	Some Proteus-like cases have mutations in the PTEN gene
CLOVES	SP	612918	PIK3CA	Phosphatidylinositol 3-kinase, catalytic, alpha	
Marfan syndrome	AD	154700	FBN1	Fibrillin 1	
Congenital contractural arachnodactyly	AD	121050	FBN2	Fibrillin 2	
Loeys–Dietz syndrome types 1A, 1B, 2A, 2B, 3, 4	AD	609192	TGFBR1	TGF beta receptor subunit 1	
		610168	TGFBR2	TGF beta receptor subunit 2	
		608967	SMAD3	SMA-related protein 3	
		610380	TGFB2	TGF beta 2	
		613795			
		614816			
Overgrowth syndrome with 2q37 translocations	SP		NPPC	Natriuretic peptide precursor C	Overgrowth probably caused by overexpression of NPPC
Overgrowth with macrodactyly and NPR2 gain of function	AD		NPR2	Natriuretic peptide receptor 2	

Overgrowth syndrome with skeletal dysplasia (Nishimura–Schmidt endochondral gigantism)	SP				Nosologic status unclear but conspicuous skeletal phenotype(s)
See also Shprintzen–Goldberg syndrome in craniosynostosis group					
31. Genetic inflammatory/rheumatoid-like osteoarthropathies					
Progressive pseudorheumatoid dysplasia (PPRD, SED with progressive arthropathy)	AR	208230	WISP3	WNT1-inducible signaling pathway protein 3	
Chronic infantile neurologic cutaneous articular (CINCA) syndrome/neonatal-onset multisystem inflammatory disease (NOMID)	AD	607115	CIAS1	Cryopyrin	
Sterile multifocal osteomyelitis, periostitis, and pustulosis (CINCA/NOMID-like)	AR	147679	IL1RN	Interleukin-1 receptor antagonist	
Chronic recurrent multifocal osteomyelitis with congenital dyserythropoietic anemia (CRMO with CDA, Majeed syndrome)	AR	609628	LPIN2	Lipin 2	
Hyperostosis/hyperphosphatemia syndrome	AR	610233	GALNT3	UDP-N-acetyl-alpha-D-galactosamine: polypeptide N-acetylgalactosaminyltransferase 3	
Hyaline fibromatosis syndrome	AR	236490	ANTXR2	Anthrax toxin receptor 2	Previously known as Infantile systemic hyalinosis, Juvenile Hyaline Fibromatosis (JHF, 228600) and Puretic syndrome

(continued)

Table 14.1 (continued)

Group/name of disorder	Inheritance	MIM No.	Locus or gene	Protein	Notes
32. Cleidocranial dysplasia and related disorders					
Cleidocranial dysplasia	AD	119600	RUNX2	Runt-related transcription factor 2	
CDAGS syndrome (craniosynostosis, delayed fontanel closure, parietal foramina, imperforate anus, genital anomalies, skin eruption)	AR	603116			
Yunis–Varon dysplasia	AR	216340	FIG4		
Parietal foramina (isolated)	AD	168500	ALX4	Aristaless-like 4	See also frontonasal dysplasia type 1 (group 34), MSX2, muscle segment homeobox 2
See also pycnodysostosis, wrinkly skin syndrome, and several others *See also metaphyseal dysplasia with maxillary hypoplasia in Group 11*					
33. Craniosynostosis syndromes					
Pfeiffer syndrome (FGFR1-related)	AD	101600	FGFR1, FGFR2	Fibroblast growth factor receptor 1 and 2	Most have FGFR1 P252R mutation Includes Jackson–Weiss syndrome (MIM 123150) and Antley–Bixler variants caused by FGFR2 mutations (see below)
Apert syndrome	AD	101200	FGFR2	Fibroblast growth factor receptor 2	
Craniosynostosis with cutis gyrata (Beare–Stevenson)	AD	123790	FGFR2	Fibroblast growth factor receptor 2	
Crouzon syndrome	AD	123500	FGFR2	Fibroblast growth factor receptor 2	
Bent bone dysplasia	AD	614592	FGFR2	Fibroblast growth factor receptor 2	
Crouzon-like craniosynostosis with acanthosis nigricans (Crouzonodermoskeletal syndrome)	AD	612247	FGFR3	Fibroblast growth factor receptor 3	Defined by specific FGFR3 A391E mutation

Craniosynostosis, Muenke type	AD	FGFR3	602849	Fibroblast growth factor receptor 3	Defined by specific FGFR3 P250R mutation
Antley–Bixler syndrome	AR	201750	POR	Cytochrome P450 oxidoreductase	Similar cases with FGFR2 mutations classified by MIM as Antley–Bixler without genital anomalies may be variants of Pfeiffer syndrome
Craniosynostosis, Boston type	AD	604757	MSX2	MSX2	Heterozygous P148H mutation in a two families
Saethre–Chotzen syndrome	AD	101400	TWIST1	TWIST	
Shprintzen–Goldberg syndrome	AD	182212	SKI	SKI	
Baller–Gerold syndrome	AR	218600	RECQL4	RECQ protein-like 4	RECQL4 might not account for all cases of Baller–Gerold
Carpenter syndrome	AR	201000	RAB23		
		614976	MEGF8		
Coronal craniosynostosis	AD	615314	TCF12	Transcription factor 12	
Complex craniosynostosis	AD	600775	ERF	ETS2 repressor factor	
See also Cole–Carpenter syndrome in group 24, CDAGS syndrome in group 29, and craniofrontonasal syndrome in group 34, and Philadelphia-type craniosynostosis (IHH duplication) in group 39					
34. Dysostoses with predominant craniofacial involvement					
Mandibulofacial dysostosis (Treacher Collins, Franceschetti–Klein)	AD, AD, AR	154500	TCOF1	Treacher Collins–Franceschetti syndrome 1	
			POLR1D	Polymerase (RNA) I polypeptide D	
			POLR1C	Polymerase (RNA) I polypeptide C	
Oral-facial-digital syndrome type 1 (OFD1)	XLR	311200	CXORF5	Chromosome X open reading frame 5	

(continued)

Table 14.1 (continued)

Group/name of disorder	Inheritance	MIM No.	Locus or gene	Protein	Notes
Weyers acrofacial (acrodental) dysostosis	AD	193530	EVC1 EVC2	Ellis-van Creveld 1 protein	See also ciliopathy group
Endocrine-cerebro-osteodysplasia (ECO)	AR	612651	ICK	Intestinal cell kinase	
Craniofrontonasal syndrome	XLD	304110	EFNB1	Ephrin-B1	
Frontonasal dysplasia, type 1	AR	136760	ALX3	Aristaless-like-3	
Frontonasal dysplasia, type 2	AR	613451	ALX4	Aristaless-like-4	
Frontonasal dysplasia, type 3	AR	613456	ALX1	Aristaless-like 1	
Hemifacial microsomia	SP/AD	164210			Includes Goldenhar syndrome and oculo–auriculo–vertebral spectrum, probably genetically heterogeneous
Miller syndrome (postaxial acrofacial dysostosis)	AR	263750	DHODH	Dihydroorotate dehydrogenase	
Acrofacial dysostosis, Nager type	AD/AR	154400	SF3B4	Splicing factor 3, subunit 4	
Acrofacial dysostosis, Rodriguez type	AR	201170			
Mandibulofacial dysostosis with microcephaly	AD	610536	EFTUD2	Elongation factor tu gtp-binding domain-containing 2	
See also oral-facial-digital syndrome type 4 in the ciliopathies with major skeletal involvement group					
35. Dysostoses with predominant vertebral with and without costal involvement					
Currarino triad	AD	176450	HLXB9	Homeobox gene HB9	
Spondylocostal dysostosis type 1 (SCDO1), type 2 (SCDO2), type 3(SCDO3), type 4 (SCDO4),	AR	277300	DLL3	Delta-like 3	
		608681	MESP2	Mesoderm posterior 2	
		609813	LFNG	Lunatic fringe	
		613686	HES7	Hairy-and-enhancer-of-split-7	

Spondylocostal dysostosis type 5 (SCDO5)	AD	122600	TBX6	T-box 6	
Spondylothoracic dysostosis (STD)	AR		MESP2	Mesoderm posterior 2	
Vertebral segmentation defect (congenital scoliosis) with variable penetrance	AD		MESP2	Mesoderm posterior 2	
			HES7	Hairy-and-enhancer-of-split-7	
Klippel–Feil anomaly with laryngeal malformation	AD	148900	GDF6	Growth and differentiation factor 6	Role of GDF6 mutations in dominant spondylothoracic dysostosis unclear
		613702	GDF3	Growth and differentiation factor 3	
	AR	214300	MEOX1	Mesenchyme homeobox 1	
Cerebro-costo-mandibular syndrome (rib gap syndrome)	AD	117650	SNRPB	Small nuclear ribonucleoprotein polypeptide B and B-prime	
Cerebro-costo-mandibular-like syndrome with vertebral defects	AR	611209	COG1	Component of oligomeric Golgi complex 1	Also classified as CDG type IIg
Diaphanospondylodysostosis	AR	608022	BMPER	Bone morphogenetic protein-binding endothelial cell precursor-derived regulator	Possibly overlaps with ischiospinal dysostosis
Spondylo-megaepiphyseal-metaphyseal dysplasia (SMMD)	AR	613330	NKX3-2	NK3 Homeobox 2	
See also spondylocarpotarsal dysplasia in group 7					
36. Patellar dysostoses					
Ischiopatellar dysplasia (small patella syndrome) AD 147891 TBX4 T-box gene 4					
Nail–patella syndrome	AD	161200	LMX1B	LIM homeobox transcription factor 1	

(continued)

Table 14.1 (continued)

Group/name of disorder	Inheritance	MIM No.	Locus or gene	Protein	Notes
Genitopatellar syndrome	AD	606170	KAT6B		
Ear-patella-short stature syndrome (Meier–Gorlin)	AR	224690	ORC1	Origin recognition complex	
		613800	ORC4		
		613803	ORC6		
		613804	CDT1		
		613805	CDC6		
See also MED group for conditions with patellar changes as well as ischiopubic-patellar dysplasia as mild expression of campomelic dysplasia					
37. Brachydactylies (without extraskeletal manifestations)					
Brachydactyly type A1	AD	112500	IHH	Indian hedgehog	
Brachydactyly type A1	AD				
Brachydactyly type A2	AD	112600	BMPR1B	Bone morphogenetic protein receptor 1B	
Brachydactyly type A2	AD	112600	BMP2	Bone morphogenetic protein type 2	Regulatory mutations
Brachydactyly type A2	AD	112600	GDF5	Growth and differentiation factor 5	
Brachydactyly type B	AD	113000	ROR2	Receptor tyrosine kinase-like orphan receptor 2	See also Robinow syndrome/ COVESDEM
Brachydactyly type B2	AD	611377	NOG	Noggin	
Brachydactyly type C	AD, AR	113100	GDF5	Growth and differentiation factor 5	See also ASPED (group 14) and other GDF5 disorders
Brachydactyly type D	AD	113200	HOXD13	Homeobox D13	
Brachydactyly type E	AD	113300	PTHLH	Parathyroid hormone-like hormone (parathyroid-hormone related peptide, PTHRP)	
Brachydactyly type E	AD	113300	HOXD13	Homeobox D13	
Brachydactyly with anonychia (Cooks syndrome)	AD	106995	SOX9		Regulatory mutations

38. Brachydactylies (with extraskeletal manifestations)					
Brachydactyly-mental retardation syndrome	AD	600430	HDAC4	Histone deacetylase 4	Some patients have microdeletions involving contiguous genes (chr. 2q37 deletion syndrome)
Hyperphosphatasia with mental retardation, brachytelephalangy, and distinct face	AR		PIGV	Phosphatidylinositol-glycan biosynthesis class V protein (GPI mannosyltransferase 2)	
Brachydactyly–hypertension syndrome (Bilginturan)	AD	112410	PDE3A	Phosphodiesterase 3A	
Microcephaly-oculo-digito-esophageal-duodenal syndrome (Feingold syndrome)	AD	164280	MYCN	nMYC oncogene	
Hand-foot-genital syndrome	AD	140000	HOXA13	Homeobox A13	
Rubinstein–Taybi syndrome	AD	180849	CREBBP	CREB-binding protein	
Rubinstein–Taybi syndrome	AD	180849	EP300	E1A-binding protein, 300-KD	
Brachydactyly, Temtamy type	AR	605282	CHSY1	Chondroitin sulfate synthase 1	
Christian-type brachydactyly	AD	112450			
Coffin–Siris syndrome 1	AR	135900			Mutations in various components of the SWI/SNF complex have been reported in patients with a diagnosis of Coffin–Siris syndrome
Adams–Oliver	AD	100300	ARHGAP31		
	AR	614219	DOCK6		
	AD	614814	RBPJ		
	AR	615297	EOGT		
Catel–Manzke syndrome	AR	616145	TGDS	TDP-glucose 4,6 dehydratase	See also chondrodysplasia gPAPP type in group 4

(continued)

Table 14.1 (continued)

Group/name of disorder	Inheritance	MIM No.	Locus or gene	Protein	Notes
See also group 20 for other conditions with brachydactyly as well as brachytelephalangic CDP					
39. Limb hypoplasia–reduction defects group					
Ulnar-mammary syndrome	AD	181450	TBX3	T-box gene 3	
de Lange syndrome	AD	122470	NIPBL	Nipped-B-like	
	XL	300590	SMC1A		
	AD	619759	SMC3		
	AD	614701	RAD21		
	XL	300882	HDAC8		
Fanconi anemia (see note below)	AR	227650	(Several)	Several complementation groups and genes	
Thrombocytopenia-absent radius (TAR)	AR	274000	RBM8A		
Thrombocythemia with distal limb defects	AD		THPO	Thrombopoietin	Distal limb defects postulated as consequence of vascular occlusions
Holt–Oram syndrome	AD	142900	TBX5	T-box gene 5	
Okihiro syndrome (Duane–radial ray anomaly)	AD	607323	SALL4	SAL-like 4	
Cousin syndrome	AR	260660	TBX15	T-box gene 15	
Roberts syndrome	AR	268300	ESCO2	Homolog of establishment of cohesion-2	
Split hand-foot malformation with long-bone deficiency (SHFLD3)	AD	612576	BHLHA9		Duplications
Tibial hemimelia	AR	275220			
Tibial hemimelia-polysyndactyly-triphalangeal thumb	AD	188740	SHH-ZRS		Also mesomelic dysplasia Werner type
Acheiropodia	AR	200500	LMBR1	Putative receptor protein	Partial LMBR1 deletion affecting expression of Sonic hedgehog (SHH) gene

Tetra-amelia	AR	273395	WNT3	Wingless-type MMTV integration site family, member 3	
Terminal transverse defect	?	102650			
Al-Awadi–Raas-Rothschild limb-pelvis hypoplasia-aplasia	AR	276820	WNT7A	Wingless-type MMTV integration site family, member 7A	
Fuhrmann syndrome	AR	228930	WNT7A	Wingless-type MMTV integration site family, member 7A	
RAPADILINO syndrome	AR	266280	RECQL4	RECQ protein-like 4	
Poland					
Femoral hypoplasia-unusual facies syndrome (FHUFS)	SP/AD?	134780			Some phenotypic overlap with FFU syndrome (below)
Femur-fibula-ulna syndrome (FFU)	SP?	228200			
Hanhart syndrome (Hypoglossia-hypodactylia)	AD	103300			
Gollop–Wolfgang	AD	228250	BHLHA9		Triplications
Scapulo-iliac dysplasia (Kosenow)	AD	169550			
See also CHILD in group 20 and the mesomelic and acromesomelic dysplasias					
40. Ectrodactyly with and without other manifestations					
Ankyloblepharon-ectodermal dysplasia cleft lip/palate (AEC)	AD	106260	P63 (TP63)	Tumor protein p63	
Ectrodactyly-ectodermal dysplasia cleft palate syndrome type 3 (EEC3)	AD	604292	P63 (TP63)	Tumor protein p63	
Ectrodactyly-ectodermal dysplasia cleft palate syndrome type 1 (EEC1)	AD	129900			

(continued)

Table 14.1 (continued)

Group/name of disorder	Inheritance	MIM No.	Locus or gene	Protein	Notes
Ectrodactyly-ectodermal dysplasia-macular dystrophy syndrome (EEM)	AR	225280	CDH3	Cadherin 3	
Limb-mammary syndrome (including ADULT syndrome)	AD	603273	P63 (TP63)	Tumor protein p63	
Split hand-foot malformation, isolated form, type 4 (SHFM4)	AD	605289	P63 (TP63)	Tumor protein p63	
Split hand-foot malformation, isolated form, type 1 (SHFM1)	AD	183600	DLX5 DLX6	Distal-less homeobox 5 Distal-less homeobox 6	
Split hand-foot malformation, isolated form, type 3 (SHFM3)	AD	246560		10q Duplications	
Split hand-foot malformation, isolated form, type 5 (SHFM5)	AD AR	606708	WNT10B	Wingless-type MMTV integration site family, member 7A	
Hartsfield syndrome	AD	615465	FGFR1	Fibroblast growth factor receptor 1	
41. Polydactyly-syndactyly-triphalangism group					
Preaxial polydactyly type 1 (PPD1)	AD	174400	SHH-ZRS	Sonic hedgehog	Regulatory mutation
Postaxial polydactyly type A	AD	174200	GLI3	GLI-Kruppel family member 3	Most cases are not GLI3 related
Postaxial polydactyly type B Complex					
Triphalangeal thumb (TPT)-polydactyly syndrome	AD	174500	SHH-ZRS	Sonic hedgehog	Regulatory mutation
Preaxial polydactyly type 3 (PPD3)	AD	174600			
Preaxial polydactyly type 4 (PPD4)	AD	174700	GLI3	GLI-Kruppel family member 3	
Greig cephalopolysyndactyly syndrome	AD	175700	GLI3	GLI-Kruppel family member 3	

Pallister–Hall syndrome	AD	146510	GLI3	GLI-Kruppel family member 3	
Synpolydactyly (complex, fibulin 1-associated)	AD	608180	FBLN1	Fibulin 1	
Synpolydactyly	AD	186000	HOXD13	Homeobox D13	
Townes–Brocks syndrome (renal-ear-anal-radial syndrome)	AD	107480	SALL1	SAL-like 1	
Lacrimo-auriculo-dento-digital syndrome (LADD)	AD	149730	FGFR2	Fibroblast growth factor receptor 2	
Lacrimo-auriculo-dento-digital syndrome (LADD)	AD	149730	FGFR3	Fibroblast growth factor receptor 3	
Lacrimo-auriculo-dento-digital syndrome (LADD)	AD	149730	FGF10	Fibroblast growth factor 10	
Acrocallosal syndrome	AR	200990	KIF7	Kinesin family member 7	
Acro-pectoral syndrome	AD	605967			
Acro-pectoro-vertebral dysplasia (F syndrome)	AD	102510	WNT6	Wingless-type mmtv integration site family, member 6	Regulatory mutations
Mirror-image polydactyly of hands and feet (Laurin– Sandrow syndrome)	AD	135750	SHH-ZRS	Sonic hedgehog	Regulatory mutations; some cases unlinked
Cenani–Lenz syndactyly	AR	212780	LRP4	Low-density lipoprotein receptorrelated protein 4	
Cenani–Lenz like syndactyly	SP (AD?)		GREM1, FMN1	Gremlin 1, Formin 1	Monoallelic duplication of both loci (observed in one case only so far)
Syndactyly, Malik–Percin type	AD	609432	BHLHA9		
STAR syndrome (syndactyly of toes, telecanthus, ano- and renal malformations)	XL	300707	FAM58A		

(continued)

Table 14.1 (continued)

Group/name of disorder	Inheritance	MIM No.	Locus or gene	Protein	Notes
Syndactyly type Lueken	AD	185900	IHH	Indian hedgehog	Regulatory mutations
Oculodentodigital dysplasia, Syndactyly type 3 (IV–V)	AD	185900	GJA1	Gap junction alpha-1 protein	
Syndactyly Haas type	AD	186200	SHH-ZRS	Sonic hedgehog	Regulatory mutations
Syndactyly with metacarpal and metatarsal fusion	AD	186300	HOXD13		
Metacarpal 4-5 fusion syndrome	XL	309630	FGF16	Fibroblast growth factor 16	
Syndactyly with craniosynostosis (Philadelphia type)	AD	185900	IHH	Indian hedgehog	Regulatory mutations
Syndactyly with microcephaly and mental retardation (Filippi syndrome)	AR	272440	CKAP2L	Cytoskeleton associated protein 2-like	
Meckel syndrome type 1,2,3,4,5,6	AR	249000	MKS1		
		603194	TMEM216		
		607361	TMEM67		
		611134	CEP290		
		611561	RPGRIP1L		
		612284	CC2D2A		
Note: The Smith–Lemli–Opitz syndrome can present with polydactyly and/or syndactyly. See also the SRPS group					
42. Defects in joint formation and synostoses					
Multiple synostoses syndrome type 3	AD	612961	FGF9	FGF9	
Proximal symphalangism type 1	AD	185800	NOG	Noggin	
Proximal symphalangism type 2	AD	185800	GDF5	Growth and differentiation factor 5	

Radioulnar synostosis with amegakaryocytic thrombocytopenia	AD	605432	HOXA11	Homeobox A11	
Liebenberg syndrome Regulatory mutations	AD	186550	PITX1	Paired-like homeodomain transcription factor 1	
Congenital club foot	AD	119800	PITX1	Paired-like homeodomain transcription factor 1	Includes forms with polydactyly/limb malformations
See also spondylo-carpal-tarsal dysplasia, mesomelic dysplasia with acral synostoses, and others					

Modified and reproduced from Ref. [25] used with permission

Achondroplasia

> [The child] *has a very unusual, peculiar appearance. It is of the female gender... It is very fat and round, but the upper and lower extremities are very much too short... The stripped bone of the forearm, elbow and wrist, I find knotty, misshapen, bent and the substance almost similar to that of a rachitic child. So that this deformity seems to me to be a true bone disease* [4].
>
> *Abbildungen und Beschreibungen Einiger Missgeburten*, 1791
> Samuel Thomas von Soemmerring (1755–1830)

Classic heterozygous achondroplasia is a common type of dwarfism and is by far the most common type of short-limb dwarfism [5]. Achondroplasia is typically evident at birth, although prenatal ultrasound can identify short femora at 24 weeks of gestation. It is characterized by rhizomelic dwarfism, trident and stubby hands, and a disproportionately large head with characteristic facies that includes a prominent forehead, mild midface hypoplasia, and depressed nasal bridge [6]. There is significant kyphosis at the thoracolumbar junction in infancy and increased pelvic tilt that leads to prominence of the buttocks and abdomen.

On radiographs, the calvarium is enlarged with shortening of the base of the skull and a small foramen magnum. Tubular bones are short with metaphyseal flaring, small sacroiliac notches, and square-shaped iliac bones. Spine films typically identify progressive caudal narrowing of interpediculate distance of lumbar vertebrae (normally, the distance increases distally) leading to narrowing of the lumbar spinal canal. Short pedicles are seen on lateral spine films [5].

Back pain is the most common complaint of both older children and adults due to the exaggerated lumbar lordosis. Nerve root compression occurs commonly in the thoracic and lumbar spine. Narrow respiratory passages can predispose patients to recurrent infections, obstructive sleep apnea, and increased risk of cardiorespiratory failure [7].

Hypochondroplasia

Hypochondroplasia is another form of dwarfism that can resemble achondroplasia. However, it has a milder phenotype and many children have body measurements within normal range and thus remain undiagnosed until school age, although prenatal diagnosis is possible. Macrocephaly sets hypochondroplasia apart from constitutional short stature [5].

Affected children can have bowed legs but they may tend to straighten spontaneously. There is mild shortening and relative squaring of tubular bones with a short and broad hip femoral neck shape. An increase in lumbar lordosis leads to a protuberant abdomen. Vertebral pedicles are short, and lumbar vertebrae have increased dorsal concavity.

Patients usually have a normal life expectancy. Mild joint pain may occur during activity in adulthood. There are reports of an increased incidence of cognitive impairment compared to the general population, but the etiology remains unclear [6].

Spondyloepiphyseal Dysplasia Congenita (SEDC)

In contrast to the above forms of short-limb dwarfism, spondyloepiphyseal dysplasia congenita (SEDC) is a form of short-trunk dwarfism characterized by a short spine and a short neck. These disorders can be detected by prenatal ultrasound and are evident at the time of birth.

Patients have an increase in the anteroposterior chest diameter and the formation of a barrel chest. Other features include a flat face, occasional cleft palate and relatively normal hands and feet except for possible equinovarus deformity. Myopia develops in up to 50% of patients [6].

Findings on radiographs are related to the patient's age and stage of development. In infancy, there is delayed ossification of the skeleton with absent ossification of the upper cervical spine. Thoracic and lumbar vertebrae are small and dorsally wedged with a characteristic "pear-shaped" appearance. Later in childhood, vertebral bodies flatten with hypoplasia of the C-2 odontoid process [5]. There continues to be slowed ossification of the hip femoral head and neck along with varying degrees of epiphyseal and metaphyseal abnormalities of long tubular bones [8]. Hands and feet are typically normal except for possible delayed appearance of ossification centers of carpal and tarsal bones. In adulthood, the spine is short with moderate kyphoscoliosis and accentuated lumbar lordosis. Due to the hypoplasia of the C-2 odontoid process and laxity of transverse ligaments, patients are predisposed to atlantoaxial subluxation and compression of the spinal cord [7].

Albright Hereditary Osteodystrophy (AHO)

Albright hereditary osteodystrophy (AHO) represents the physical findings of patients with pseudohypoparathyroidism (PHP) . It is characterized by short stature, obesity, cognitive impairment, and round facies with a possible depressed nasal bridge. The classic presentation also includes short fingers, often asymmetric, due to underlying short metacarpals, particularly affecting the fourth and fifth digits. When a fist is made, the affected digit(s) will have the appearance of a dimple instead of a knuckle. Other hand bones are less frequently affected in AHO. Subcutaneous calcifications occur in up to 50% of patients with basal ganglia calcification in some, as well as occasional exostoses and generalized coarse skeletal trabeculations [5, 9].

PHP type IA includes the AHO phenotype and end-organ resistance to parathyroid hormone. Resistance to other hormones can also occur, presenting frequently as hypothyroidism and occasionally as hypogonadism. Pseudopseudohypoparathyroidism (PPHP) shares the same *GNAS* coding region mutation with PHP type IA but has normal end-organ response to parathyroid hormone and thus normal calcium homeostasis and normal serum calcium. Individuals within the same family could have different phenotypes due to genetic imprinting [10].

Biochemical features of PHP, if present, rarely occur before the third year of life, whereas skeletal osteodystrophy can develop at various stages and as late as adolescence and typically more severe in females. A short proximal phalanx of the great toe may be the only sign of PHP in an affected male. PHP is discussed in further detail in Chap. 6.

Ellis-van Creveld Syndrome (Chondroectodermal Dysplasia)

Ellis-van Creveld syndrome is a form of disproportionate short-limb dwarfism that is diagnosed at birth but can be detected as early as 15 weeks' gestation due to the presence of polydactyly and short extremities. Affected individuals have hypoplastic or absent nails, dental abnormalities such as enamel hypoplasia and small teeth, a short upper lip connected to the alveolar ridge, a narrow thorax leading to pulmonary hypoplasia, and congenital heart defects (up to 60%) with atrial septal defect being the most common. Hydrocephalus and renal abnormalities may also be present [6].

Developmentally, there is progressive acromesomelic shortening of the extremities as well as genu valgum. Polydactyly occurs with or without fusion of metacarpals and cone-shaped epiphyses of middle and distal phalanges. Furthermore, there is premature ossification of femoral capital epiphyses and a characteristic appearance of the tibia (i.e., hypoplastic lateral aspect of proximal tibia with medial diaphyseal exostoses).

This disease is autosomal recessive and results from the founder effect such as seen in the Amish community. There is a high rate of infant mortality due to cardiac or pulmonary complications. Individuals may have significant disability in ambulation due to the knock-knee deformity [7].

Osteopetrosis

Osteopetrosis is a group of disorders characterized by defective bone resorption due to a decrease in the number and/or function of osteoclasts. They are often associated with widened metaphyses of the tubular bone. The delayed onset adult type of osteopetrosis is autosomal dominant and is separated into two types. Type 1 has pronounced sclerosis and widening of the cranial vault with only mild hyperdensity of vertebral bodies, whereas in type 2 disease sclerosis can occur with a typical "bone-in-bone" appearance primarily involving the base of the skull, vertebral end plates, and iliac crest. Radiographically, both types share highly variable degrees of asymmetric increases in bone density, a normal trabecular skeletal pattern and signs of fluctuating activity of the sclerotic process (such as transverse bands) [6, 11].

Clinically, type 1 osteopetrosis can be relatively asymptomatic with occasional bone pain or hearing loss. In contrast, fractures occur in up to 80% of patients with type 2 osteopetrosis, and patients may also have cranial nerve impingement (commonly VII or VIII), osteomyelitis of the mandible, anemia, and extramedullary erythropoiesis, the latter which may reduce life expectancy [11].

Melorheostosis

Melorheostosis has a very wide range of clinical manifestations. Patients rarely are diagnosed at birth. Children may be asymptomatic or have localized pain with sclerotic dermal changes and joint contractures. Disease involvement can occur in a single bone (monostotic), a whole limb (monomelic), or multiple bones (polyostotic) and can lead to discrepant limb length with increased circumference and curving or angulation of affected limbs [12].

Affected joints can develop swelling and chronic pain and may be misdiagnosed as arthritis. Skin overlying affected joints may be tense, shiny, and erythematous, and the subcutaneous tissue can be indurated and edematous. Skin abnormalities can appear prior to the bone changes [7].

Radiographically, bone lesions are unilateral, irregular linear areas of increased density that follow sclerotomes and appear to be flowing down the long axes of the tubular bones to give the appearance of "dripping candle wax." These osteophytic periosteal excrescences tend to progress and can cause significant muscle weakness and atrophy as well as joint disability [6].

Osteogenesis Imperfecta

Osteogenesis imperfecta is discussed separately in Chap. 10.

Hypophosphatasia

Hypophosphatasia is discussed separately in Chap. 9.

Hypophosphatemic Rickets

Hypophosphatemic rickets is discussed separately in Chap. 4.

Multicentric Carpotarsal Osteolysis Syndrome (MCTO)

Multicentric carpotarsal osteolysis syndrome (MCTO) with or without nephropathy is an autosomal dominant disorder, familial or sporadic, that typically arises in early childhood with pain and swelling of peripheral joints and may be misdiagnosed as arthritis. Joint involvement may be asymmetric, and deformities affect primarily the wrists and feet with possible later progression to the elbows and knees [13].

Characteristic radiographic signs include destructive lesions starting at carpal and tarsal bones with possible extension to adjacent portions of the proximal metacarpals and metatarsals diaphysis. Imaging typically shows progressive erosive destruction and distortion of bones [14, 15].

MCTO is a noninflammatory osteolytic process characterized by missense mutations in the *MAFB* gene; the latter has been shown to be involved in negative downstream regulation of RANKL-mediated osteoclast differentiation [16]. Furthermore, *MAFB* is expressed in the kidney and responsible for the nephropathy present in a large proportion of patients with MCTO.

Fibrous Dysplasia

Fibrous dysplasia is discussed separately in Chap. 13.

Fibrodysplasia Ossificans Progressiva (FOP)

Fibrodysplasia ossificans progressiva (FOP) is a rare autosomal dominant disease, with an estimated prevalence of about 1:1,000,000. Heterotopic ossifications occur and typically proceed in a direction from axial to appendicular, dorsal to ventral, cranial to caudal, and proximal to distal, leading to widespread rigidity and profound disability. There is preferential involvement of the paraspinal, limb girdle, and mastication ligaments and muscles. Furthermore, exostosis at ligamentous insertions appears with progressive fusion across apophyseal joints of the cervical spine. Ossifications are noted clinically as soft-tissue swelling that might be mistaken as an inflammatory process; however, biopsy for diagnostic purposes is contraindicated as it exacerbates the disease process [6, 17].

The pathognomonic feature of FOP is a short great first toe with a short or absent proximal phalanx and short metatarsal. A similar process can involve the thumb but is less common and may not be clinically prominent [7].

FOP is progressive and debilitating with at least some form of restrictive ossification occurring in up to 80% of individuals by age 7. By young adulthood, most patients are chair-bound, and respiratory function may be impaired [6].

Camurati–Engelmann Disease (Diaphyseal Dysplasia)

Generalized and bilateral symmetrical dysplasia of bone characterizes Camurati–Engelmann disease. Age of onset is variable, although symptoms usually become manifest after the second year of life. Mild forms of the disease can present in adulthood. There is wide variability in the clinical expression of the disease, even within the same family of affected individuals [6].

Prepubertal muscular pain and weakness are associated with characteristic tubular-shaped legs leading to a broad-based waddling gait and difficulty running. Patients develop failure to thrive with loss of body fat and muscle mass leading to a thin body habitus and progressive disability. Rarely, macrocephaly and a prominent forehead are present [11].

Skeletal imaging shows cortical bone thickening and narrowing of medullary cavities. Sclerosis occurs in the diaphyses of long bones with endosteal and, to a lesser extent, periosteal proliferation and sparing of the epiphyses. Osteosclerosis is irregular and heterogeneous with variable involvement of the base of the skull. Occasionally, there is spontaneous improvement during adolescence, while others have progression to include cranial nerve impingement and sequelae, notably optic atrophy and impaired hearing [5].

Approach to the Patient with Skeletal Dysplasia

Most of the skeletal dysplasias present during early development, either in utero or during infancy or childhood. Prenatal ultrasounds can detect defects in skeletal development, sometimes leading to recognition of specific entities or groups of disorders based on pathognomonic features. During infancy and childhood, a clinical presentation with short stature, bony deformities, or fractures should raise suspicion of an underlying skeletal defect. The pattern and progression of prenatal and postnatal growth and development is essential for the clinician to narrow the list of differential diagnoses for skeletal dysplasias [18, 19].

Obtaining an accurately detailed and extensive family history pedigree (at times in consultation with a clinical geneticist) is also essential. This includes all history of skeletal defects and fractures as well as related disorders such as retinal or renal diseases. This detailed history is not only important for diagnosis but also provides clues as to the prognosis of the phenotypic gene expression in a particular family. Some genetic defects can manifest differently clinically, but generally speaking, the prognosis of an individual can be predicted from the history of affected family members [19, 20].

A thorough medical examination is a cornerstone in the appropriate evaluation of a patient with suspected skeletal dysplasia. Body measurements should include limb measurements to determine discrepancies and disproportions, chest measurements to identify abnormal anteroposterior dimensions, and skull measurements to detect micro- or macrocephaly. Skeletal examination aims at documenting the presence or absence of polydactyly and brachydactyly, joint hypermobility, widening of metaphyses and growth plates, bowing of extremities, and spinal deformities such as scoliosis or kyphosis [18, 19].Other areas important to examine include facial features, the nasal bridge, and fingernails; the latter can be hypoplastic or absent in such disorders as nail–patella syndrome or Ellis-van Creveld syndrome [18].

A full skeletal survey is extremely useful in patients with suspicion of skeletal dysplasia. Despite advances in bone imaging and micro-architectural assessment, plain radiographs remain the foundation for skeletal evaluation of these patients. Historically, radiographic features have been essential to identify and classify these disorders; many well-known "identifiers" and pathognomonic features can provide a radiographic "spot diagnosis." It thus becomes important to visualize the complete skeleton (i.e., skull, entire spine, pelvis, all long bones, hands and feet) to examine all bone structures and growth plates [21].

Diagnosing the specific type of skeletal dysplasia is important from therapeutic and prognostic standpoints. With molecular advancement, targeted treatments for a number of these disorders are increasingly available with the potential to significantly reduce disability and possibly improve survival. However, for many patients, treatment is at best supportive or directed to symptom relief. Still, accurate identification of the disorder and the underlying genetic defect provides insight for patient prognosis and life expectancy as well as genetic transmission and progeny counseling [22].

Many of these disorders remain poorly understood and have limited treatment options. Nonetheless, experiential expertise in rare bone diseases can lead to accurate and earlier diagnosis, provide both proficient and empathic patient care, and help direct early access to available state-of-the-art therapeutic options and clinical trials. Patient care may overlap disciplines in pediatric/adult endocrinology and rheumatology, medical genetics, molecular biology, radiology, and one or more surgical subspecialties depending on the underlying disease. For these reasons, referral to medical centers with providers having multidiscipline expertise in bone disorders and skeletal dysplasias is recommended for most patients in an effort to limit disabilities and improve quality of life.

Case Management and Discussion

The patient described in this clinical vignette underwent genetic consultation (see Fig. 14.2 for family pedigree) and testing that confirmed the presence of a heterozygous c.161C>T (p.Ser54Leu) mutation in the *MAFB* gene consistent with MCTO syndrome. Interestingly, this patient's mutation has been previously reported in two unrelated families that had MCTO without nephropathy [23, 24].

There are very limited treatment venues for patients with MCTO, particularly for skeletal disease modification. One could postulate that increased RANK signaling due to the missense mutations in *MAFB* would be reduced using RANKL monoclonal antibodies (such as denosumab) and significantly limit osteoclastogenesis and restore, to some extent, the balance in bone remodeling [16]. However, there have been no reports to date of denosumab use in patients with MCTO.

The patient received four courses of pamidronate (45 mg infusion for 3 days each) 3 months apart, and treatment was then switched to zoledronic acid (5 mg infusion) of which she received two infusions 12 months apart. She noted a significant decrease in pain following zoledronic acid infusions.

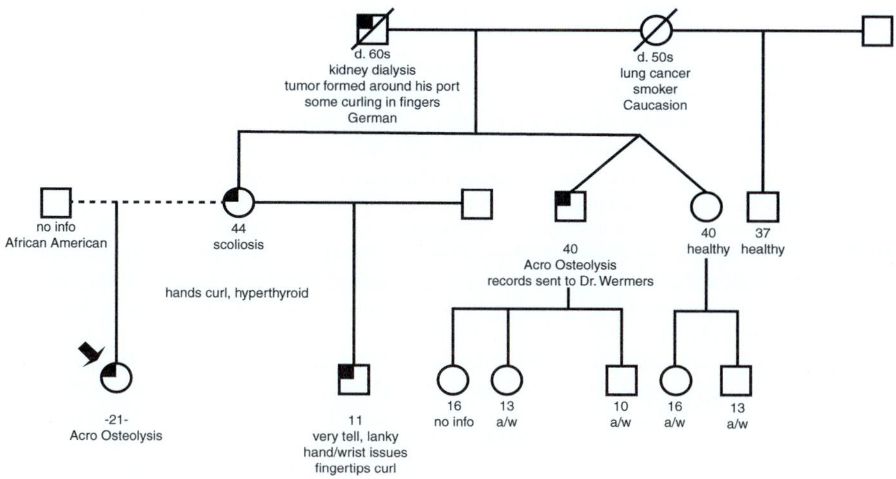

Fig. 14.2 Family pedigree with descriptive details on involved family members (index patient identified by black arrow)

References

1. Baitner AC, Maurer SG, Gruen MB, Di Cesare PE. The genetic basis of the osteochondrodysplasias. J Pediatr Orthop. 2000;20(5):594–605.
2. Alanay Y, Rimoin DL. Osteochondrodysplasia. In: Rosen CJ, American Society for Bone and Mineral Research, editors. Primer on the metabolic bone diseases and disorders of mineral metabolism. 8th ed. Ames: Wiley-Blackwell; 2013. p. xxvi, 1078 p.
3. Warman ML, Cormier-Daire V, Hall C, Krakow D, Lachman R, LeMerrer M, et al. Nosology and classification of genetic skeletal disorders: 2010 revision. Am J Med Genet A. 2011;155A(5):943–68.
4. Huth EJ, Murray TJ. Medicine in quotations: views of health and disease through the ages. 2nd ed. Philadelphia: American College of Physicians; 2006. p. xvi, 581 p.
5. McAlister WH, Herman TE. Osteochondrodysplasias, dysostoses, chromosomal aberrations, mucopolysaccharidoses, and mucolipidoses. In: Resnick DLAK, Mark J, editors. Bone and joint imaging. 3rd ed. Philadelphia: Elsevier; 2005.
6. Spranger JW, Spranger JW. Bone dysplasias: an atlas of genetic disorders of skeletal development. 3rd ed. Oxford: Oxford University Press; 2012. p. xxiii, 802 p.
7. Kozlowski K, Beighton P. Gamut index of skeletal dysplasias. London: Springer; 2001.
8. Sheridan BD, Gargan MF, Monsell FP. The hip in osteochondrodysplasias: general rules for diagnosis and treatment. Hip Int. 2009;19(Suppl 6):S26–34.
9. Rubin MR, Levine MA. Hypoparathyroidism and pseudohypoparathyroidism. In: Rosen CJ, Bouillon R, Compston J, Rosen V, Bauer DC, American Society for Bone and Mineral Research, editors. Primer on the metabolic bone diseases and disorders of mineral metabolism. 8th ed. Ames: Wiley-Blackwell: ASBMR; 2013. p. xxvi, 1078 pages.
10. Jüppner H, Batsepe M. Pseudohypoparathyroidism. In: Rosen CJ, Bouillon R, Compston J, Rosen V, Bauer DC, American Society for Bone and Mineral Research, editors. Primer on the metabolic bone diseases and disorders of mineral metabolism. 8th ed. Ames: Wiley-Blackwell: ASBMR; 2013. p. xxvi, 1078 pages.
11. Whyte MP. Hereditary disorders of the skeleton. In: Jameson JL, LJ DG, De Kretser DM, Giudice L, Grossman A, Melmed S, et al., editors. Endocrinology: adult and pediatric. 7th ed: W.B. Saunders; 2016. p. 1173–1183.e4. https://doi.org/10.1016/B978-0-323-18907-1.00068-8.

12. Kotwal A, Clarke BL. Melorheostosis: a rare sclerosing bone dysplasia. Curr Osteoporos Rep. 2017;15(4):335–42.
13. Hardegger F, Simpson LA, Segmueller G. The syndrome of idiopathic osteolysis. Classification, review, and case report. J Bone Joint Surg Br. 1985;67(1):88–93.
14. Castriota-Scanderbeg A, Dallapiccola B. Hands. In: Castriota-Scanderbeg A, Dallapiccola B, SpringerLink (Online service), editors. Abnormal skeletal phenotypes from simple signs to complex diagnoses. Berlin: Springer-Verlag Berlin Heidelberg; 2005.
15. Thomas CW, Bisset AJ, Sampson MA, Armstrong RD. Case report: multicentric carpal/tarsal osteolysis: imaging review and 25-year follow-up. Clin Radiol. 2006;61(10):892–5.
16. Cuevas VD, Anta L, Samaniego R, Orta-Zavalza E, Vladimir de la Rosa J, Baujat G, et al. MAFB determines human macrophage anti-inflammatory polarization: relevance for the pathogenic mechanisms operating in multicentric carpotarsal osteolysis. J Immunol. 2017;198(5):2070–81.
17. Kaplan FS, Pignolo RJ, Shore EM. Fibrodysplasia ossificans progressiva. In: Rosen CJ, Bouillon R, Compston J, Rosen V, Bauer DC, American Society for Bone and Mineral Research, editors. Primer on the metabolic bone diseases and disorders of mineral metabolism. 8th ed. Ames: Wiley-Blackwell: ASBMR; 2013. p. xxvi, 1078 pages.
18. Krakow D, Rimoin DL. The skeletal dysplasias. Genet Med. 2010;12(6):327–41.
19. Unger S, Andrea S-F, Rimoin DL. A diagnostic approach to skeletal dysplasias. In: Glorieux FH, Pettifor JM, Jüppner H, editors. Pediatric bone. 2nd ed. London: Elsevier/Academic Press; 2012. p. 1.. online resource (volume).
20. Offiah AC. Skeletal dysplasias: an overview. Endocr Dev. 2015;28:259–76.
21. Alanay Y, Lachman RS. A review of the principles of radiological assessment of skeletal dysplasias. J Clin Res Pediatr Endocrinol. 2011;3(4):163–78.
22. Ireland P, Johnston LM. Measures of self-care independence for children with osteochondrodysplasia: a clinimetric review. Phys Occup Ther Pediatr. 2012;32(1):80–96.
23. Zankl A, Duncan EL, Leo PJ, Clark GR, Glazov EA, Addor MC, et al. Multicentric carpotarsal osteolysis is caused by mutations clustering in the amino-terminal transcriptional activation domain of MAFB. Am J Hum Genet. 2012;90(3):494–501.
24. Temtamy SA, Ismail S, Aglan MS, Ashour AM, Hosny LA, El-Badry TH, et al. A report of three patients with MMP2 associated hereditary osteolysis. Genet Couns. 2012;23(2):175–84.
25. Bonafe L, Cormier-Daire V, Hall C, Lachman R, Mortier G, Mundlos S, et al. Nosology and classification of genetic skeletal disorders: 2015 revision. Am J Med Genet A. 2015;167A(12):2869–92.

Chapter 15
Malignancies of the Bone

Megan R. Crawford, Susan E. Williams, Leila Khan, and Angelo Licata

Abbreviations

ASCO	American Society of Clinical Oncology
BAP	Bone-specific alkaline phosphatase
BMI	Body mass index
Bpm	Beats per minute
CT	Computed tomography
CTX	Carboxy-terminal telopeptide of type I collagen or C-telopeptide
dL	Deciliter
DPD	Deoxypyridinoline
EBCTCG	Early Breast Cancer Trialists' Collaborative Group
ESR	Erythrocyte sedimentation rate
FDA	Food and drug administration
G	Gram
GFR	Glomerular filtration rate
h	Hour
IGF	Insulin-like growth factor
IL	Interleukin
IV	Intravenous

M. R. Crawford · S. E. Williams · L. Khan · A. Licata (✉)
Department of Endocrinology, Diabetes and Metabolism, Cleveland Clinic Foundation, Cleveland, OH, USA
e-mail: CRAWFOM@CCF.ORG; WILLIAS9@CCF.ORG; KHANL@CCF.ORG; LICATAA@CCF.ORG

P. M. Camacho (ed.), *Metabolic Bone Diseases*,
https://doi.org/10.1007/978-3-030-03694-2_15

K	Thousand
L	Liter
Lb	Pounds
mg	Milligram
MGUS	Monoclonal gammopathy of undetermined significance
mmHg	Millimeters of mercury
mmol	Millimoles
MRI	Magnetic resonance imaging
Ng	Nanogram
NTX	Amino-terminal telopeptide of type I collagen or N-telopeptide
ONJ	Osteonecrosis of the jaw
P1CP	Procollagen type I intact C-terminal propeptide
P1NP	Procollagen type I intact N-terminal propeptide
PET	Positron emission tomography
Pg	Picogram
POEMS	Polyneuropathy, organomegaly, endocrinopathy, monoclonal proteins, and skin findings
PTH	Parathyroid hormone
PTHrP	Parathyroid hormone-related peptide
RANKL	Receptor activator of nuclear factor κB ligand
RECIST	Response Evaluation Criteria in Solid Tumors
SPECT	Single-positron emission tomography
TGF-β	Tumor growth factor-β
TRACP5b	Isoform 5b of the osteoclast enzyme tartrate-resistant acid phosphatase
U	Unit

Case

A 70-year-old man is referred for hypercalcemia. His past medical history is pertinent for hypertension and hyperlipidemia, and he takes a beta-blocker and a statin, respectively. During consultation, he reports a history of severe back pain that awakens him from sleep for the past 2 weeks, with only minimal improvement with ibuprofen. The patient denies any traumatic accidents or injuries and denies fevers or chills. There was a confirmed weight loss of 7 lb in 2 months and decreased appetite. He denies a history of nephrolithiasis or parathyroid disease and has no known family history of calcium disorders.

On exam, the patient appears ill and weighs 157 lb BMI is 21.9 kg/m^2. He has had a 3 in. height loss since college. Heart rate is 85 bpm and blood pressure is 135/81 mmHg. Lungs are clear to auscultation bilaterally and cardiac exam is unremarkable. The abdomen is soft and non-tender without any evidence of hepatosplenomegaly. There is point tenderness on palpation of the spine at T6–T7. His joints do not appear arthritic. Neurologic exam is grossly normal.

Laboratory testing reveals the following:

Laboratory test	Reference range	11 months ago	Present day
Sodium	136–144 mmol/L	138	134
Potassium	3.7–5.1 mmol/L	3.6	3.8
Blood urea nitrogen	9–24 mg/dL	11	32
Serum creatinine	0.73–1.22 mg/dL	1.21	2.11
Estimated GFR	>60 mL/min/1.73 m^2	59	33
Serum total protein	6–8.4 g/dL	8.2	11.0
Albumin	3.9–4.9 g/dL	3.4	3.2
Serum calcium	8.6–10.5 mg/dL	8.7	11.1
ALT	10–54 U/L	27	38
AST	14–40 U/L	20	24
25-hydroxyvitamin D	31.0–80.0 ng/mL	19.8	20.1
White blood count	3.70–11.00 k/uL	5.12	6.51
Hemoglobin	13.0–17.0 g/dL	12.2	8.9
Hematocrit	39.0–51.0%	39	28
Platelet count	150–400 k/uL	206	250
Intact PTH	15–65 pg/mL	–	8
Erythrocyte sedimentation rate (ESR)	0–22 mm/h	–	41

X-ray of the spine subsequently showed a wedge-shaped compression fracture of T7 vertebra as shown in Fig. 15.1. Baseline densitometry shows a T-score of −2.7 in the vertebral spine and −2.0 in the left total hip.

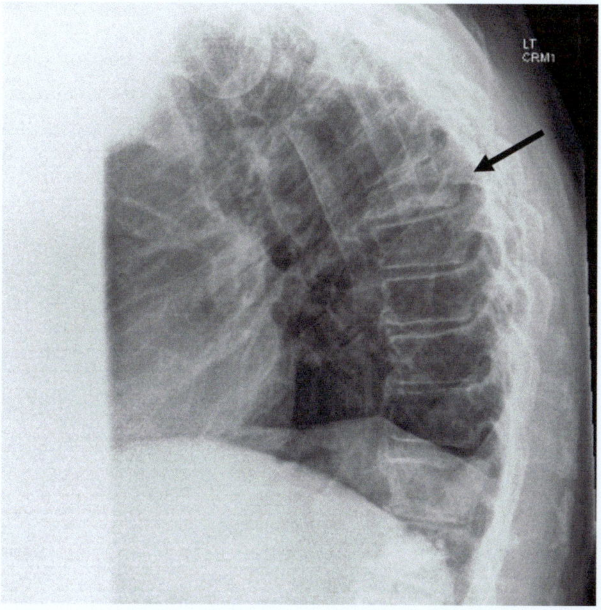

Fig. 15.1 Radiograph of thoracic spine, lateral view, demonstrating compression fracture of T7 vertebra

What are the diagnostic considerations that need to be made in this patient with new metabolic findings and bony lesions on imaging? What treatment options should be considered with regard to his vertebral fractures and pain symptoms?

Introduction

Skeletal malignancy may take the form of hematologic malignancy with bone involvement, primary bone tumors, or metastatic bone lesions from extraskeletal primary cancers. Both cortical and trabecular bone can be involved in malignancy of bone in both a primary and metastatic fashion. Skeletal involvement from a malignancy often leads to significant morbidity and carries a worrisome prognosis.

In the case described above, the patient has new-onset PTH-independent hypercalcemia, anemia, an elevated protein gap, an elevated ESR, and worsening renal function. These lab abnormalities were discovered in the setting of painful vertebral fractures of recent onset and associated red flags of weight loss and pain that wakes him from sleep. This constellation of findings is characteristic for the presentation multiple myeloma, and thus, the patient requires further oncologic workup. Important considerations regarding malignancy of bone, including multiple myeloma, will be discussed herein.

Discussion

Initial workup of skeletal lesions includes thorough clinical history, physical exam, imaging, and laboratory testing. The differential diagnosis of bone pain and/or pathologic fracture (Table 15.1) is broad, but certain lab abnormalities and skeletal imaging characteristics enable the clinician to narrow the list. The age of the patient may also provide clues to diagnosis, given that bone tumors often have a

Table 15.1 Differential diagnosis: causes of painful fractures (list not comprehensive)

Trauma
Osteoporosis
Hyperparathyroidism
Primary bone malignancy
Hematologic or lymphoproliferative malignancies involving bone
Skeletal metastases
Osteogenesis imperfecta
Tumor-induced osteomalacia
Hypophosphatasia
Nutritional deficiencies/osteomalacia

characteristic age-related distribution. The optimal approach to patients diagnosed with malignancy that involves bone includes a multidisciplinary approach with a variety of subspecialists including pathologists, radiologists, oncologists, radiation oncologists, surgeons, physical and occupational therapists, and palliative medicine. Presence of skeletal metastases may prompt a shift in focus of oncologic therapy from curative to palliative approach, as there is generally a poor prognosis when metastatic skeletal involvement is present.

Hypercalcemia in Malignancy of Bone

Hypercalcemia from osteolysis is described in cases of multiple myeloma and other solid tumors which become locally invasive or metastatic or cause paraneoplastic syndromes. In fact, up to 30% of patients with a malignancy may develop hypercalcemia at some point during their disease [1]. Hypercalcemia from neoplastic bone resorption is often acute and severe, as in our patient's case. Severe hypercalcemia may lead to hypercalciuria, volume contraction, and impaired GFR. It is believed that the mechanism of osteolysis in multiple myeloma and solid tumors stems from the production of inflammatory cytokines (i.e., IL-11, IL-6, macrophage inflammatory protein-1α) that increase expression of receptor activator of nuclear factor κB ligand (RANKL) and its effects to increase differentiation and activity of osteoclasts.

Myeloma cells are also often found proximally located to sites of bone resorption suggesting that some direct cell-cell mechanisms may be involved as well in the dysregulation of bone metabolism [2, 3]. Increased bone resorption and impaired bone formation result in a net loss of bone via uncoupling of the normal balanced osteoclastic and osteoblastic function [4]. Not surprisingly, bone formation markers have been shown to be decreased in subjects with multiple myeloma [5].

Another contributor to hypercalcemia in hematologic malignancies including lymphoma is the extrarenal production of 1,25-dihydroxyvitamin D via α-hydroxylase produced by tumor cells. This vitamin leads to increased osteoclastic activity, increased urinary calcium excretion, and increased intestinal absorption of calcium [1].

Certain malignant cells, including squamous cell carcinoma and breast cancer cells, also produce parathyroid hormone-related protein (PTHrP). Increased PTHrP may further stimulate renal resorption and intestinal absorption of calcium by mimicking the actions of PTH. PTHrP may play a local role in bone resorption when produced by neoplastic cells within metastatic bony lesions as well [6, 7]. (Please refer to the chapter on parathyroid hormone-independent hypercalcemia for additional considerations regarding this subject). Rarely, undifferentiated tumor cells can produce ectopic PTH, which has been described in case reports of squamous cell lung cancer, papillary thyroid carcinoma, renal cell carcinoma, and ovarian cancer among others [1]. Additionally, a patient with cancer may have pre-existing primary hyperparathyroidism that may worsen in the setting of dehydration or renal dysfunction and further aggravate the hypercalcemia in these patients.

Role of Imaging in Skeletal Malignancy

Imaging is imperative for diagnosis, surveillance, staging, and therapeutic monitoring in the setting of malignancy of bone. Imaging also aids in differentiating fractures of skeletal malignancy from those due to metabolic bone diseases.

All bone lesions that have features of malignancy may warrant further evaluation with biopsy; but plain radiograph remains the initial recommended imaging modality in patients who present with skeletal-related pain symptoms. Radiograph is usually readily available, is cost-effective, and can provide information regarding bone formation/destruction, margin of the lesion, and periosteal changes. Other forms of imaging including computed tomography (CT) and magnetic resonance imaging (MRI) are also used if additional anatomical detail is required. Advanced imaging modalities including whole-body skeletal scintigraphy (bone scan), single-positron emission computed tomography with fused CT (SPECT/CT), and positron emission tomography with fused CT (PET/CT) are also employed in certain cases for staging, surveillance, and posttreatment monitoring purposes.

To ascertain the degree of involvement of the medullary cavity and for presurgical planning regarding the relation of tumor to local soft tissue structures, MRI is often done on patients with skeletal malignancies. Bone tumors in treatment-naïve patients appear isointense to muscle, have low signal intensity compared with adjacent bone marrow, and often enhance with gadolinium-based intravenous contrast on T1-weighted MR images (Fig. 15.2) [8]. Normal bone cortex itself appears black due to lack of MR-responsive protons in heavily mineralized material. Bone scan employs technetium-labeled diphosphonates to evaluate a large anatomic area, but it is important to note that uptake of this tracer can be seen in both benign and malignant lesions; thus this imaging modality is most useful when evaluating for presence of skeletal metastases or multifocal primary lesions in the presence of a known malignancy [8].

PET/CT exploits the metabolically active nature of malignant cells to provide functional imaging of neoplasms and can be used as an alternative to bone scintigraphy to diagnose and monitor therapeutic response in skeletal malignancies. Both bone-specific (^{18}F-sodium fluoride) and tumor-specific (^{18}F-fluorodeoxyglucose or ^{18}F-fluorocholine) tracers are currently available, and new gallium-labeled tracers that bind to somatostatin receptors are currently under investigation to see if they will have utility in bone malignancies (^{68}Ga-DOTA-D-Phe^{1}-Tyr^{3}-octreotide) [9]. Though PET/CT can provide information regarding response to therapy given its improved spatial resolution over bone scan, it is costly, and standardization between institutions can be difficult. Also, current therapy-response protocols, such as Response Evaluation Criteria in Solid Tumors (RECIST), rely heavily on tumor size changes which are better ascertained via CT or MRI, than PET/CT [10].

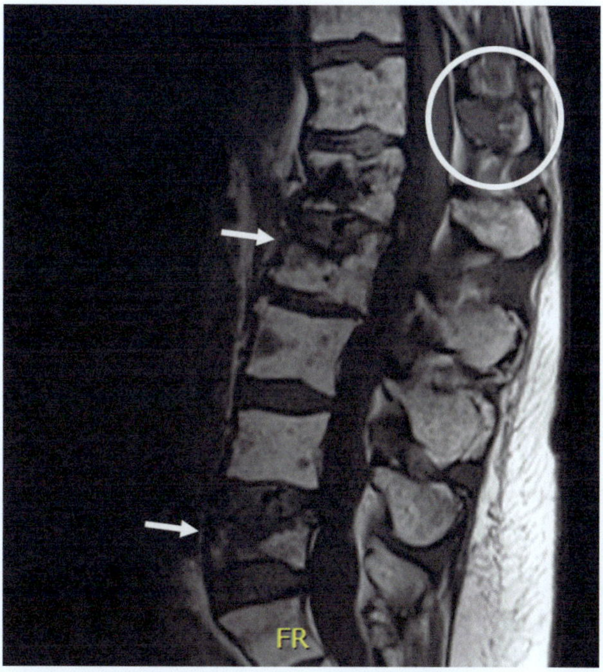

Fig. 15.2 T1-weighted sagittal MR image of lumbar spine depicting multiple metastatic lesions involving T12 spinous process (white circle) and L1–L5 vertebrae demonstrating low signal intensity compared with bone marrow; also shown is compression fracture in L2 and L5 vertebrae as a result of lytic lesions (white arrows). Note the thin black link surrounding the vertebral bodies which depicts bone cortex

When evaluating positive response of a bone malignancy to chemotherapy and/or radiation on imaging, most tumors also become more mineralized on radiograph and CT and exhibit decreased T2 signal intensity and IV contrast enhancement on MRI [11].

Pathologic Fractures in Malignancy of Bone

Pathological fractures lead to significant reduction in quality of life for patients due to severe pain. Primary bone malignancies predispose to fracture when they exhibit significant destruction of the local skeletal and alteration of local supportive structure, thereby compromising the integrity of bone and ability to self-repair. The cytokine cascade that has been described in multiple myeloma leads to weakening of the bone structure from upregulated bone resorption and concomitant suppression of Wnt signaling pathways for bone formation [12, 13]. Compromised bone integrity as a result of multiple myeloma can decrease bone mineral density and cause fracture that can mimic primary osteoporosis. Malignant bony lesions alter the ability of the bone to withstand compression, torsion, and tensile forces that would otherwise be tolerated. Malignant lesions of skeleton are classically described as an osteolytic or osteoblastic, which result from alternative pathways of osteoblast and osteoclast dysfunction; however malignant bone tumors often exhibit some degree of overlap of these two destructive processes. Predominantly osteoblastic metastases – such as those seen in metastatic prostate cancer – involve pathologic bone formation attributed to factors including platelet-derived growth factor, insulin-like growth factors, adrenomedullin, and endothelin-1 [14]. Osteolytic bony metastases are more so associated with hypercalcemia and painful pathologic fracture via cytokine profiles described above and unfortunately are the more common type of metastatic bone lesion.

Pathologic fractures due skeletal malignancy are often characterized by acute onset, pain at presentation, and tenderness and swelling in the vicinity of the lesion. Up to 67% of patients with skeletal metastases have associated pain symptoms [15]. History of malignancy led to a 33% posttest probability that new-onset low back pain was related to malignant vertebral lesions in an emergency care setting [16]. Bony destruction and fracture may also be associated with nerve compression depending on the location. Spinal cord impingement resulting in symptoms of weakness or paralysis can occur if a vertebral body metastasis exhibits epidural extension and can occur in up to 20% of patients with spinal metastases [17].

Interventions to address pain and to prevent overt fracture where possible may lead to better quality of life. Several definitions of impending fracture exist, with recent criteria by Memorial Sloan Kettering as follows: (a) a painful lytic lesion of the medullary cavity resulting in endosteal reabsorption of >50% cortical thickness; (b) a painful lytic lesion greater than the cross-sectional diameter of the bone, involving the cortex; (c) a painful cortical lesion that is >2.5 cm in length; or (d) a lesion that exhibits functional pain after irradiation [18]. Treatment goals for pathologic fractures include pain control and optimization of function. Surgical intervention (i.e., tumor excision, internal fixation, joint replacement) is often indicated in the setting of impending or existing pathologic fracture – which can be present in 9–29% of cases with bone metastases – or threatened neurologic compromise from a metastasis [19, 20]. Surgical intervention provides joint stabilization, improved function, and pain control, though ultimately the type of tumor and time of survival are likely the largest contributors to fracture healing. Kyphoplasty (insufflation of balloon device sometimes followed by cement injection in compressed intravertebral space) and vertebroplasty (injection of cement into compressed intravertebral space alone) are percutaneous procedures shown in several studies to restore height and decrease pain associated with vertebral compression fracture [21, 22].

Some surgical materials are able to be impregnated with chemotherapeutic agents to control local residual metastatic skeletal disease following surgery; and postsurgical adjuvant radiation therapy is often indicated for primary bone malignancies [18]. Pathologic fractures due to multiple myeloma may have a better chance of healing during a patient's lifetime than a fracture due to metastatic breast carcinoma [23]. Bone pain, fracture incidence, and hypercalcemia in patients with multiple myeloma and some metastatic malignancies are improved with adequate bisphosphonate therapy; however this class of medication does not promote bone formation which is inherently impaired in these patients. The use of bisphosphonates in skeletal malignancy is discussed later in this chapter in further detail.

Glucocorticoids, adjuvant hormonal therapies, and gonadal ablation procedures (i.e., oophorectomy, orchiectomy) indicated for certain malignancies may contribute to premature bone loss in these patients, placing them at increased risk of fracture. Hormonal therapies given for treatment of breast and prostate cancers, including aromatase inhibitors, selective estrogen receptor modulators, and androgen deprivation, lead to hypogonadism which in turn promotes bone resorption, increased risk of osteoporosis, and fragility fracture [14]. Patients undergoing cancer-related therapy who are at increased risk for bone loss and fracture should have calcium and vitamin D status assessed and optimized as possible. Screening bone densitometry should be done in cancer patients at the time of initiation of hormonal interventions and at regular intervals thereafter to allow for timely treatment with antiresorptive therapy [14].

Primary Malignancy of Bone

In discerning the differential diagnosis for neoplastic skeletal lesions, the age of the patient and the location of the lesion may provide important clues. For example, knowing that Ewing's sarcoma occurs primarily in children and adolescents, but that osteosarcoma has peaks of incidence in both childhood and adulthood may provide some historical clues for the diagnosis [24, 25]. Other primary bone malignancies seen more commonly in adulthood include chondrosarcoma, fibrosarcoma, and malignant fibrous histiocytoma. Imaging features often also provide considerable clues. Primary malignancy of bone is often characterized by a single, large soft tissue mass with extension into surrounding tissue that has a lytic pattern of destruction, while metastases may be multiple, often are contained within the bone itself, and demonstrate various degrees of margin definition. Ewing's sarcoma usually involves the shaft of long bones, while osteosarcoma primarily involves the metaphyseal portions of long bones. Chondrosarcomas and malignant fibrous histiocytomas involve the pelvis and bones of the lower extremity (i.e., femur) most commonly. Diagnosis and treatment of primarily bone malignancy require timely interventions by a multidisciplinary team.

Hematologic Malignancy and Bone

On the spectrum of plasma cell dyscrasias, the diagnosis of multiple myeloma signifies the presence of ≥10% clonal plasma cells on bone marrow biopsy and associated end-organ disease manifestations including low bone density for age, lytic bone lesions, PTH-independent hypercalcemia, renal dysfunction, and cytopenias (except smoldering myeloma which is primarily asymptomatic). Monoclonal gammopathy of undetermined significance (MGUS) is diagnosed when <10% of clonal plasma cells are seen on bone marrow examination and elevated serum M protein (<3 g/dL) is present and by definition does not lead to disease-specific signs and symptoms [26]. However, patients with MGUS are at increased risk of bone loss and vertebral fractures, and intermittent bone densitometry is warranted [27]. Patients with MGUS have 0.25–3% per year risk of progression to symptomatic disease, so adequate follow-up with monitoring is currently recommended [26].

Solitary plasmacytomas are rare, comprising 5–10% of plasma cell neoplasms, and present as a single destructive osteolytic lesion without the systemic manifestations or marrow involvement associated with multiple myeloma [28]. About half of reported cases of solitary plasmacytomas involve vertebral bodies [29]. These patients may not present with the typical monoclonal gammopathy features of myeloma, though many will progress to overt myeloma without timely intervention and occasionally progress despite appropriate therapy [30]. Another entity is osteosclerotic myeloma which results from clonal plasma cell proliferation. Osteosclerotic myeloma can be seen as a component of the paraneoplastic POEMS syndrome (polyneuropathy, organomegaly, endocrinopathy, monoclonal proteins, and skin findings). Indeed, the diagnosis of POEMS syndrome requires presence of monoclonal gammopathy and polyneuropathy [31]. Over 95% of patients with POEMS have bony involvement, and lesions can appear lytic, sclerotic, or mixed on radiograph [31].

Other plasma cell dyscrasias are not often directly associated with bone-related manifestations. Leukemia has also not been shown to have significant direct skeletal manifestations, likely due to a different profile of cytokine/chemokine production in these malignancies than in multiple myeloma or lymphoma. An exception to this is plasma cell leukemia, seen in 2–5% of advanced myeloma cases, which is characterized by aggressive bone marrow involvement and poor prognosis [32].

In the realm of hematopoietic malignancies that affect bone, lymphomas have also been shown to have the capacity for bone resorption and can present with osteolytic lesions associated with pain, palpable mass, hypercalcemia, and/or pathologic fracture. Both primary bone lymphomas, defined as lymphoma arising in bone at least 4–6 months prior to extraskeletal manifestation, and secondary bony involvement following diagnosis of extraskeletal lymphoma have been shown to occur [33]. Primary bone lymphoma is a rare clinical entity, accounting for 3–7% of primary bone malignancies and <2% of lymphomas in adults [34, 35]. Primary bone lymphoma is largely comprised of non-Hodgkin's histopathological features, most commonly diffuse large B cell lymphomas; however rare cases of Hodgkin's lymphoma have also been described as primarily arising in bone [35–37]. Lymphoma has also been shown to demonstrate metastatic infiltration of the bone marrow and lead to compromised bone architecture in advanced stage disease; however lymphomas often demonstrate less focal destruction than sarcomas on bone [38, 39].

Metastatic Involvement of Bone

Metastases are the most common form of malignant bone tumor. Given the robust vascular supply to bone, metastatic carcinomas often find their way to the skeletal system via hematogenous spread. Once malignant cells arrive in the bone marrow, they can express adhesive, angiogenic and bone-resorbing factors to promote their ongoing survival in the bone microenvironment [40]. Tumor growth factor-β (TGF-β) is a bone-derived factor which has been found to be integral to the destructive cycle of metastases within bone from breast, prostate, and lung cancers among others [41]. TGF-β inhibits epithelial cell growth as part of physiologic homeostasis; however this inhibition is lost in the case of neoplastic infiltration in bone [42]. The bone matrix itself also houses many growth factors including insulin-like growth factors (IGF) I and II, which have the potential to induce further proliferation of tumor in the bony environment and contribute to development of hypercalcemia in patients with skeletal metastases [43].

Clinically apparent bone metastases are common in the axial or proximal appendicular skeleton. They are often locally destructive of bone cortices and extend into adjacent soft tissues where new bone formation may cause sclerotic lesions on imaging. Virtually every carcinoma has been documented as metastasizing to the skeleton, but the most common are breast, prostate, renal cell, and pancreatic carcinoma [44]. In addition, melanomas and extraskeletal sarcomas can exhibit skeletal metastasis. A focused history and exam, imaging, and immunohistochemical analysis of a pathology specimen may be of significant help in identifying the primary neoplasm.

Bone metastases present unique and multifaceted challenges in the management of patients with cancer. The presence of metastases to bone may prompt a shift from curative treatment options to palliative management as survival is poor, with the median survival time being around 24 months [45]. Goals of therapy include pain control, maintenance or improvement of function, bone stabilization, and tumor control; and the means employed to obtain these goals should be undertaken with life expectancy in mind.

Role of Bone-Modifying Agents in Management of Malignant Bone Lesions

Bisphosphonates inhibit osteoclastic resorption and curtail hypercalcemia of malignancy. Structurally they resemble the naturally occurring inhibitor of bone metabolism pyrophosphate but are not catabolized by endogenous pyrophosphatases; they also affect cholesterol synthesis of osteoclasts, their longevity, and perhaps local vascular activity [46]. More recently, another type of antiresorptive drug has emerged which mediates osteoclast activity by inhibiting its regulator RANKL. Denosumab is an injectable agent, and several trials have demonstrated that it may be more efficacious than zoledronic acid in preventing skeletal-related events in certain metastatic solid tumors [47–49]. Both medications are considered relatively safe and have very few reports of associated osteonecrosis of the jaw (ONJ), though the risk is likely higher with use of high-dose IV bisphosphonates.

Bisphosphonates are a key component of pain management for skeletal metastases of solid tumors alongside radiation, chemotherapy, and analgesic medications, but major guidelines do not currently recommend sole use of bisphosphonates for the purpose of bone pain in malignancy. Many phase III trials have shown that intravenous pamidronate is able to reduce pain related to bone metastases in patients with metastatic breast cancer and multiple myeloma [46]. In 2002, the FDA also expanded the indications for zoledronic acid to include its use in skeletal-related pain from multiple myeloma and metastatic breast cancer after a study demonstrated non-inferiority to pamidronate [50]. While oral bisphosphonates appear to reduce skeletal-related adverse events in patients with metastatic breast cancer compared with placebo, a phase III trial demonstrated superiority of IV bisphosphonates over oral ibandronate [51, 52].

The American Society of Clinical Oncology (ASCO) currently recommends use of intravenous pamidronate or zoledronic acid every 3–4 weeks in patients with multiple myeloma who have radiographic evidence of lytic bone destruction or vertebral compression fracture even in the presence of osteopenia [53]. Appropriate reduction in dose of zoledronic acid per package insert should be adhered to for patients with renal dysfunction, though the reduction of intravenous pamidronate is not as well-studied. It is recommended that these patients be evaluated for albuminuria every 3–6 months while on bisphosphonate therapy, with interruption of therapy recommended in the setting of unexplained albuminuria. Treatment should typically be given for at least 2 years, with consideration for further treatment depending on stability/responsiveness of disease and clinical judgment [53]. Ideally, bone-targeted therapy is initiated soon after discovery of metastatic bone involvement to avoid development of skeletal-related adverse events (i.e., pathologic fracture).

The American Society of Clinical Oncology (ASCO) recommends treatment with denosumab, pamidronate, or zoledronic acid every 3–4 weeks if there is evidence of bony destruction or metastasis-related bone pain from breast cancer [54]. The most recent guidelines do not recommend denosumab over bisphosphonate therapy in this cohort; however when creatinine clearance is <30 ml/min or patient is on dialysis, denosumab is preferred as it does not exhibit renal clearance. Renal function should be monitored prior to each dose of bisphosphonate. Though professional societies do recommend regular monitoring of serum calcium, phosphate, and electrolytes for patients receiving bone-modifying therapy, there is no consensus on the optimal frequency of such monitoring. ASCO also recommends dental examination and optimal dental health prior to administration of either class of agent, and a similar recommendation also is noted in multiple myeloma patients [54].

Controversy still exists about whether bisphosphonates have inherent antitumor properties, and studies on this subject are lacking. Two large trials using clodronate (currently commercially unavailable in the USA) in patients with metastatic breast cancer showed no difference in skeletal or visceral metastasis burden after long-term follow-up in treatment versus placebo arms [55]. The Early Breast Cancer Trialists' Collaborative Group (EBCTCG) performed a recent meta-analysis including over 18,000 patients to ascertain if bisphosphonate therapy had an adjuvant role in breast cancer therapy. This study showed that bisphosphonate therapy reduced breast cancer recurrence in bone and improved survival for postmenopausal women only [56]. Current guidelines do not routinely recommend use of bisphosphonates in metastatic breast cancer without clear evidence of skeletal involvement [54].

RANKL is thought to play a role in tumor cell migration which has led to the hypothesis that denosumab may have the potential to decrease metastatic potential of cancer cells [57]. A recent prospective, randomized controlled phase III trial in postmenopausal breast cancer patients receiving aromatase inhibitors demonstrated improved disease-free survival in patients receiving denosumab versus placebo at a median follow-up of 4 years, which was deemed similar to the disease-free survival for bisphosphonates in similar cohorts [58]. Further, high-quality studies are needed to evaluate the use of bone-directed drugs as adjuvant therapies for preventing skeletal metastasis in patients with extraskeletal malignancy.

Role of Bone Turnover Markers in Skeletal Malignancy

Various urine and serum measures of bone turnover are now commercially available and may provide insight into treatment efficacy with antiresorptive therapy [59–61]. Bone formation markers include osteocalcin, bone-specific alkaline phosphatase (BAP), and peptide cleavage products from the amino (PINP)- and carboxy (PICP)-terminal ends of procollagen 1 [62]. Bone resorption markers that are commonly used include deoxypyridinoline (DPD), isoform 5b of the osteoclast enzyme tartrate-resistant acid phosphatase (TRACP5b), amino-terminal telopeptide of type I collagen or N-telopeptide (NTX), and carboxy-terminal telopeptide of type I collagen or C-telopeptide (CTX).

Prospective studies regarding the use of bone turnover markers to quantify skeletal tumor burden prior to antiresorptive therapy, detection of early bony metastases that are not visible on imaging, or progression of metastatic bone disease are scant. However, the use of bone turnover markers for early detection, prognosis, and monitoring is increasingly an area of study. Several studies have demonstrated increased bone resorption markers in the presence of metastatic disease to bone, and perhaps even a correlation with degree of tumor burden, primarily for urinary marker NTX [62–64]. A recent review of the literature also notes that NTX may be the most accurate single marker for determining extent of bone involvement in malignancy and most closely correlates with antiresorptive therapy response and clinical outcomes in patients with skeletal malignancy [52]. One prospective study evaluating 50 postmenopausal women with early stage luminal-type invasive ductal carcinoma of the breast showed that the combination of BAP + PINP + TRACP5b predicted the development of bone metastases with 82% accuracy over the course of 50-month follow-up [65].

The use of bone turnover markers in patients with known bone metastases on bisphosphonate therapy has been evaluated in several studies, however, and suggests these markers may have implications for prognosis in certain patient populations. A recent retrospective analysis of phase III trials comparing IV zoledronic acid to denosumab in over 5000 patients with metastatic bone involvement of a solid primary tumor showed that urine NTX and serum BAP levels elevated above median levels for the cohort after 3 months of antiresorptive therapy were associated with decreased overall survival and increased risk of disease progression compared with individuals who exhibited values less than the median for either assay [66]. There are no current standard recommendations for the use of bone turnover markers in the diagnosis or prognosis of metastatic bony lesions; imaging studies remain the preferred diagnostic tools. Future research may carve out a role for bone turnover markers as diagnostic or prognostic markers; however, their routine clinical use for such purposes is not recommended at present.

References

1. Clines GA, Guise TA. Hypercalcaemia of malignancy and basic research on mechanisms responsible for osteolytic and osteoblastic metastasis to bone. Endocr Relat Cancer. 2005;12(3):549–83.
2. Edwards CM, Zhuang J, Mundy GR. The pathogenesis of the bone disease of multiple myeloma. Bone. 2008;42(6):1007–13.
3. Mundy GR, Raisz LG, Cooper RA, Schechter GP, Salmon SE. Evidence for the secretion of an osteoclast stimulating factor in myeloma. N Engl J Med. 1974;291(20):1041–6.
4. Bataille R, Chappard D, Marcelli C, Dessauw P, Baldet P, Sany J, Alexandre C. Recruitment of new osteoblasts and osteoclasts is the earliest critical event in the pathogenesis of human multiple myeloma. J Clin Investig. 1991;88(1):62–6.
5. Woitge HW, Horn E, Keck AV, Auler B, Seibel MJ, Pecherstorfer M. Biochemical markers of bone formation in patients with plasma cell dyscrasias and benign osteoporosis. Clin Chem. 2001;47:686–93.
6. Guise TA, Yin JJ, Taylor SD, Kumagai Y, Dallas M, Boyce BF, Yoneda T, Mundy GR. Evidence for a causal role of parathyroid hormone-related protein in the pathogenesis of human breast cancer-mediated osteolysis. J Clin Investig. 1996;98(7):1544–9.
7. Henderson MA, Danks JA, Slavin JL, Byrnes GB, Choong PF, Spillane JB, Hopper JL, Martin TJ. Parathyroid hormone-related protein localization in breast cancers predict improved prognosis. Cancer Res. 2006;66(4):2250–6.
8. Lecouvet FE, Larbi A, Pasoglou V, Omoumi P, Tombal B, Michoux N, Malghem J, Lhommel R, Vande Berg BC. MRI for response assessment in metastatic bone disease. Eur Radiol. 2013;23(7):1986–97.
9. Cook GJ. PET and PET/CT imaging of skeletal metastases. Cancer Imaging. 2010;10(1):101–8.
10. Eisenhauer EA, Therasse P, Bogaerts J, Schwartz LH, Sargent D, Ford R, Dancey J, Arbuck S, Gwyther S, Mooney M, Rubinstein L, Shankar L, Dodd L, Kaplan R, Lacombe D, Verweij J. New response evaluation criteria in solid tumours: revised RECIST guideline (version 1.1). Eur J Cancer. 2009;45(2):228–47.
11. Ueda T, Naka N, Araki N, Ishii T, Tsuchiya H, Yoshikawa H, et al. Validation of radiographic response evaluation criteria of preoperative chemotherapy for bone and soft tissue sarcomas: Japanese Orthopaedic Association Committee on musculoskeletal tumors cooperative study. J Orthop Sci. 2008;13(4):304–12.
12. Guise TA. Molecular mechanisms of osteolytic bone metastases. Cancer. 2000;88(S12):2892–8.
13. Tian E, Zhan F, Walker R, Rasmussen E, Ma Y, Barlogie B, Shaughnessy JD. The role of the Wnt-signaling antagonist DKK1 in the development of osteolytic lesions in multiple myeloma. N Engl J Med. 2003;349(26):2483–94.

14. Guise TA, Mohammad KS, Clines G, Stebbins EG, Wong DH, Higgins LS, et al. Basic mechanisms responsible for osteolytic and osteoblastic bone metastases. Clin Cancer Res. 2006;12(20 Pt 2):6213s–6s.
15. Bonica JJ. Management of cancer pain. Acta Anaest Scand Suppl. 1982;74:75–82.
16. Downie A, Williams CM, Henschke N, Hancock MJ, Ostelo RW, de Vet HC, et al. Red flags to screen for malignancy and fracture in patients with low back pain: systematic review. BMJ. 2013;347:f7095.
17. Schaberg J, Gainor BJ. A profile of metastatic carcinoma of the spine. Spine. 1985;10(1):19–20.
18. Healey JH, Brown HK. Complications of bone metastases: surgical management. Cancer. 2000;88(12 Suppl):2940–51.
19. Buggay D, Jaffe K. Metastatic bone tumors of the pelvis and lower extremity. J Surg Orthop Adv. 2004;12(4):192–9.
20. Biermann JS, Holt GE, Lewis VO, Schwartz HS, Yaszemski MJ. Metastatic bone disease: diagnosis, evaluation, and treatment. J Bone Joint Surg Am. 2009;91(6):1518–30.
21. Papanastassiou ID, Filis AK, Gerochristou MA, Vrionis FD. Controversial issues in kyphoplasty and vertebroplasty in malignant vertebral fractures. Cancer Control. 2014;21(2):151–7.
22. Health Quality Ontario. Vertebral augmentation involving vertebroplasty or kyphoplasty for cancer-related vertebral compression fractures: a systematic review. Ont Health Technol Assess Ser. 2016;16(11):1–202.
23. Gainor BJ, Buchert P. Fracture healing in metastatic bone disease. Clin Orthop. 1983;178:297–302.
24. Harting MT, Lally KP, Andrassy RJ, Vaporciyan AA, Cox CS, Hayes-Jordan A, Blakely ML. Age as a prognostic factor for patients with osteosarcoma: an analysis of 438 patients. J Cancer Res Clin Oncol. 2010;136(4):561–70.
25. Lee J, Hoang BH, Ziogas A, Zell JA. Analysis of prognostic factors in Ewing sarcoma using a population-based cancer registry. Cancer. 2010;116(8):1964–73.
26. Kyle RA, Durie BGM, Rajkumar SV, Landgren O, Blade J, Merlini G, Kröger N, Einsele H, Vesole DH, Dimopoulos M, San Miguel J, Avet-Loiseau H, Hajek R, Chen WM, Anderson KC, Ludwig H, Sonneveld P, Pavlovsky S, Palumbo A, Richardson PG, Barlogie B, Greipp P, Vescio R, Turesson I, Westin J, Boccadoro M. Monoclonal Gammopathy of Undetermined Significance (MGUS) and smoldering (asymptomatic) multiple myeloma: IMWG consensus perspectives risk factors for progression and guidelines for monitoring and management. Leukemia. 2010;24(6):1121–7.
27. Piot JM, Royer M, Schmidt-Tanguy A, Hoppé E, Gardembas M, Bourrée T, et al. Factors associated with an increased risk of vertebral fracture in monoclonal gammopathies of undetermined significance. Blood Cancer J. 2015;5:e345.
28. Kyle RA, Durie BG, Rajkumar SV, Landgren O, Blade J, Merlini G, et al. Criteria for the classification of monoclonal gammopathies, multiple myeloma and related disorders: a report of the international myeloma working group. Br J Haematol. 2003;121(5):749–57.
29. Wiltshaw E. The natural history of extramedually plasmacytoma and its relation to soliray myeloma of bone and myelomatosis. Medicine. 1976;55(3):217–38.
30. Kilciksiz S, Karakoyun-Celik O, Agaoglu FY, Haydaroglu A. A review for solitary plasmacytoma of bone and extramedullary plasmacytoma. Sci World J. 2012;2012:895765.
31. Dispenzieri A. POEMS syndrome: 2014 update on diagnosis, risk-stratification, and management. Am J Hematol. 2014;89(2):213–23.
32. Dimopoulos M, Kyle R, Fermand J-P, Rajkumar SV, San Miguel J, Chanan-Khan A, Ludwig H, Joshua D, Mehta J, Gertz M, Avet-Loiseau H, Beksac M, Anderson KC, Moreau P, Singhal S, Goldschmidt H, Boccadoro M, Kumar S, Giralt S, Munshi NC, Jagannath S. Consensus recommendations for standard investigative workup: report of the international myeloma workshop consensus panel 3. Blood. 2011;117(18):4701–5.
33. Fletcher CD, Brigde JA, Hogendoorn PC, Mertens F. World Health Organization classification of tumours of soft tissue and bone. Lyon: IARC Press; 2013.
34. Dubey P, Ha CS, Besa PC, Fuller L, Cabanillas F, Murray J, Hess MA, Cox JD. Localized primary malignant lymphoma of bone. Int J Radiat Oncol Biol Phys. 1997;37(5):1087–93.

35. Limb D, Dreghorn C, Murphy JK, Mannion R. Primary lymphoma of bone. Int Orthop. 1994;18(3):180–3.
36. Ramadan K, Shenkier T, Sehn L, Gascoyne R, Connors J. A clinicopathological retrospective study of 131 patients with primary bone lymphoma: a population-based study of successively treated cohorts from the British Columbia Cancer Agency. Ann Oncol. 2006;18(1):129–35.
37. Zhang X, Zhu J, Song Y, Ping L, Zheng W. Clinical characterization and outcome of primary bone lymphoma: a retrospective study of 61 Chinese patients. Sci Rep. 2016;6:28834.
38. Freeman C, Berg JW, Cutler SJ. Occurrence and prognosis of extranodal lymphomas. Cancer. 1972;29(1):252–60.
39. Rudders RA, Ross ME, Delellis RA. Primary extranodal lymphoma. Response to treatment and factors influencing prognosis. Cancer. 1978;42(2):406–16.
40. Van Der Pluijm G, Sijmons B, Vloedgraven H, Deckers M, Papapoulos S, Löwik C. Monitoring metastatic behavior of human tumor cells in mice with species-specific polymerase chain reaction: elevated expression of angiogenesis and bone resorption stimulators by breast cancer in bone metastases. J Bone Miner Res. 2001;16(6):1077–91.
41. Juárez P, Guise TA. TGF-Î^{2} in cancer and bone: implications for treatment of bone metastases. Bone. 2011;48(1):23–9.
42. Takai H, Kanematsu M, Yano K, Tsuda E, Higashio K, Ikeda K, Watanabe K, Yamada Y. Transforming growth factor-Î^{2} stimulates the production of osteoprotegerin/osteoclastogenesis inhibitory factor by bone marrow stromal cells. J Biol Chem. 1998;273(42):27091–6.
43. Mohan S, Baylink DJ. Bone growth factors. Clin Orthop Relat Res. 1991;263:30–48.
44. Coleman RE, Rubens RD. The clinical course of bone metastases from breast cancer. Br J Cancer. 1987;55(1):61–6.
45. Rubens RD, Mundy GR, editors. Bone metastases- incidence and complications. Cancer and the skeleton. London: Martin Dunitz; 2000. p. 33–42.
46. Fulfaro F, Casuccio A, Ticozzi C, Ripamonti C. The role of bisphosphonates in the treatment of painful metastatic bone disease: a review of phase III trials. Pain. 1998;78(3):157–69.
47. Fizazi K, Carducci M, Smith M, Damiao R, Brown J, Karsh L, et al. Denosumab versus zoledronic acid for treatment of bone metastases in men with castration resistant prostate cancer: a randomised, double-blind study. Lancet. 2011;377:813–22.
48. Henry DH, Costa L, Goldwasser F, Hirsh V, Hungria V, Prausova J, Scagliotti GV, Sleeboom H, Spencer A, Vadhan-Raj S, von Moos R, Willenbacher W, Woll PJ, Wang J, Qi J, Jun S, Dansey R, Yeh H. Randomized, double-blind study of denosumab versus zoledronic acid in the treatment of bone metastases in patients with advanced cancer (excluding breast and prostate cancer) or multiple myeloma. J Clin Oncol. 2011;29(9):1125–32.
49. Stopeck AT, Lipton A, Body J-J, Steger GG, Tonkin K, de Boer RH, Lichinitser M, Fujiwara Y, Yardley DA, Viniegra M, Fan M, Jiang Q, Dansey R, Jun S, Braun A. Denosumab compared with zoledronic acid for the treatment of bone metastases in patients with advanced breast cancer: a randomized, double-blind study. J Clin Oncol. 2010;28(35):5132–9.
50. Rosen LS, Gordon D, Kaminski M, Howell A, Belch A, MacKey J, et al. Zoledronic acid versus pamidronate in the treatment of skeletal metastases in patients with breast cancer or osteolytic lesions of multiple myeloma: a phase III, double-blind, comparative trial. Cancer J. 2001;7:377–87.
51. Barrett-Lee P, Casbard A, Abraham J, Hood K, Coleman R, Simmonds P, Timmins H, Wheatley D, Grieve R, Griffiths G, Murray N. Oral ibandronic acid versus intravenous zoledronic acid in treatment of bone metastases from breast cancer: a randomised, open label, non-inferiority phase 3 trial. Lancet Oncol. 2014;15(1):114–22.
52. Irelli A, Cocciolone V, Cannita K, Zugaro L, Di Staso M, Baldi PL, Paradisi S, Sidoni T, Ricevuto E, Ficorella C. Bone targeted therapy for preventing skeletal-related events in metastatic breast cancer. Bone. 2016;87:169–75.
53. Kyle RA, Yee GC, Somerfield MR, Flynn PJ, Halabi S, Jagannath S, Orlowski RZ, Roodman DG, Twilde P, Anderson K. American Society of Clinical Oncology 2007 clinical practice guideline update on the role of bisphosphonates in multiple myeloma. J Clin Oncol. 2007;25(17):2464–72.

54. Van Poznak CH, Temin S, Yee GC, Janjan NA, Barlow WE, Biermann JS, Bosserman LD, Geoghegan C, Hillner BE, Theriault RL, Zuckerman DS, Von Roenn JH. American Society of Clinical Oncology executive summary of the clinical practice guideline update on the role of bone-modifying agents in metastatic breast cancer. J Clin Oncol. 2011;29(9):1221–7.
55. Powles T, Paterson S, Kanis JA, McCloskey E, Ashley S, Tidy A, Rosenqvist K, Smith I, Ottestad L, Legault S, Pajunen M, Nevantaus A, Männistö E, Suovuori A, Atula S, Nevalainen J, Pylkkänen L. Randomized, placebo-controlled trial of clodronate in patients with primary operable breast cancer. J Clin Oncol. 2002;20(15):3219–24.
56. Coleman R, Powles A, Paterson M, Gnant S, Anderson I, Diel J, et al. Early Breast Cancer Trialists' Collaborative Group (EBCTCG). Adjuvant bisphosphonate treatment in early breast cancer: meta-analyses of individual patient data from randomised trials. Lancet. 2015;386(10001):1353–61.
57. Jones DH, Nakashima T, Sanchez OH, Kozieradzki I, Komarova SV, Sarosi I, Morony S, Rubin E, Sarao R, Hojilla CV, Komnenovic V, Kong Y-Y, Schreiber M, Dixon SJ, Sims SM, Khokha R, Wada T, Penninger JM. Regulation of cancer cell migration and bone metastasis by RANKL. Nature. 2006;440(7084):692–6.
58. Gnant M, Pfeiler G, Dubsky PC, Hubalek M, Greil R, Jakesz R, Wette V, Balic M, Haslbauer F, Melbinger E, Bjelic-Radisic V, Artner-Matuschek S, Fitzal F, Marth C, Sevelda P, Mlineritsch B, Steger GG, Manfreda D, Exner R, Egle D, Bergh J, Kainberger F, Talbot S, Warner D, Fesl C, Singer CF. Adjuvant denosumab in breast cancer (ABCSG-18): a multicentre, randomised, double-blind, placebo-controlled trial. Lancet. 2015;386(9992):433–43.
59. Blomqvist C, Risteli L, Risteli J, Virkkunen P, Sarna S, Elomaa I. Markers of type I collagen degradation and synthesis in the monitoring of treatment response in bone metastases from breast carcinoma. Br J Cancer. 1996;73(9):1074–9.
60. Koizumi M, Matsumoto S, Takahashi S, Yamashita T, Ogata EM. Bone metabolic markers in the evaluation of bone scan flare phenomenon in bone metastases of breast cancer. Clin Nucl Med. 1994;24(1):15–20.
61. Maeda H, Koizumi M, Yoshimura K, Yamauchi T, Kawai T, Ogata E. Correlation between bone metabolic markers and bone scan in prostatic cancer. J Urol. 1997;157(2):539–43.
62. Demers LM, Costa L, Lipton A. Biochemical markers and skeletal metastases. Cancer. 2000;88(12 Suppl):2919–26.
63. Costa L, Demers LM, Speicher T, Gouveia T, Curley E, Harvey H, et al. Biochemical markers of bone turnover correlate with the extent of metastatic bone disease. Cancer. 2000;88(12 Suppl):2919–26.
64. Withold W, Friedrich W, Reinauer H. Comparison of biochemical markers of bone resorption in patients with metabolic and malignant bone diseases. Ann Clin Biochem. 1996;33(Pt 5):421–7.
65. Lumachi F, Basso SMM, Camozzi V, Tozzoli R, Spaziante R, Ermani M. Bone turnover markers in women with early stage breast cancer who developed bone metastases. A prospective study with multivariate logistic regression analysis of accuracy. Clin Chim Acta. 2016;460:227–30.
66. Lipton A, Smith MR, Fizazi K, Stopeck AT, Henry D, Brown JE, et al. Changes in bone turnover marker levels and clinical outcomes in patients with advanced cancer and bone metastases treated with bone antiresorptive agents. Clin Cancer Res. 2016;22(23):5713–21.

Correction to: Metabolic Bone Diseases

Pauline M. Camacho

Correction to: P. M. Camacho (ed.), Metabolic Bone Diseases, https://doi.org/10.1007/978-3-030-03694-2

The book was inadvertently published with an incorrect Author name in chapter 1 "Michael Lewiecki, E". The correct name is "Lewiecki, E. Michael"

The book was inadvertently published with an incorrect Author name in chapter 3 "Gregory Charnogursky". The correct name is "Gerald Charnogursky"

The updated online version of these chapters can be found at
https://doi.org/10.1007/978-3-030-03694-2_1
https://doi.org/10.1007/978-3-030-03694-2_3

P. M. Camacho (ed.), *Metabolic Bone Diseases*,
https://doi.org/10.1007/978-3-030-03694-2_16

Index

P. M. Camacho (ed.), *Metabolic Bone Diseases*,
https://doi.org/10.1007/978-3-030-03694-2

MIX
Papier aus verantwortungsvollen Quellen
Paper from responsible sources
FSC® C105338

If you have any concerns about our products,
you can contact us on
ProductSafety@springernature.com

In case Publisher is established outside the EU,
the EU authorized representative is:
Springer Nature Customer Service Center GmbH
Europaplatz 3, 69115 Heidelberg, Germany

Printed by Libri Plureos GmbH
in Hamburg, Germany